GERIATRIC MENTAL HEALTH CARE

Lessons From a Pandemic

GERIATRIC MENTAL HEALTH CARE

Lessons From a Pandemic

Edited by
Robert P. Roca, M.D., M.P.H., M.B.A.
Micheline Dugué, M.D.
Maria D. Llorente, M.D., FAPA

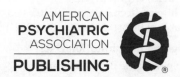

AMERICAN
PSYCHIATRIC
ASSOCIATION
PUBLISHING

Copyright © 2022 American Psychiatric Association Publishing
ALL RIGHTS RESERVED
First Edition
Manufactured in the United States of America on acid-free paper
26 25 24 23 22   5 4 3 2 1
American Psychiatric Association Publishing
800 Maine Avenue SW
Suite 900
Washington, DC 20024-2812
www.appi.org

Library of Congress Cataloging-in-Publication Data
Names: Roca, Robert, editor. | Dugué, Micheline, editor. | Llorente, Maria D., editor. | American Psychiatric Association, issuing body.
Title: Geriatric mental health care : lessons from a pandemic / edited by Robert P. Roca, Micheline Dugué, Maria D. Llorente.
Other titles: Geriatric mental health care (Roca)
Description: First edition. | Washington, DC : American Psychiatric Association Publishing, [2022] | Includes bibliographical references and index.
Identifiers: LCCN 2021059068 (print) | LCCN 2021059069 (ebook) | ISBN 9781615374656 (paperback ; alk. paper) | ISBN 9781615374663 (ebook)
Subjects: MESH: Mental Disorders | Aged | Mental Health | Health Services for the Aged | Mental Health Services | COVID-19 | United States
LC Classification: RC451.4.A5 (print) | LCC RC451.4.A5 (ebook) | NLM WT 150 | DDC 618.97/689—dc23/eng/20211228
LC record available at https://lccn.loc.gov/2021059068
LC ebook record available at https://lccn.loc.gov/2021059069

British Library Cataloguing in Publication Data
A CIP record is available from the British Library.

CONTENTS

I Pandemics and Mental Health
Epidemiology and Public Health. . . . .

Joshua C. Morganstein, M.D.
Holly B. Herberman Mash, Ph.D.
Madeline B. Teisberg, D.O.
Shannon C. Ford, M.D.
Carol S. Fullerton, Ph.D.
Robert J. Ursano, M.D.

2 Historical Overview of Pandemics. . . . .

Matthew L. Edwards, M.D.
Yolonda R. Pickett, M.D.
Maria D. Llorente, M.D., FAPA

3 Emergency Psychiatric Care for Older Adults During the COVID-19 Pandemic
Workflow, Common Presentations, and Overall Trends . . . .

Dwight Kemp, M.D., M.S.
Neha N. Sharma, M.D.
Alan Akira, M.D.
Eitan Z. Kimchi, M.D.

CONTRIBUTORS

Marc Agronin, M.D., DFAPA, DFAAGP
Senior Vice President for Behavioral Health, Miami Jewish Health;
Chief Medical Officer, MIND Institute at Miami Jewish Health; Affiliate
Associate Professor of Psychiatry and Neurology, University of Miami
Miller School of Medicine, Miami, Florida

Iqbal "Ike" Ahmed, M.D., FRCPsych (UK)
Faculty Psychiatrist, Tripler Army Medical Center; Clinical Professor of
Psychiatry, Uniformed Services University of Health Sciences; Clinical
Professor of Psychiatry and Geriatric Medicine, University of Hawai'i,
Honolulu, Hawaii

Alan Akira, M.D.
Chief Resident of Emergency Psychiatry and Medical Student Education, Department of Psychiatry and Behavioral Sciences, Rush University Medical Center, Chicago, Illinois

Janet Baek, M.D.
Child and Adolescent Psychiatry Fellow, Stanford University School of
Medicine, Palo Alto, California

Magdalena Bednarczyk, M.D.
Assistant Professor, Rush University Medical College, Chicago, Illinois

Laura Bevilacqua, M.D., Ph.D.
Psychiatrist, private practice, Brooklyn, New York

O. Joseph Bienvenu, M.D., Ph.D.
Professor, Psychiatry and Behavioral Sciences, Johns Hopkins University School of Medicine, Baltimore, Maryland

Shehan Chin, LMSW
Director, Caregiver Support Program, Alzheimer's Disease Research Center, Icahn School of Medicine at Mount Sinai, New York, New York

Daniel C. Dahl, M.D.
Psychiatrist, private practice, Birmingham, Alabama

Jonathan M. DePierro, Ph.D.
Clinical and Research Director, Mount Sinai Center for Stress, Resilience, and Personal Growth, Icahn School of Medicine at Mount Sinai, New York, New York

Ebony Dix, M.D.
Assistant Professor, Yale School of Medicine; Unit Chief, Inpatient Geriatric Psychiatry, Interventional Psychiatric Services, Yale-New Haven Hospital, Saint Raphael Campus, New Haven, Connecticut

Micheline Dugué, M.D.
Attending Psychiatrist, Department of Mental Health, VA Pacific Islands Healthcare Systems, Maui, Hawaii

Matthew L. Edwards, M.D.
Fellow in Forensic Psychiatry, Psychiatry and Law Service, Department of Psychiatry and Behavioral Sciences, Emory University School of Medicine, Atlanta, Georgia

Shannon C. Ford, M.D.
Program Director, Consultation-Liaison and Geriatric Psychiatry Fellowship, Walter Reed National Military Medical Center, Bethesda, Maryland

Carol S. Fullerton, Ph.D.
Research Professor of Psychiatry and Scientific Director, Center for the Study of Traumatic Stress, School of Medicine, Uniformed Services University, Bethesda, Maryland

Rebecca Grossman-Kahn, M.D.
Resident Physician, Department of Psychiatry and Behavioral Sciences, University of Minnesota, Minneapolis, Minnesota

Rita Hargrave, M.D., FAPA
Geriatric Psychiatrist, VA Northern California Systems of Clinics, Martinez Behavioral Health Clinic, Martinez, California; Consultant to University of California, Davis Alzheimer's Disease Center, Walnut Creek, California

Holly B. Herberman Mash, Ph.D.
Research Associate Professor of Psychiatry and Research Psychologist/Program Manager III, Center for the Study of Traumatic Stress, and Contractor, Henry M. Jackson Foundation for the Advancement of Military Medicine, School of Medicine, Uniformed Services University, Bethesda, Maryland

Paul B. Hill, M.D.
Assistant Professor and Geriatric Psychiatry Fellowship Director, Department of Psychiatry, University of Tennessee Health Science Center, Memphis, Tennessee

Donald M. Hilty, M.D., M.B.A.
Associate Chief of Staff, Mental Health, Northern California Veterans Affairs Health Care System; Professor and Vice-Chair of Veterans Affairs, Department of Psychiatry and Behavioral Sciences, University of California, Davis School of Medicine, Sacramento, California

Sharwat Jahan, M.D.
Resident, Department of Psychiatry, George Washington University Hospital, Washington, D.C.

Dwight Kemp, M.D., M.S.
Resident, Department of Psychiatry and Behavioral Neurobiology, University of Alabama at Birmingham School of Medicine, Birmingham, Alabama

Raya E. Kheirbek, M.D., M.P.H.
Professor of Medicine and Division Head, Gerontology, Geriatrics and Palliative Medicine, University of Maryland School of Medicine, Baltimore, Maryland

Eitan Z. Kimchi, M.D.
Assistant Professor, Associate Resident Training Director, Medical Director of Emergency Psychiatry, and Associate Medical Director of Geriatric Psychiatry, Department of Psychiatry and Behavioral Sciences, Rush University Medical Center, Chicago, Illinois

Sarah E. LaFave, Ph.D., M.P.H., R.N.
Postdoctoral Fellow, Johns Hopkins University School of Nursing and
Bloomberg School of Public Health, Baltimore, Maryland

Susan W. Lehmann, M.D.
Clinical Director, Division of Geriatric Psychiatry and Neuropsychiatry,
Director, Geriatric Psychiatry Fellowship, Director, Geriatric Psychiatry
Day Hospital, and Associate Professor, Department of Psychiatry and
Behavioral Sciences, Johns Hopkins University School of Medicine, Bal-
timore, Maryland

Maria D. Llorente, M.D., FAPA
Deputy to Assistant Undersecretary for Health, Patient Care Services,
Department of Veterans Affairs and Professor of Psychiatry, George-
town University School of Medicine, Washington, D.C.

Maria Loizos, Ph.D.
Assistant Professor, Department of Psychiatry, Icahn School of Medicine at Mount Sinai, New York, New York

Joshua C. Morganstein, M.D.
Associate Professor of Psychiatry and Deputy Director, Center for the
Study of Traumatic Stress, and Vice Chair, Department of Psychiatry,
School of Medicine, Uniformed Services University, Bethesda, Mary-
land

Kanya Nesbeth, M.D.
Resident, Department of Psychiatry, Howard University Hospital,
Washington, D.C.

Judith Neugroschl, M.D.
Associate Professor, Department of Psychiatry, Icahn School of Medicine at Mount Sinai, New York, New York

Linda Nix, M.D, M.P.H.
Psychiatry Resident, Rush University Medical Center, Chicago, Illinois

Donna M. Norris, M.D.
Assistant Professor (PT), Harvard Medical School; Assistant Professor
of Psychiatry, Department of Psychiatry, Beth Israel Deaconess Medical
Center, Boston, Massachusetts

Yolonda R. Pickett, M.D.
Associate Professor, Department of Psychiatry and Behavioral Health, Hackensack Meridian School of Medicine, Hackensack University Medical Center, Hackensack, New Jersey

Marilyn Price, M.D.
Assistant Professor, Harvard Medical School; Assistant Professor of Psychiatry, Law and Psychiatry Service, Department of Psychiatry, Massachusetts General Hospital, Boston, Massachusetts

Samara E. Rainey, B.A.
Research Consultant, Maple Key Consulting, Danbury, Connecticut

Badr Ratnakaran, M.B.B.S.
Fellow in Geriatric Psychiatry, Carilion Clinic, Virginia Tech Carilion School of Medicine, Roanoke, Virgina

Col. (Ret.) Elspeth Cameron Ritchie, M.D., M.P.H.
Chair, Department of Psychiatry, Medstar Washington Hospital Center; Vice Chair, Psychiatry, Georgetown University School of Medicine, Washington, D.C.

Robert P. Roca, M.D., M.P.H., M.B.A.
Vice Chair, Department of Psychiatry, The Johns Hopkins University School of Medicine, Baltimore, Maryland

Neha N. Sharma, M.D.
Resident, Department of Psychiatry and Behavioral Sciences, Rush University Medical Center, Chicago, Illinois

Shilpa Srinavasan, M.D., DFAPA, DFAAGP
Professor, Department of Neuropsychiatry and Behavioral Science, Prisma Health—University of South Carolina School of Medicine, Greenville, South Carolina

Karla Steinberg, LMSW
Formerly at Mount Sinai Morningside Geriatric Clinic, New York, New York

Sandra Swantek, M.D., FAPA
Associate Professor, Department of Psychiatry and Behavioral Sciences, Rush University Medical College, Chicago, Illinois

Farah Tabaja, M.D.
Psychiatry Resident, Institute of Living, Hartford Hospital, Hartford, Connecticut

Emily Tan, B.A.
Program Coordinator, Depression Clinical and Research Program, Department of Psychiatry, Massachusetts General Hospital, Boston, Massachusetts

Madeline B. Teisberg, D.O.
Assistant Professor of Psychiatry, School of Medicine, Uniformed Services University, Bethesda, Maryland

Nhi-Ha Trinh, M.D., M.P.H.
Director, Department of Psychiatry Center for Diversity, Massachusetts General Hospital, Boston, Massachusetts; Assistant Professor of Psychiatry and Associate Director, William Augustus Hinton Society, Harvard Medical School, Cambridge, Massachusetts

Mari Umpierre, Ph.D., LCSW
Director, Community Relations and Partnerships, Alzheimer's Disease Research Center, Icahn School of Medicine at Mount Sinai, New York, New York

Robert J. Ursano, M.D.
Professor of Psychiatry and Neuroscience and Director, Center for the Study of Traumatic Stress, School of Medicine, Uniformed Services University, Bethesda, Maryland

Antoinette M. Valenti, M.D.
Special Advisor to Deputy Assistant Under Secretary for Health for Patient Care Services, Veterans Health Administration; Assistant Professor in Psychiatry, Uniformed Services University of the Health Sciences F. Edward Hébert School of Medicine; Assistant Professor, Psychiatry, Georgetown University School of Medicine; Clinical Assistant Professor, Psychiatry, George Washington University School of Medicine, Washington, D.C.

Yee Xiong, M.D.
Addiction Psychiatry Fellow, Department of Psychiatry, School of Medicine and Public Health, University of Wisconsin–Madison, Madison, Wisconsin

DISCLOSURES

The following contributor to this book has indicated a financial interest in or other affiliation with a commercial supporter, a manufacturer of a commercial product, a provider of a commercial service, a nongovernmental organization, and/or a government agency, as listed below:

Robert P. Roca, M.D., M.P.H., M.B.A. *Honorarium:* Maryland Board of Physicians

The following contributors have indicated that they have no financial interests or other affiliations that represent or could appear to represent a competing interest with their contributions to this book:

Alan Akira, M.D.; Magdalena Bednarczyk, M.D.; Laura Bevilacqua, M.D., Ph.D.; Daniel C. Dahl, M.D.; Jonathan M. DePierro, Ph.D.; Ebony Dix, M.D.; Micheline Dugué, M.D.; Paul B. Hill, M.D.; Sharwat Jahan, M.D.; Dwight Kemp, M.D., M.S.; Eitan Z. Kimchi, M.D.; Maria D. Llorente, M.D., FAPA; Badr Ratnakaran, M.B.B.S.; Col. (Ret.) Elspeth Cameron Ritchie, M.D., M.P.H.; Neha N. Sharma, M.D.; Shilpa Srinivasan, M.D., DFAPA, DFAAGP; Antoinette M. Valenti, M.D.

FOREWORD

Time magazine called 2020 the "worst year in memory," and it was indeed so for many people, especially younger ones. As of November 2021, more than 5.1 million people have died from coronavirus SARS-CoV-2 disease (COVID-19) worldwide; about 15% of these deaths occurred in the United States. The age group with the highest risk of serious physical illness and mortality has been people older than age 65. Naturally, the COVID-19 pandemic should be of major concern for geriatric psychiatry.

No rational person would question the need and timeliness of a book titled *Geriatric Mental Health Care: Lessons from a Pandemic*. However, what sets this book apart is much more than that. This is an outstanding compilation of highly thoughtful, comprehensive, and balanced reviews of various relevant topics, with pragmatic and evidence-based recommendations for clinicians, educators, researchers, administrators, and policy makers. Having read numerous books on different topics over the decades, I can truthfully call this one of the finest works I have read. The major credit goes to the three coeditors, Drs. Roca, Dugué, and Llorente, all distinguished geriatric psychiatrists and national leaders, who put together a superb list of relevant topics, chose the best possible authors, and offered an optimal balance between a formal structure and individuality of style for individual chapters. Of course, all the authors of these chapters share the credit, given their expertise and scholarship combined with an ability to write in a reader-friendly manner. The outcome is a book that is both comprehensive and succinct and describes real science using a lucid writing style.

This book is exemplary in more ways than one. Each chapter has sections that readers will find helpful, including an abstract and an illustrative vignette at the beginning and chapter summary, key take-home messages, review questions, and resources at the end. The total number of chapters—that is, 17—may seem high for a book on such a specific topic, yet not a single chapter would be considered unnecessary. The authors come from varied professional backgrounds, and I was also struck by the fact that the first authors of several chapters are trainees or junior faculty members. What is most impressive, however, is the content of the chapters.

The authors have highlighted countless fascinating facts in their chapters. For example, although everyone knows what a terrible toll a pandemic takes on a society, the longer-term effects can be unexpectedly positive, sometimes for the wrong reason. In Chapter 2, "Historical Overview of Pandemics," the authors quote a study that showed that bubonic plague, which led to a 30%–50% depopulation of Europe, was followed by higher overall standards of living, longer life expectancy, and lower mortality in the postpandemic years. The likely and unfortunate reason for the good outcome was plague's putative role as an agent of natural selection, removing the weakest persons from the genetic pool.

The authors of Chapter 1, "Pandemics and Mental Health," and Chapter 3, "Emergency Psychiatric Care for Older Adults During the COVID-19 Pandemic," describe how COVID-19 pulled at the fault lines of society, exacerbating divisions already present because of socioeconomic disparities, race, religion, and other factors. However, older adults did surprisingly better than their younger counterparts in terms of mental health despite far worse physical health risks and poor access to technology. The incidence of anxiety, depression, and perceived stress was several folds lower in adults older than age 65 than in those younger than age 25. The likely reason is the greater wisdom and resilience that are commonly associated with aging. Thus, older adults served as role models for younger ones in terms of facing crises with emotional regulation, positivity, self-reflection, empathy, compassion, and decisiveness in the midst of uncertainty—all of which are components of wisdom, which tends to increase with aging and experience.

In Chapter 15, "Neuropsychiatric Manifestations of COVID-19," the authors lists the plethora of acute as well as longer-lasting behavioral and neurological signs and symptoms that have been reported in individuals infected with the coronavirus. For practicing clinicians, the authors of Chapter 16, "Psychopharmacological Challenges of Treating Older Adults With COVID-19," urge caution in safely prescribing psychotropic medications in older adults with COVID-19 infection because of multiorgan involvement of the virus and potential drug-drug interactions with medications used for treatment of the infection.

With the need for social distancing in order to stem the spread of coronavirus infection, use of telehealth became widespread for outpatient care. Many older adults had considerable difficulty at the beginning of the pandemic in terms of accessing and properly using videoconferencing or even telephone visits. The authors of Chapter 7, "Telehealth Models of Care for Geriatric Behavioral Health During a Pandemic," offer specific suggestions for preparation and support so that older adults can use and benefit from telepsychiatry. This chapter shows how ongoing clinical experience, teaching, and professional development facilitate telepsychiatry skills and attitudes, ensuring high quality of care and improved outcomes.

No less important is caring for the care providers. The authors of Chapter 8, "Managing Health Care Staff Concerns During Pandemics," discuss how the COVID-19 pandemic added considerable strain to health care workers and brought about a multitiered psychosocial support approach incorporating basic needs, mental health services, education and outreach, and clear messaging. The authors present evidence from one New York–based hospital system to suggest strategies for improving staff utilization of mental health treatment and spiritual care services. They also make an important point that staff support efforts should include ancillary staff, who are often members of historically disadvantaged groups.

As a researcher, I found Chapter 11, "The Effect of COVID-19 on Research," compelling. The authors describe how conducting research during a pandemic has presented serious challenges on multiple levels of clinical research, including enrollment, retention, patient safety, the conduct of research itself, outcome measures, and future research. It will likely take years to fully understand COVID-19's long-term impact on research. At the same time, I share the authors' optimism that the determination and creativity of researchers and study participants have led to and will continue to lead to creation of innovative protocols with largely continuous collection of excellent data.

Chapter 10, "Social Determinants of COVID-19 Morbidity and Mortality," is of special significance because research in the past two decades has clearly established that these social factors have greater impact on health and longevity than traditionally studied risk factors such as obesity, sedentary behavior, poor nutrition, and substance abuse. The pandemic has exacerbated the impact of social determinants of health (SDOH) on medical and psychiatric morbidity and mortality, especially among marginalized and vulnerable communities. Therefore, in moving toward a postpandemic world, it is important to implement necessary strategies in communities most affected by SDOH. For instance, COVID-19 vaccine distribution should be prioritized among communities with limited access to health care and/or technology. Two of the most important SDOH are social isolation/loneliness and racial/ethnic disparities in health care. Chapter 12, "Social Isolation and Loneliness in Older Adults During the COVID-19 Pandemic," and Chapter 9, "Geriatric Psychiatry Among Older Adults From Diverse Backgrounds in the Age of COVID-19," provide excellent discussion on both these topics.

In Chapter 12, the authors suggest that technology can create opportunities for social connectedness, although many older adults do not have the digital literacy skills, the hardware, and/or the infrastructure to use technology as a resource. Fortunately, a growing number of local and national organizations, including community-based agencies, have focused on teaching older adults to become comfortable with technology use by providing digital literacy services in addition to traditional care and case management services. The authors recommend that clinical providers become familiar with local senior service organizations in the communities in which they practice so as to provide a combination of personalized and comprehensive clinical and psychosocial care to this vulnerable group of patients.

Chapter 9 shows that the COVID-19 pandemic has disproportionately affected the economic stability as well as physical and mental health of racial/ethnic minority communities in the United States. The authors recommend coordinated interventions by faith-based organizations, community agencies, and health care systems to improve COVID-19-related public education, engagement, and access to culturally competent care for older adults from racial/ethnic minority communities.

Chapter 13, "The COVID-19 Economy," highlights the fact that older adults, particularly ethnic and racial minorities and those with the least wealth, have been especially vulnerable to economic downturns. However, such adverse impact has been somewhat softened in recent decades by federal programs such as Social Security and Medicare for those fortunate to have access to them, although these programs have not kept pace with the rising cost of living for those for whom they are a primary income source. In Chapter 14, "Ethical Dilemmas and Resource Scarcities During Pandemics," the authors stress how ethical issues permeate virtually all aspects of pandemic and disaster response. The American Psychiatric Association has encouraged psychiatrists to seek consultation with colleagues and ethics resources to navigate these challenging times.

In sum, I want to compliment the editors and chapter authors on jointly producing an exceptional monograph on a topic of great public health significance. Although a pandemic is not a pleasant subject area, this book presents a forward-looking and optimistic approach to coping with it in positive ways. A societal-level trauma need not be followed by posttraumatic stress disorder. Instead, posttraumatic growth can be an outcome if we pursue appropriately balanced strategies as described in *Geriatric Mental Health Care: Lessons from a Pandemic*.

Dilip V. Jeste, M.D.
Departments of Psychiatry and Neurosciences, Sam and Rose Stein Institute for Research on Aging, University of California San Diego, San Diego, California

PREFACE

Everybody knows that pestilences have a way of recurring in the
world, yet somehow we find it hard to believe in ones that crash
down on our heads from a blue sky. There have been as many
plagues as wars in history, yet always plagues and wars take people
equally by surprise.

—Albert Camus, *The Plague*

By mid-March 2020, it was clear that a highly transmissible and potentially fatal disease caused by a new coronavirus had spread rapidly
from China to the United States and Europe and around the world. Very
little was known about the virus in those early days, but public health
experts understood that measures to contain transmission of coronavirus
SARS-CoV-2 disease (COVID-19) needed to be implemented as quickly
as possible. The tactics adopted—lockdowns, quarantines, masking—
resembled those that had been used over the centuries to arrest the
spread of other pandemic illnesses, and they were somewhat effective.
But the pandemic raged on, taking its toll in lives, forcing us to stay put
and stay apart, straining health care resources everywhere, highlighting
health care disparities, exposing supply chain vulnerabilities, and
strangling the global economy. And although everyone suffered, those
most likely to be hospitalized, need ICU care, and die—and those most
vulnerable to the isolating impact of measures to prevent contagion—
were older adults, particularly those with chronic physical and mental
health conditions.

It was the recognition that older mentally ill persons were among
those most susceptible to harm—and in need of services tailored to address their special needs—that led the American Psychiatric Association (APA) Council on Geriatric Psychiatry to assemble this volume. We

understood that we would be writing about experiences and real-world trial-and-error efforts that were occurring as we wrote and that we would be documenting the early stages of treatment and care models that likely would evolve over time. But we were struck by how quickly the field sensed the needs of our patients and took effective steps both to protect our patients and employees from infection and to mitigate the unfortunate adverse psychosocial impact of infection control measures. Mental health clinicians working on inpatient units discovered ways to screen prospective patients, cohort those who might be infected, and prevent the spread of infection to staff and other patients. Consultation-liaison clinicians developed methods for safely evaluating medical in-patients who might be infected and for treating patients who would typically warrant psychiatric hospitalization on medical-surgical units because COVID-19-adapted psychiatric inpatient beds were no longer available.

Mental health professionals working in many clinical environments, particularly outpatient settings, rapidly adapted their practices to make the most of videoconferencing technology, and even the telephone, as means of reaching and serving patients who would have otherwise lost their connection to care. We were discovering a lot about how to support older adults with mental illnesses in the new and challenging circumstances of a pandemic, and there was a great opportunity—and a great need—for us to learn from one another.

It is the intent of this book to contribute to this effort to learn from one another. The chapter authors have all been in the trenches since the onset of the pandemic and are able to provide firsthand accounts of care in the age of COVID-19 that readers can compare with their own experiences. The fact that they were personally laboring in the trenches makes their accounts compelling and remarkable—remarkable not least of all because the author-clinicians managed to make the time to research and write their chapters while spending long days in the clinics, on medical and psychiatric wards, and in long-term care settings, daily providing care under unprecedented and stressful conditions. We cannot thank them enough for putting in the time and effort required to create this volume and share what they were learning. We also owe a special debt of gratitude to Sejal Patel for her tireless and spot-on efforts to support the authors and coeditors throughout the process of creating the manuscript. And we would be remiss if we failed to thank the staff of APA Publishing for their guidance throughout the publication process and of course Laura Roberts, M.D., for her belief in the project and her confidence in us to pull it off.

As we write this preface, the pandemic is not over. Despite the development, rigorous testing, and approval of COVID-19 vaccines at a previously unheard-of pace, thousands of people are still becoming infected and dying. The persistence of the virus in the community and the emergence of variants, exacerbated by the unwillingness of many people to accept vaccination, compel us to continue keeping our distance, wearing masks in many settings, and limiting our travel. The elderly and marginalized remain the most vulnerable to the manifold effects of the pandemic.

The lessons learned about how to care for older adults with mental illness under these circumstances remain relevant. We hope that this book will assist our colleagues who are caring for seniors and will inspire others to share their experiences and insights about how to do it better. In keeping with principles of high reliability, we need to continue learning from one another to improve our approaches to providing care under the trying conditions of pandemics. After all, we are still in the midst of one. And, if the experts are correct, this one will not be the last. We want to be prepared.

CHAPTER 1

PANDEMICS AND MENTAL HEALTH

Epidemiology and Public Health

Joshua C. Morganstein, M.D.
Holly B. Herberman Mash, Ph.D.
Madeline B. Teisberg, D.O.
Shannon C. Ford, M.D.
Carol S. Fullerton, Ph.D.
Robert J. Ursano, M.D.

Coronavirus SARS-CoV-2 disease (COVID-19) has caused injury, death, and distress in millions around the globe. Adverse mental health effects are substantial, with distress, health risk behaviors, and mental disorders exacerbating the threat of morbidity and mortality related to infection itself. The unique impacts of COVID-19, as well as the measures required to control the spread of infection, have buffered against some aspects of psychological and behavioral risk for older adults in disasters. Established principles of interventions must be adapted to the unique needs

The views expressed are those of the authors and do not necessarily reflect the views of the Department of Defense, the Uniformed Services University, the Department of Health and Human Services, or the U.S. Public Health Service.

of older adults, with particular attention to effective methods of implementation within the context of an infectious disease outbreak.

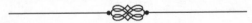

Vignette

In February 2020, COVID-19 infections began to spread around the
United States. An assisted living facility in Seattle, Washington, began
to receive calls from concerned family members of the residents. Some
residents also asked questions about the virus and expressed concerns
about their health and safety. As COVID-19 began to dominate the media
cycle and infections in Washington State rapidly increased, the health
care workers at the facility talked with the leadership team and director
frequently, noting concerns about the safety of residents and themselves. The leadership team sensed the escalating distress among residents and workers and initially responded with efforts to downplay the
significance and provide persistent reassurance in an effort to prevent
people from panicking. This response led to increased distress and a
growing mistrust between workers, residents, and the leadership at the
facility, as well as a higher volume of calls from concerned family members. Over the subsequent days, the leadership team at this assisted living
facility, like others around the world, would come to better understand
the range of psychological and behavioral responses and developmental
concerns of older adults during a crisis event. They would also learn
about the unique impacts of infectious disease outbreaks on risk perception and public health behaviors, as well as ways of supporting older
adults to reduce distress, enhance resilience, and reduce adverse psychological outcomes during a global pandemic.

Pandemics are extreme, disruptive global events that overwhelm
health systems, create financial crises, and can lead to civil unrest. Although infectious disease outbreaks are not new, the COVID-19 pandemic
that began in 2019 led to catastrophic illness and death unprecedented
since the pandemic influenza of 1918. Like other disasters, COVID-19
pulled at the fault lines of society, exacerbating divisions already present
because of socioeconomic disparities, race, religion, and other factors.
Measures required to control the spread of the disease were perceived
by some as restricting individual liberties, creating conflict among citizens and leaders.

Pandemics require considering psychological and behavioral effects
that are both the same and different from those observed after other disasters, such as hurricanes, wildfires, and even mass violence (Morganstein
et al. 2017). Infectious disease outbreaks generate concerns as a result of
isolation and quarantine, stay-at-home orders and physical distancing,
and apprehension about scarcity of medical treatment and vaccines.

The prolonged nature of COVID-19 led to financial crisis and civil strife as society struggled to balance issues of physical and economic health amid rapidly spreading disinformation and the inherently political landscape characterizing all disasters. As a result, COVID-19 was marked by significant fear, uncertainty, and anger, which greatly influenced the perception of risk and the willingness of individuals and communities to engage in recommended health behaviors necessary to control the pandemic.

As is common with disasters, COVID-19 has disproportionately affected various populations, often those who were already living on the margins, which serves as an important reminder that risk is not distributed equitably. Historically, older adults are often at elevated risk for adverse mental health outcomes in disasters, typically related to the conditions of aging (e.g., cognitive impairment, mobility limitations, reliance on systems of care, living situations) as well as the medical comorbidities associated with age itself. Not all people at a specific age share the same level of risk. Aging also confers significant benefits through past experiences, learning how to adapt, and stress tolerance, at times creating a unique capacity for resilience. In the COVID-19 pandemic, although older adults are the highest-risk age group for illness and death, they often report lower adverse mental health symptoms, including depression, anxiety, psychological stress, and suicidal thoughts, as well as lower rates of health risk behaviors, such as substance use (Czeisler et al. 2021). These findings suggest that the protective effects of aging may have buffered some of the pandemic stressors of COVID-19.

The scope, magnitude, and duration of a global pandemic necessitate the use of public mental health approaches to augment and target social and clinical interventions. Public health focuses on prevention, wellness, enhancing adaptive coping mechanisms, and promoting resilience for individuals and communities, as well as identifying those at risk and targeting the best interventions for population-level health. These approaches require an understanding of the population, including where people reside, factors affecting their well-being, and the systems in which they receive care and support. Effective interventions to address infectious disease necessitate an appreciation of what works and what does not and how it works in actual practice (e.g., masks, isolation, vaccination programs). In addition, interventions should address the unique needs of older adults regarding communication, information dissemination, access to and delivery of resources, and age-related factors affecting response and recovery.

DEFINING AND UNDERSTANDING THE POPULATION

The composition and needs of the older adult population have changed significantly over the past few centuries. Global life expectancy in the United States has increased by approximately 50 years since 1800 (Xu et al. 2020); 9% of the world's population is currently older than age 65. In contrast, 25% are younger than age 15 (Statista 2020). The percentage of older adults is expected to rise to 12% by 2030 and 17% by 2050 (Roberts et al. 2018). Because life expectancy has increased and the spectrum of developmental needs and tasks evolves across various ages, it is important to refine and distinguish subcategories of older adults. Importantly, age is currently defined by a combination of factors, including actual age in years, living situation, longevity in the work force, social supports, functional capacity, and physical and mental illnesses and disability.

Presently, 25% of Americans older than age 65 live in California, Florida, or Texas, and another 25% are in Georgia, Illinois, Michigan, New York, North Carolina, Ohio, and Pennsylvania. However, older adults are increasingly residing in geographically diverse locations, with at least 27 states predicted by 2040 to have demographic profiles closer to Florida and Maine, where 20% of the population are currently older than 65 (Himes and Kilduff 2019).

Access to care for older adults is increasingly challenged by global shortages of geriatric medicine and mental health providers. For example, estimates suggest that there will be only 1 geriatric psychiatrist per 5,682 older adults by 2030, when upward of 5,000 or more additional psychiatrists will be required to meet the anticipated need (American Association for Geriatric Psychiatry 2008). In light of the fact that more than 20% of adults ages 60 and over have a mental or neurological disorder and 6.6% of all disability within this age group is attributed to these health conditions (World Health Organization 2017), shortages of mental health providers will serve as further barriers to care.

Cultural and socioeconomic factors also affect vulnerability to COVID-19 in this population. Some older adults require assistance through physical contact with family, friends, or other caretakers; the inability to live independently increases the risk of infection. Caretaking relationships may enhance social connections but increase risk during a pandemic in which physical distancing is a critical health measure.

When younger family is providing for older adults with cognitive impairment and other illnesses, this living arrangement can create significant emotional and financial stress for caregivers, furthering the community burden of distress.

IMPACT OF DISASTERS AND UNDERSTANDING RISK

Psychological and Behavioral Impact of Disasters in the General Population

Disasters of all types can overwhelm the resources of a community. Disasters may be natural events such as floods, hurricanes, and earthquakes or human-generated events such as mass violence and critical infrastructure failings (Morganstein and Ursano 2020). The initial impact of a disaster may last moments or extend over many months as in a pandemic. Regardless of duration, the resulting adverse mental health effects can be substantial, and some are long-lasting, exceeding the physical effects (Shultz et al. 2017). An understanding of the psychological and behavioral health impacts of disasters is essential to optimize public mental health response in supporting community preparedness and recovery.

Following a disaster, distress reactions, health risk behaviors, and psychological disorders occur (Figure 1–1) (Ursano et al. 2017). After a disaster, distress reactions are common and often manifest as insomnia, decreased sense of safety, and somatic symptoms. Distress reactions are typical responses to abnormal events; however, prolonged symptoms may develop into psychiatric disorders such as PTSD, depression, anxiety, and complicated grief. Insomnia and decreased sense of safety are associated with higher rates of depression and PTSD after a disaster (Fan et al. 2017; Fullerton et al. 2015), indicating that distress reactions also increase risk for psychiatric disorders. Health risk behaviors, such as family conflict and difficulty balancing work and home life, are also common following disasters, as are increased use of tobacco and alcohol, which have significant adverse public mental health effects. For example, regardless of whether or not someone develops alcohol use disorder, increased use of alcohol is associated with increased falls, accidents, family violence, assaults, and exacerbation of underlying health conditions, increasing the overall burden of risk for older adults (Barry and Blow 2016). Psychological disorders such as PTSD, depres-

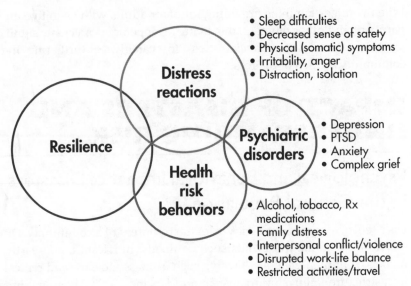

- Sleep difficulties
- Decreased sense of safety
- Physical (somatic) symptoms
- Irritability, anger
- Distraction, isolation

- Depression
- PTSD
- Anxiety
- Complex grief

- Alcohol, tobacco, Rx medications
- Family distress
- Interpersonal conflict/violence
- Disrupted work-life balance
- Restricted activities/travel

FIGURE 1–1. **Psychological and behavioral effects of disasters.**

sion, and anxiety develop and can emerge weeks or months after exposure to a disaster.

Pandemics are one of the deadliest ecological disasters. Mass migration and international travel have aided the global spread of numerous infectious diseases in just the past two decades, including H1N1, Ebola, Zika, and COVID-19. During COVID-19, as with other pandemics, fear and uncertainty have driven public responses, including anger, scapegoating, and blaming. Perceptions of risk have been shaped by evolving health guidance; isolation and quarantine; concerns about scarcity and shortages of jobs, food, and vaccines; and conflicting messages from government leaders and public health experts. Importantly, risk perception affects the willingness of the public to engage in recommended health behaviors required to control a pandemic, such as compliance with vaccination. For example, in Japan, people who perceived the COVID-19 health risk as low were less likely to engage in risk reduction behaviors such as handwashing and mask wearing in public (Shiina et al. 2020).

Pandemics such as COVID-19 have both acute and longer-term mental health outcomes that span the globe. Increased depression in the United States was disproportionately seen in individuals who lost employment, housing, and health care, particularly older adults (Ettman et al. 2020), and anxiety increased to twice prepandemic levels (Kwong et al. 2020). Bereavement is, and will be, profound for the loved ones of older adults, with 80% of deaths occurring among those older than age 65 (Centers for Disease Control and Prevention 2021) and an estimated nine people affected for every COVID-19 death (Verdery et al. 2020).

Ultimately, most people recover following disasters, with many reporting an increased sense of ability to handle future stressors. Interventions to address early adverse psychological and behavioral responses are intended to restore well-being, improve functioning, and enhance adaptive coping in order to improve the trajectory of individual and community recovery.

Impact of Disasters on Older Adults

Many older adults are at increased risk for adverse outcomes following disasters because of, in part, chronic medical conditions, cognitive impairments, limited mobility, and fixed low income. Lower-income and minority older adults may encounter systemic barriers to effectively preparing for disasters, resulting in greater losses and adverse effects (Cox and Kim 2018).

In order to understand the impact of disasters on older adults, it is important to examine risk factors across disaster events. Table 1–1 compares the impact of three different disasters on older adults.

Table 1–1. Factors affecting older adults across disaster types

	Pandemic	Hurricane	Mass violence
Socioeconomic status	++	++	+
Limited mobility	++	+++	++
Cognitive impairment	+++	++	+
Group living	++	+	0
Limited technology use	+++	++	0
Dependence on health systems	++	+++	0

Note. The extent of impact is denoted by +, with the extent of impact increasing with the number of pluses; 0 denotes no specific impact.

Decreased mobility can be life-threatening following disasters that necessitate evacuation or relocation, such as a hurricane or flood or in a mass violence situation. Cognitive impairment may lead to confusion, particularly in unfamiliar surroundings or when routines are disrupted, making it difficult for older adults to find safe emergency shelter if evacuation is needed or to follow disaster-related public health guidance. Health conditions increase the reliance of older adults on health care systems, including the need for dialysis, chemotherapy, medical devices, and pharmacotherapy modifications. Facilities such as assisted living or nursing homes are often disrupted following a disaster and may be uniquely vulnerable during pandemics.

Communication is critical for effective public health messaging after a disaster, with mobile devices and social media playing an increased role in the past two decades. Although older adults are increasingly online, their adoption of this technology lags behind that of younger adults, with more than 25% of those over 65 not using smartphones or the internet (Pew Research Center 2019a, 2019b). In addition, older adults have higher rates of hearing and vision impairments and may be less alert to public messaging. These factors increase the risk that older adults will not have access to important health recommendations and the systems in which health is increasingly delivered, such as online distribution of vaccination appointments during COVID-19.

Risks to Mental Health for Older Adults During COVID-19

Understanding the unique facets of aging across the older adult spectrum and the extent to which they enhance risk or serve as protective factors is important for anticipating mental health care needs after a pandemic as well as planning for future disasters. The COVID-19 pandemic brought increased risk for illness and death with advanced age, and numerous factors account for the psychological impact of COVID-19 and pandemics on older adults, such as cumulative health burden, living situation, financial stability, and health disparities for minority and other marginalized communities.

Residential living facilities, such as nursing homes, offer potential benefits to residents and their families but have conferred significant risks during the COVID-19 pandemic. In the United States, nursing home residents account for less than 0.5% of the population but experienced 7% of confirmed COVID-19 cases and about one-third of deaths (Chen et al. 2021). One of the first cases of SARS-CoV-2 in the United States was documented in a Washington State nursing home and was followed by more than 200 infections, putting older friends, relatives, and caregivers at significant risk. In nursing homes, visitors and staff were vectors for disease transmission, leading to catastrophic outbreaks. Separating or isolating residents, including from their families, was feasible in some facilities but led to isolation and loneliness, an increasing concern in the older adult population associated with a variety of adverse health effects and lower perceived quality of life (O'Súilleabháin et al. 2019). Cognitive impairment or dementia put some older adults at risk because of difficulty remembering and following social distancing and mask guidelines.

Requirements to limit movement and stay at home increased some health risks for older adults, including decreased utilization of health care early in the pandemic (Mehrotra et al. 2020), decreased physical activity, and less healthy nutritional intake (Omura et al. 2020). In addition, limited mobility and cognitive impairment increase the risk that older adults will be the victim of abuse. In the United States, during the first 2 months of the COVID-19 pandemic, there was an 83.6% increase in rates of elder abuse compared with prepandemic levels, with financial stress increasing risk and social connections and physical distancing being associated with decreased risk of abuse (Chang and Levy 2021). Difficulty accessing medical care and increased alcohol use by caregivers are factors that may also increase the risk that older adults will be abused and experience falls. These factors are a reminder that efforts to reduce certain health risks, such as risk of infection, can increase risk in other areas.

During the COVID-19 pandemic, the percentage of Americans older than age 65 who continued to work past retirement age increased from less than 4% in 2008 to about 8% in 2020 (U.S. Bureau of Labor and Statistics 2020), possibly reflecting financial instability or uncertainty. Remaining employed offered protection from some risks associated with finances but created fears of financial hardship if a job was lost, as well as increased exposure to infection through proximity to other people. On the positive side, employment provided a sense of purpose, social connection, and physical activity, which were protective.

Lack of access to and limited comfort with technology reduced access to lifesaving public health information by older adults during the COVID-19 pandemic. Online information and scheduling of COVID-19 vaccine appointments made this critical health intervention inaccessible to some older adults. Inability to access technology also limited access to general health and mental health care more broadly as appointments were canceled and medical offices limited visits before telehealth became more accessible.

Protective Factors for Older Adults During COVID-19

Although older adults are physically at a higher risk of infection and death, Centers for Disease Control and Prevention surveys in the

United States during the COVID-19 pandemic reported that the older population had less anxiety compared with younger age groups (Vahia et al. 2020), with wisdom and empathy thought to be factors contributing to the higher rates of well-being. Importantly, a longitudinal Swedish study found that early in the COVID-19 pandemic, individuals older than age 65 rated their overall well-being higher currently than for the previous 5 years, and they rated their well-being higher than did young cohorts (Kivi et al. 2021). As additional research emerges, it will be important to better understand the trajectory of well-being and associated protective factors for older adults during the COVID-19 pandemic.

Individuals older than age 65 who were retired and living on fixed incomes were less affected by the marked rise in unemployment during COVID-19, which contributed to stress for working younger and middle-age adults. Older adults are also less likely to have small children in their homes, eliminating the stressors of work-home imbalance and altered family dynamics that emerged when school- and college-age children were abruptly transitioned to extended virtual learning.

It is important to consider older adults as a nuanced and multifaceted population. Early fears that age was directly related to decreased chance of survival during the COVID-19 pandemic led some overburdened health care systems to ration care solely on the basis of age. If health care is rationed by age, then age itself, independent of health, becomes a risk factor.

INTERVENTIONS DURING PANDEMICS

Disaster-related interventions for older adults should consider age-specific comorbidities and vulnerabilities and needs in the context of disaster preparedness, risk communication, and early and longer-term postdisaster interventions. It is important to empower older adults, recognize their strengths and lifetime of experience, and avoid marginalization of this heterogeneous population during each stage of a disaster (Deeny et al. 2010). Further, disaster planning and intervention must consider the special challenges for the older population in the various types of disaster (e.g., pandemics, such as COVID-19, vs. climate-related disasters, such as hurricanes). Although limited research exists on disaster interventions to support the needs of older adults, established principles can serve as a useful guide for developing interventions in the unique context of COVID-19 and other public health emergencies.

Pandemic-Related Mental Health and Behavioral Interventions

Maintaining social relationships with loved ones through technology can be protective by decreasing loneliness and social isolation that may develop during stay-at-home orders, lockdowns, and quarantine (Vahia et al. 2020). Caregivers should gauge the availability of diverse resources that will help older adults manage pandemic-related stress and foster resilience, including technology access and skills, social connections, ability to engage in physical activity, and opportunities for spiritual or religious involvement.

Older adults decreased their use of mental health services during the COVID-19 pandemic, in part because of stay-at-home requirements and fear of contamination. Telehealth interventions can be more readily implemented during a pandemic than other forms of health care delivery and can enhance access to mental health care for older adults (Colle et al. 2020). In a nursing home for older adults with different levels of cognitive functioning, despite some difficulties in using technology, a telematics psychological service used during the COVID-19 pandemic was well received and appreciated by 75% of patients involved in the intervention, demonstrating good feasibility (Renzi et al. 2020). However, lack of comfort with technology, preference for in-person interaction around issues of mental health, and limited access to the internet may serve as barriers for some older adults.

Public health interventions and behavioral practices learned from the 2003 severe acute respiratory syndrome (SARS) epidemic (e.g., strict governmental measures, mask wearing, maintaining social distance, handwashing practices) were important factors in maintaining low incidence of COVID-19-related infection and deaths in Hong Kong (Lum et al. 2020). After the SARS epidemic, the Hong Kong government required all residential programs to appoint an infection control officer to oversee all infection control measures according to established guidelines. It was determined that during the epidemic, most nursing home infections were due to hospital visits; therefore, during the COVID-19 pandemic, nonessential visits and care from visiting doctors were suspended, and centers limited capacity and suspended day care services to address the spread of infection. However, limited day care services for older adults with no care at home were maintained, as were meal delivery, assistance with medication administration, and travel to doctor's appointments. In-person visits were also suspended, but remote visits by teleconference were coordinated to maintain social connections. Each of these actions helped limit infection transmission (Lum et al. 2020).

Disaster Preparedness, Resources, and Screening

Preparedness education can reduce disaster- and evacuation-related concerns (Lach et al. 2005). However, only one-third of older adults have established disaster emergency plans (Bhalla et al. 2015), which can have a substantial impact on responses during pandemics. Public health assistance for older adults is often found through community resources, such as churches and community and neighborhood centers, making them important partners in public health planning to support the needs of older adults. Further, disaster plans that include local registries and emergency contact information of older adults who are homebound can increase outreach, with postdisaster recovery plans providing critical support (Wyte-Lake et al. 2017). Including independent older adults in the design of preparedness and response resources builds collaboration, enhances trust, and improves the likelihood plans will be maintained over time (Kamau et al. 2018).

Personal disaster preparedness can be promoted through organizations that support older adults by providing education and training (e.g., lectures, videos). Further, educational materials and resources can be distributed at doctors' offices and grocery stores. Designing systems for medical and psychiatric medication distribution to the older population can be a very important and fear-reducing intervention in communities.

Access to reliable sources of public health information is critical during a prolonged public health emergency. During the COVID-19 pandemic, evolving health recommendations from public health experts, confusing and contradictory messaging from political figures and other community leaders, and the emergence of disinformation campaigns made it difficult for adults of all ages to make informed health choices (National Academies of Science, Engineering, and Medicine 2020). Trusted and credible messengers within communities can assist older adults by delivering public health messages at settings in which older adults gather, assisting with access to technology needed to acquire recommended health interventions (such as vaccinations), and educating community members on trusted sources of information. Establishing community helpers who can reach out to older members of a community (in houses or apartment buildings) can foster support, limit loneliness and depression, identify health needs, and provide education and information of critical importance.

Preventive interventions, such as treatments to prevent falls among frail older adults, can minimize injury risk during a disaster, especially if older adults are isolated during a pandemic. These interventions include strength and balance training, modification of home hazards, and decreasing use of psychotropic medications to reduce risk of falls and improve overall health and safety (Gates et al. 2008). Similarly, home visit programs coordinated by emergency response agencies and volunteer community groups can educate older adults about safety measures, how to recognize hazards, and how to develop a clear, easy-to-implement safety plan that can reduce risk of injury (Tannous and Agho 2019). Nursing home staff should be trained for disaster response and receive disaster preparedness resources (e.g., care of patients with emerging disaster-related medical conditions, evacuation processes, educational materials for families) (Lach et al. 2005). In order to coordinate residents' medical and physical needs, plans need to ensure that adequate supplies and medications are available for periods when residents must restrict movement for extended periods of time.

Particular attention is needed for older adults with mild cognitive impairment, who may reside in independent housing without a caregiver. These older adults may not understand or may become confused by communication of disaster-related information (e.g., content, instructions, and future risk communication via broadcasted news), which may complicate disaster response (Akanuma et al. 2016). Predisaster outreach can increase preparedness among this subgroup, and news broadcasts that rely primarily on photos and slower presentation of the news may help older adults with cognitive impairments process information.

Early Interventions

Early interventions focusing on older adults' emotional response during a disaster may help mitigate adverse psychological consequences (Wilson-Genderson et al. 2018).

Psychological First Aid

Psychological First Aid (PFA) is a widely used intervention for providing acute psychological care that is effective in enhancing well-being, reducing distress, and improving functioning immediately postdisaster (Hobfoll et al. 2007). Older adults are often especially responsive to natural spontaneous discussions with peers during this period, which can help establish feelings of calm and normalcy (Langan and Palmer 2012) and provide social support for those who are isolated. Although most disaster-exposed individuals do not develop psychiatric disorders, PFA addresses the distress that many people experience after a disaster. PFA materials have been modified to address the specific needs of older adults who live in residential facilities to assist nursing home staff in providing mental and medical health care while ensuring physical safety (Brown et al. 2009).

The goals of PFA are accomplished by 1) establishing a sense of safety as well as actually having a physically safe environment, 2) promoting social connectedness, 3) maintaining community and individual self-efficacy (a sense that one can accomplish the task and ensuring one has the skills to do so) through emergency response guidance and policies and self-care (e.g., healthy nutrition, adequate sleep, rest, exercise), 4) increasing calmness by using arousal reduction methods (e.g., relaxation training), and 5) fostering optimism and hope in the context of ongoing disaster-related risks. Other immediate disaster interventions involve screening, which can be administered by individuals without special training, such as public health workers and volunteers. For example, Seniors Without Families Team (SWiFT) is an important screening tool for identifying older adults who require immediate care (Dyer et al. 2008).

Crisis Counseling

Older individuals who need additional mental and behavioral health assistance may benefit from crisis counseling in the initial postdisaster period (Gibson et al. 2018). Care provision may be particularly complicated during pandemics, when access to health care is significantly altered and the recovery period may be greatly prolonged. Rapid community assessment can help with identification of older adults' needs and in planning appropriate and timely services (Lach et al. 2005), which may be implemented through informal community support systems (e.g., religious organizations) or local agencies. Although many older adults will not need intervention following PFA and crisis counseling, for those with severe, prolonged adverse outcomes, formal treatment administered by licensed clinicians may be recommended. Because of long-standing mental health stigma, older adults may underreport distress and/or present with somatic complaints instead of psychological symptoms, which merit particular attention. Although it is suggested that psychological interventions be individualized to the older adult's specific needs, relatively few available interventions have been specifically adapted for this population (Gibson et al. 2018). Cognitive decline, which may interfere with older adults' ability to remember therapeutic material, may not be accounted for in psychotherapy; therefore, multimodal methods in therapy and psychoeducation are suggested.

Prevention of functional decline and recovery among older adults during a pandemic can be promoted by attention to medical care access, which has been facilitated effectively by mobile medical teams for treatment and provision of essential medications, and efforts to develop and maintain opportunities for social engagement and physical activity during disasters (Tsuboya et al. 2017). Pandemic-related stressors, such as loss of in-person social contact and difficulties with health care access, may be additional risk factors for psychological and behavioral difficulties, such as sleep problems (Li et al. 2018), among older adults and should be targeted in recovery efforts to prevent exacerbation of chronic physical and mental health problems (Pietrzak et al. 2013).

Postdisaster Interventions

Overall, there may be long-term decreases in disaster-related health care use among older adults, in part because of overburdened community systems postdisaster and logistical and emotional challenges that may occur as older adults attempt to reestablish health care behaviors (Quast and Feng 2019). Although enhancing telehealth services may offer improved access, reduced health care use is particularly problematic for older adults, for whom the physical impact of disasters may be greater, chronic conditions may be exacerbated, and the risk of developing new medical problems is higher. It is critical for local governments to establish public health clinics and coordinate medical outreach for this population.

After Hurricane Sandy, the Sandy Mobilization, Assessment, Referral, and Treatment for Mental Health (SMART-MH) program was developed as a systematic assessment and evidence-based intervention and administered with a multilingual, culturally sensitive approach to identifying older adults needing assistance and increasing and improving mental health service delivery (Sirey et al. 2017). It provides critical postdisaster services, including case identification, community outreach in homes and senior centers, and needs assessment, and coordinates social services. For those with mental health problems, short-term psychotherapy is provided at no cost. Establishing trust and bonds with the community was accomplished by involving residents in program development and application. Although COVID-19 created challenges to face-to-face health care interactions, adapting effective community outreach programs within the environment of a pandemic can improve access to care, particularly for older adults with mobility limitations, cognitive difficulties, and lower engagement with technology.

Among older disaster survivors without mobility impairment, interventions that incorporate frequent physical activity, such as group exercise and daily walking, were associated with less depression in (Tsuji et al. 2017). Social engagement and stress reduction experienced during active group activities may have positive preventive and intervention effects on mental health. Participation in an exercise program for older adults, particularly if initiated early, was associated with lower long-term functional disability (i.e., psychological and physical problems and reduced quality of life) (Kuroda et al. 2018).

Home-Based Primary Care

Home-based primary care programs, such as the one developed by the U.S. Department of Veterans Affairs, have a primary role in promoting patients' safety and well-being and enhancing social support for isolated older adults. In these programs, health care practitioners visit older veterans to provide medical care and have effectively individualized preparedness and recovery efforts (Wyte-Lake et al. 2019). Early and consistent efforts to monitor patients postdisaster can reveal opportunities to foster resilience and treat early psychiatric illness such as depression, alcohol use disorders, and anxiety disorders. A home-based primary care evidence-based tool kit, which has been administered to health providers who deliver home care and act as liaisons with the community health care system, is helpful in preparing care providers to assist older adults with disaster-related hazards (Wyte-Lake et al. 2017).

Informal Social Supports

Disaster preparedness is associated with greater community membership and informal social support, with emergency preparedness information exchanged through these important connections (Kim and Zakour 2017). Predisaster community cohesion and attention to strategies that promote neighbors helping each other are important for ensuring support during disasters (Deeny et al. 2010; Ursano et al. 2014). Opportunities for frequent communication with familiar neighbors and friends that are adapted for pandemics using virtual resources and health protection guidelines can help older adults receive or provide needed support, reduce isolation, manage stress, and instill a sense of belonging, security, and self-efficacy, enhancing disaster resilience (Sasaki et al. 2020).

SUMMARY

COVID-19 adversely affected health, economic, and social systems and led to human suffering on a scale not seen from a health crisis in more than a century. An appreciation of adverse mental health effects for older adults has been informed by previous disaster literature and early research during the pandemic. Although older adults have borne a disproportionate burden of illness and death during the pandemic, some of the actions required to manage COVID-19 have protected older adults against certain social and economic adversities associated with worsened mental health. Emerging research will further our understanding of risk and protective factors that allow for optimized and targeted preparedness, response, and recovery interventions during future pandemics. Public health interventions that target community-level factors, such as preparedness, technology use, communication, and access to care, while addressing the essential elements of early interventions, show the greatest promise for enhancing the trajectory of recovery for older adults after the COVID-19 pandemic.

KEY POINTS

- Pandemics are global disasters that produce fear, uncertainty, loss, and threats of death that alter perceptions of risk and result in psychological and behavioral distress and disorders.

- The risk-mitigating behaviors required by a society to control a pandemic can add additional stress for older adults, some of which may be buffered by psychosocial aspects of advanced age.

- Interventions to support individuals and communities throughout a pandemic should be tailored to address the needs, strengths, and challenges of older adults.

QUESTIONS FOR REVIEW

1. Which of the following is *not* a common and early psychological or behavioral response after disasters?

   A. PTSD
   B. Insomnia
   C. Irritability
   D. Decreased sense of safety

Answer: A. PTSD takes at least 30 days before a diagnosis can be made. By contrast, the other responses listed can occur immediately following exposure to a disaster and will affect far more people, even in a transient capacity.

2. Which of the following is *not* one of the essential elements that are critical to enhance following exposure to trauma to reduce distress and enhance well-being?

    A. Safety
    B. Calming
    C. Enlightenment
    D. Social connectedness
    E. Self-efficacy

Answer: C. The five essential elements are safety, calming, self-efficacy or community efficacy, social connectedness, and hope or optimism.

3. Which statement is *least* accurate about older adults and disaster planning?

    A. Needs and concerns change across the age spectrum.
    B. Risk is typically associated with diseases of aging rather than age itself.
    C. Age can bring unique protective factors related to stress tolerance and prior lived experiences.
    D. The same interventions can be used for all age groups.

Answer: D. Interventions should be tailored to address the unique needs of older adults and all populations across the age spectrum.

REFERENCES

Akanuma K, Nakamura K, Meguro K, et al: Disturbed social recognition and impaired risk judgement in older residents with mild cognitive impairment after the Great East Japan Earthquake of 2011: the Tome Project. Psychogeriatrics 16(6):349–354, 2016 26756451

American Association for Geriatric Psychiatry: IOM study on mental health workforce of older adults fact sheet. McLean, VA, American Association for Geriatric Psychiatry, 2008. Available at: www.aagponline.org/index.php?src=gendocs&ref=FactSheetIOMStudyonMentalHealthWorkforceof OlderAdults&category=Advocacy&link=FactSheetIOMStudyonMental HealthWorkforceofOlderAdults. Accessed June 23, 2021.

Barry KL, Blow FC: Drinking over the lifespan: focus on older adults. Alcohol Res 38(1):115–120, 2016 27159818

Bhalla MC, Burgess A, Frey J, et al: Geriatric disaster preparedness. Prehosp Disaster Med 30(5):443–446, 2015 26369366

Brown LM, Bruce ML, Hyer K, et al: A pilot study evaluating the feasibility of psychological first aid for nursing home residents. Clin Gerontol 32(3):293–308, 2009 20592947

Centers for Disease Control and Prevention: Weekly updates by select demographic and geographic characteristics. Atlanta, GA, Centers for Disease Control and Prevention, March 10, 2021. Available at: www.cdc.gov/nchs/nvss/vsrr/covid_weekly/index.htm. Accessed March 11, 2021.

Chang ES, Levy BR: High prevalence of elder abuse during the COVID-19 pandemic: risk and resilience factors. Am J Geriatr Psychiatry Jan 19, 2021 33518464Epub ahead of print

Chen Y, Klein SL, Garibaldi BT, et al: Aging in COVID-19: vulnerability, immunity and intervention. Ageing Res Rev 65:101205, 2021 33137510

Colle R, Ait Tayeb AEK, de Larminat D, et al: Short-term acceptability by patients and psychiatrists of the turn to psychiatric teleconsultation in the context of the COVID-19 pandemic. Psychiatry Clin Neurosci 74(8):443–444, 2020 32511825

Cox K, Kim B: Race and income disparities in disaster preparedness in old age. J Gerontol Soc Work 61(7):719–734, 2018 29979948

Czeisler MÉ, Lane RI, Wiley JF, et al: Follow-up survey of US adult reports of mental health, substance use, and suicidal ideation during the COVID-19 pandemic, September 2020. JAMA Netw Open 4(2):e2037665, 2021 33606030

Deeny P, Vitale CT, Spelman R, et al: Addressing the imbalance: empowering older people in disaster response and preparedness. Int J Older People Nurs 5(1):77–80, 2010 20925761

Dyer CB, Regev M, Burnett J, et al: SWiFT: a rapid triage tool for vulnerable older adults in disaster situations. Disaster Med Public Health Prep 2 (suppl 1):S45–S50, 2008 18769267

Ettman CK, Abdalla SM, Cohen GH, et al: Prevalence of depression symptoms in US adults before and during the COVID-19 pandemic. JAMA Netw Open 3(9):e2019686, 2020 32876685

Fan F, Zhou Y, Liu X: Sleep disturbance predicts posttraumatic stress disorder and depressive symptoms: a cohort study of Chinese adolescents. J Clin Psychiatry 78(7):882–888, 2017 27574834

Fullerton CS, Herberman Mash HB, Benevides KN, et al: Distress of routine activities and perceived safety associated with post-traumatic stress, depression, and alcohol use: 2002 Washington, DC, sniper attacks. Disaster Med Public Health Prep 9(5):509–515, 2015 26045212

Gates S, Fisher JD, Cooke MW, et al: Multifactorial assessment and targeted intervention for preventing falls and injuries among older people in community and emergency care settings: systematic review and meta-analysis. BMJ 336(7636):130–133, 2008 18089892

Gibson A, Walsh J, Brown LM: Disaster mental health services review of care for older persons after disasters. Disaster Med Public Health Prep 12(3):366–372, 2018 28851475

Himes CL, Kilduff L: Which U.S. states have the oldest populations? Washington, DC, Population Reference Bureau, March 16, 2019. Available at: www.prb.org/which-us-states-are-the-oldest. Accessed February 28, 2021.

Hobfoll SE, Watson P, Bell CC, et al: Five essential elements of immediate and mid-term mass trauma intervention: empirical evidence. Psychiatry 70(4):283–315, discussion 316–369, 2007 18181708

Kamau PW, Ivey SL, Griese SE, et al: Preparedness training programs for working with deaf and hard of hearing communities and older adults: lessons learned from key informants and literature assessments. Disaster Med Public Health Prep 12(5):606–614, 2018 29041996

Kim H, Zakour M: Disaster preparedness among older adults: social support, community participation, and demographic characteristics. Journal of Social Service Research 43(4):498–509, 2017

Kivi M, Hansson I, Bjälkebring P: Up and about: older adults' well-being during the COVID-19 pandemic in a Swedish longitudinal study. J Gerontol B Psychol Sci Soc Sci 76(2):e4–e9, 2021 32599622

Kuroda Y, Iwasa H, Orui M, et al: Risk factor for incident functional disability and the effect of a preventive exercise program: a 4-year prospective cohort study of older survivors from the Great East Japan Earthquake and nuclear disaster. Int J Environ Res Public Health 15(7):1430, 2018 29986471

Kwong ASF, Pearson RM, Adams MJ, et al: Mental health before and during the COVID-19 pandemic in two longitudinal UK population cohorts. Br J Psychiatry Nov 24, 2020 33228822 Epub ahead of print

Lach HW, Langan JC, James DC: Disaster planning: are gerontological nurses prepared? J Gerontol Nurs 31(11):21–27, 2005 16317991

Langan JC, Palmer JL: Listening to and learning from older adult Hurricane Katrina survivors. Public Health Nurs 29(2):126–135, 2012 22372449

Li X, Buxton OM, Hikichi H, et al: Predictors of persistent sleep problems among older disaster survivors: a natural experiment from the 2011 Great East Japan earthquake and tsunami. Sleep (Basel) 41(7):zsy084, 2018 29726979

Lum T, Shi C, Wong G, et al: COVID-19 and long-term care policy for older people in Hong Kong. J Aging Soc Policy 32(4–5):373–379, 2020 32476597

Mehrotra A, Chernew M, Linetsky D, et al: The impact of the COVID-19 pandemic on outpatient visits: a rebound emerges. New York, Commonwealth Fund, May 19, 2020. Available at: www.commonwealthfund.org/publications/2020/apr/impact-covid-19-outpatient-visits. Accessed March 7, 2021.

Morganstein JC, Ursano RJ: Ecological disasters and mental health: causes, consequences, and interventions. Front Psychiatry 11:1, 2020 32116830

Morganstein JC, Fullerton CS, Ursano RJ, et al: Pandemics: health care emergencies, in Textbook of Disaster Psychiatry, 2nd Edition. Edited by Ursano RJ, Fullerton CS, Weisaeth L, et al. New York, Cambridge University Press, 2017, pp 270–284

National Academies of Science, Engineering, and Medicine: Addressing Health Misinformation With Health Literacy Strategies: Proceedings of a Workshop—in Brief. Washington, DC, National Academies Press, 2020

Omura T, Araki A, ShigemotoK, et al: Geriatric practice during and after the COVID-19 pandemic. Geriatr Gerontol Int 20(7):735–737, 2020 32428997

O'Súilleabháin PS, Gallagher S, Steptoe: Loneliness, living alone, and all-cause mortality: the role of emotional and social loneliness in the elderly during 19 years of follow-up. Psychosom Med 81(6):521–526, 2019 31094903

Pew Research Center: Internet/broadband fact sheet. Washington, DC, Pew Research Center, June 12, 2019a. Available at: www.pewresearch.org/internet/fact-sheet/internet-broadband. Accessed March 11, 2021.

Pew Research Center: Mobile fact sheet. Washington, DC, Pew Research Center, June 12, 2019b. Available at: www.pewresearch.org/internet/fact-sheet/mobile/. Accessed March 11, 2021.

Pietrzak RH, Van Ness PH, Fried TR, et al: Trajectories of posttraumatic stress symptomatology in older persons affected by a large-magnitude disaster. J Psychiatr Res 47(4):520–526, 2013 23290559

Quast T, Feng L: Long-term effects of disasters on health care utilization: Hurricane Katrina and older individuals with diabetes. Disaster Med Public Health Prep 13(4):724–731, 2019 30621803

Renzi A, Verrusio W, Messina M, et al: Psychological intervention with elderly people during the COVID-19 pandemic: the experience of a nursing home in Italy. Psychogeriatrics 20(6):918–919, 2020 32770596

Roberts A, Ogunwole SU, Blakeslee L, et al: The population 65 years and older in the United States: 2016: American community survey reports. Washington, DC, U.S. Census Bureau, October 2018. Available at: www.census.gov/content/dam/Census/library/publications/2018/acs/ACS-38.pdf. Accessed June 23, 2021.

Sasaki Y, Tsuji T, Koyama S, et al: Neighborhood ties reduced depressive symptoms in older disaster survivors: Iwanuma study, a natural experiment. Int J Environ Res Public Health 17(1):337, 2020 31947798

Shiina A, Niitsu T, Kobori O, et al: Relationship between perception and anxiety about COVID-19 infection and risk behaviors for spreading infection: a national survey in Japan. Brain Behav Immun Health 6:100101, 2020 32835297

Shultz JM, Espinola M, Rechkemmer A, et al: Prevention of disaster impact and outcome cascades, in The Cambridge Handbook of International Prevention Science. Edited by Israelashvili M, Romano JL. New York, Cambridge University Press, 2017, pp 492–519

Sirey JA, Berman J, Halkett A, et al: Storm impact and depression among older adults living in Hurricane Sandy–affected areas. Disaster Med Public Health Prep 11(1):97–109, 2017 27995840

Statista: Proportion of selected age groups of world population in 2020, by region. New York, Statista, July 2020. Available at: www.statista.com/statistics/265759/world-population-by-age-and-region. Accessed March 18, 2021.

Tannous WK, Agho K: Domestic fire emergency escape plans among the aged in NSW, Australia: the impact of a fire safety home visit program. BMC Public Health 19(1):872, 2019 31272445

Tsuboya T, Aida J, Hikichi H, et al: Predictors of decline in IADL functioning among older survivors following the Great East Japan earthquake: a prospective study. Soc Sci Med 176:34–41, 2017 28122269

Tsuji T, Sasaki Y, Matsuyama Y, et al: Reducing depressive symptoms after the Great East Japan Earthquake in older survivors through group exercise participation and regular walking: a prospective observational study. BMJ Open 7(3):e013706, 2017 28258173

Ursano RJ, McKibben JBA, Reissman DB, et al: Posttraumatic stress disorder and community collective efficacy following the 2004 Florida hurricanes. PLoS One 9(2):e88467, 2014 24523900

Ursano RJ, Fullerton CS, Weisaeth L, et al: Individual and community responses to disasters, in Textbook of Disaster Psychiatry, 2nd Edition. Edited by Ursano RJ, Fullerton CS, Weisaeth L, et al. New York, Cambridge University Press, 2017, pp 1–26

U.S. Bureau of Labor and Statistics: US civilian labor force, by age, sex, race, and ethnicity 1999, 2008, 2019 and projected 2029. Washington, DC, U.S. Bureau of Labor and Statistics, September 1, 2020. Available at: www.bls.gov/emp/tables/civilian-labor-force-summary.htm. Accessed March 2, 2021.

Vahia IV, Jeste DV, Reynolds CF III: Older adults and the mental health effects of COVID-19. JAMA 324(22):2253–2254, 2020 33216114

Verdery AM, Smith-Greenaway E, Margolis R, et al: Tracking the reach of COVID-19 kin loss with a bereavement multiplier applied to the United States. Proc Natl Acad Sci USA 117(30):17695–17701, 2020 32651279

Wilson-Genderson M, Heid AR, Pruchno R: Long-term effects of disaster on depressive symptoms: type of exposure matters. Soc Sci Med 217:84–91, 2018 30296694

World Health Organization: Mental health of older adults. Geneva, World Health Organization, December 12, 2017. Available at: www.who.int/news-room/fact-sheets/detail/mental-health-of-older-adults. Accessed March 11, 2021.

Wyte-Lake T, Claver M, Der-Martirosian C, et al: Developing a home-based primary care disaster preparedness toolkit. Disaster Med Public Health Prep 11(1):56–63, 2017 27839522

Wyte-Lake T, Claver M, Johnson-Koenke R, et al: Home-based primary care's role in supporting the older old during wildfires. J Prim Care Community Health 10:2150132719846773, 2019 31088255

Xu JQ, Murphy SL, Kochanek KD, et al: Mortality in the United States, 2018. Hyattsville, MD, National Center for Health Statistics, 2020. Available at: www.cdc.gov/nchs/data/databriefs/db355-h.pdf. Accessed June 23, 2021.

CHAPTER 2

HISTORICAL OVERVIEW OF PANDEMICS

Matthew L. Edwards, M.D.
Yolonda R. Pickett, M.D.
Maria D. Llorente, M.D., FAPA

Pandemics have existed throughout the history of humankind and have wrought fear, economic devastation, and, in many cases, death with associated societal impacts. In some cases, whole populations were eliminated. Older adults are often, although not always, more vulnerable to morbidity and mortality associated with the causes of these pandemics. Multiple factors can contribute to an infectious agent moving from being infective to causing an epidemic and then to worldwide pandemic spread. With technological advances, more treatments are available to mitigate morbidity and mortality, as well to develop vaccines and treatments more quickly. In this chapter, we provide a historical overview of pandemics and their impact on older populations. We focus primarily on rapidly emerging communicable diseases that have had large and lasting impacts on society and public health.

Vignette

"OK now, Grandma. Your family is not here. So we are your family now" (Wu and Tsien 2020). The young nurse was trying to comfort an elderly woman who would soon die without relatives nearby. In January 2020, the hospitals, doctors, and nurses of Wuhan, China, were the first to witness and care for, and become overwhelmed by, an unknown respiratory illness that the world would come to call COVID-19. At the time of this writing, more than 263 million people worldwide are confirmed to have been infected, and more than 5.3 million have died. Like in Wuhan, other health care systems soon would become overwhelmed, and ethical dilemmas regarding whom to admit, whom to place on a ventilator, and for whom to offer only comfort care as they died have, unfortunately, become all too commonplace. The unique features of each infectious agent, as well as the characteristics of the host, confer greater morbidity and mortality for some and protection for others. Coronavirus SARS-CoV-2 disease (COVID-19) preferentially attacks and kills older adults. And because of the highly contagious nature of this virus, older adults are often isolated and/or die alone. When all scientific and medical recourses are exhausted, however, the one remaining thing every health care provider can offer is comfort. That was what the nurse in Wuhan did. That was what Dr. Joseph Varon did on his 252nd consecutive day of caring for COVID-19 patients in the intensive care unit of a Texas hospital: It was Thanksgiving. An elderly man was trying to escape, crying and saying he wanted to be with his wife. "So I just grab him and I hold him…I was feeling very sad, just like him. Eventually he felt better and he stopped crying" (NDTV 2020).

BRIEF OVERVIEW

The World Health Organization designated COVID-19 a pandemic on March 11, 2020. As of December 3, 2021, it has caused more than 5.23 million deaths worldwide, more than 777,000 of which were in the United States. The rapid emergence of the COVID-19 pandemic has exposed weaknesses in our public health response system, led some people to blame ethnic groups for the virus, and revealed cultural, social, and political tensions in American society. Although these events may appear unique to this moment in history, physician-historian Howard Markel's work suggests that they represent broader patterns common to many epidemics. These leitmotifs include responses shaped by a society's understanding of infection and disease, behaviors strongly influenced by the degree of economic devastation of the pandemic, attempts to conceal the disease, and scapegoating of specific groups (Institute of Medicine 2007). Developing processes of globalization have also contributed to the spread of the disease and possibly facilitated the emergence of more contagious variants.

OVERVIEW AND TIMELINE OF PANDEMICS

Table 2–1 provides a broad overview of pandemics throughout the history of humankind. Both viruses and bacteria have been causative agents; humans, mammals, and insects have all served as vectors, and multiple means of transmission have occurred. As we are starting to see with COVID-19, many pandemics are also associated with long-term sequelae.

CHANGING DEMOGRAPHICS

For most of the history of humankind, communicable diseases were the primary cause of death, and often, the very old and the very young were most affected. By 2030, as the population worldwide ages, one in eight of Earth's inhabitants will be age 65 or older (National Institute of Aging 2017); 2030 will also mark the first time in U.S. history when the population older than 65 will outnumber the population younger than 18 (U.S. Census Bureau 2018).

The agents that cause pandemics are highly infectious, often with high mortality rates and with long-lasting impacts on populations. The infectious diseases associated with the deadliest pandemics include bubonic plague, smallpox, cholera, and influenza. These pandemics affected ages and populations differently.

Bubonic Plague

The Black Death, which resulted in a 30%–50% depopulation of Europe during the fourteenth century, preferentially killed elderly individuals and those who were already in poor health (DeWitte 2010; DeWitte and Wood 2008), leading some researchers to suggest that the plague acted as an agent of natural selection, removing the weakest persons from the genetic pool. This massive loss of population resulted in labor shortages but also led to increased resources. As a result, the system of serfdom ended; wages and payments in kind (extra food and clothing) rose; and prices for food, goods, and housing fell (Bailey 1996; Munro 2004). These changes resulted in higher overall standards of living, higher life expectancy, and lower mortality in the postpandemic years (DeWitte 2014). One study has found that before the plague, only 10% of Europeans reached age 70, whereas in the centuries following the plague, 20% of Europeans lived past age 70 (DeWitte 2014).

Table 2–1. Pandemics throughout history

Disease	Agent	Vector	Type	Transmission	Global disease burden[a]	Mortality	Geography	Sequelae
Smallpox[b]	Variola major virus	Human	Virus	Airborne, physical contact	Eradicated	30%	Europe, Latin America, Africa, Asia	Scarring, pockmarks, vision problems, blindness, encephalitis, osteomyelitis, infertility
Diphtheria[c]	Corynebacterium diphtheriae	Human	Bacterium	Aerosol, skin exudates	16,000	5%–10%	Africa, India, Indonesia	Heart, nerve, and other damage
Measles[d]	Measles virus, rubeola	Human	Virus	Airborne, physical contact	870,000	10%	Africa, Asia	Subacute sclerosing panencephalitis
Cholera[e]	Vibrio cholerae	Human	Bacterium	Fecal-oral	2.8 million	1%–60%	Africa, Southeast Asia	Fatal complications include electrolyte abnormalities and profound hypovolemic loss
Tuberculosis[f]	Mycobacterium tuberculosis	Human	Bacterium	Airborne	10 million	0.20%	Worldwide	Pulmonary and neurological deficits

Table 2–1. Pandemics throughout history *(continued)*

Disease	Agent	Vector	Type	Transmission	Global disease burden[a]	Mortality	Geography	Sequelae
Influenza[g]	Influenza	Human	Virus	Airborne, physical contact	1 billion	Varies	Worldwide	Complications include inflammation, myocarditis, encephalitis, rhabdomyolysis, and multisystem organ failure
Bubonic plague[h]	Yersinia pestis	Rodents, fleas	Bacterium	Fleabites, aerosols	1–17	30%–100%	Africa, Asia, South America	Fatal complications include meningitis, pneumonia, septicemia, and DIC
Yellow fever[i]	Yellow fever virus	Mosquito	Virus	Insect bite	200,000	1.50%	South America, Africa	Bleeding, kidney issues
Poliomyelitis[j]	Polio virus	Human	Virus	Fecal-oral	200	2%–30%	Africa, South Asia	Paralysis

Table 2–1. Pandemics throughout history *(continued)*

Disease	Agent	Vector	Type	Transmission	Global disease burden[a]	Mortality	Geography	Sequelae
HIV[k]	Human immunodeficiency virus	Human	Virus	Bodily fluids	38 million	4.70%	Worldwide	AIDS, psychiatric disorders, HAND, chronic inflammation and associated conditions
SARS[l]	SARS-CoV-1	Palm civets, bats	Virus	Airborne, physical contact	8,422	11%	Asia, North America, Europe	Pulmonary fibrosis, femoral head necrosi
Zika[m]	Zika virus	Mosquito	Virus	Insect bite, sexual, vertical (pregnancy/childbirth), blood-borne	None	Unknown	Brazil, United States, Africa, Asia	Guillain-Barré syndrome, fetal abnormalities
Ebola[n]	Ebola virus	Fruit bats	Virus	Contact with human fluids, animals	Varies	25%–90%	Africa, United States	Paresthesia, headache, sensory hearing loss, myalgias, arthralgias, vision problems

Table 2–1. Pandemics throughout history *(continued)*

Disease	Agent	Vector	Type	Transmission	Global disease burden[a]	Mortality	Geography	Sequelae
COVID-19[o]	SARS-CoV-2	Human	Virus	Airborne, physical contact	263 million	Unknown	Worldwide	Neurological, pulmonary, and multiorgan dysfunction

Note. COVID-19= coronavirus SARS-CoV-2 disease; DIC=disseminated intravascular coagulation; HAND=HIV-associated neurocognitive disorders; SARS=severe acute respiratory syndrome.

[a]Global disease burden represents the best available estimate of the number of cases reported to the World Health Organization. The number may not be the true incidence or prevalence but represents the most recent estimates of the reported worldwide cases.

[b]Centers for Disease Control and Prevention 2016; World Health Organization 2021b.

[c]Centers for Disease Control and Prevention 2020b.

[d]Gastanaduy et al. 2020; Tanne 2020.

[e]Ali et al. 2012.

[f]Centers for Disease Control and Prevention 2020e; American Lung Association 2013.

[g]Centers for Disease Control and Prevention 2021b, 2021b; Hall 2021; World Health Organization 2019.

[h]Mead 2015; World Health Organization 2000.

[i]Centers for Disease Control and Prevention 2018.

[j]Estivariz et al. 2020.

[k]U.S. Department of Health and Human Services 2020.

[l]World Health Organization 2003; Zhang et al. 2020.

[m]Hall et al. 2018.

[n]Tozay et al. 2020; World Health Organization 2021a

[o]Johns Hopkins University and Medicine 2021.

Smallpox

Smallpox, with a mortality rate of 30% (World Health Organization 2021b), preferentially affected children where it was endemic because only two outcomes could occur following infection: death or lifelong immunity. In communities never previously exposed, however, smallpox affected all ages. These types of outbreaks were periodically seen in Africa, Asia, and Europe but were most deadly in the Americas, wiping out as many as 90% of Indigenous peoples (Koch et al. 2019). In fact, smallpox, along with other infectious agents (diphtheria, measles, influenza, and typhus), killed so many Indigenous peoples that a recent study showed that it caused Earth's climate to cool prior to the Industrial Revolution (Koch et al. 2019). With the introduction of vaccination programs, smallpox cases and deaths rapidly declined until smallpox was eradicated in 1980, leading several researchers to single out vaccination as a major contributor to increased life expectancy (Ochmann and Roser 2018).

Cholera

Cholera remains a significant cause of epidemics, most commonly in areas where disasters, war, or severe poverty lead to crowded living conditions with poor hygiene and sanitation (Centers for Disease Control and Prevention 2020a; National Organization for Rare Disorders 2009). Although it is highly treatable, primarily with rehydration solution, if left untreated, cholera may result in mortality within hours. Children younger than age 5 are most susceptible to adverse impacts, but other groups at risk include those with achlorhydria, blood type O, and chronic medical conditions, as well as health care workers sent to manage cholera epidemics and those who have no access to rehydration therapies. Cases in the United States are rare, but because natural reservoirs for the bacteria exist in warm coastal waters, eradication is unlikely. According to the Centers for Disease Control and Prevention (2020a), a global pandemic has been ongoing for the past six decades in Asia, Africa, and South America, with the highest case fatality rates in Africa.

Influenza

For at least the past 150 years, influenza has had a U-shaped death-by-age curve, preferentially killing children under age 5 and adults older than 65, with relatively low numbers of deaths in the ages in between (Centers for Disease Control and Prevention 2021b). The one exception was the 1918 epidemic, which exhibited a W-shaped curve: a distinct additional peak of deaths in adults 20–40 years old. Influenza-related deaths in those

15–34 years old during the 1918 pandemic were more than 20 times higher than in previous years, and nearly half of influenza-related deaths were in people ages 20–40 years, such that the absolute risk of death in those younger than 65 was higher than in those 65 and older (Simonsen et al. 1998). More than 99% of excess influenza-related deaths in the 1918 pandemic were among persons younger than 65. For comparison, this same group accounted for only 36% of excess influenza-related deaths in the 1957 H2N2 pandemic and less than half in the 1968 H3N2 pandemic (Grove and Hetzel 1968; Viboud et al. 2016). The lower-than-predicted mortality in older adults was thought to be due to immunity that resulted from previous exposure to influenza A–containing surface proteins shared with the 1918 virus (Taubenberger et al. 2006). Of interest, the 1918 pandemic has had a long-lasting impact in that all influenza A pandemics since then have been caused by descendants of that 1918 virus (Taubenberger et al. 2006).

COVID-19

As noted, the population of the world is aging, with the proportion ages 85 years and older being the fastest-growing group in many nations (National Institute of Aging 2017). Throughout history, children and young people have outnumbered older adults, such that prior pandemics, although often preferentially affecting seniors, could theoretically have been even deadlier had more elderly people been alive. The COVID-19 pandemic is the first to test this hypothesis and seems to be bearing it out. In fact, COVID-19 is now the leading cause of death in the United States (Cox and Amin 2021). As of this writing, deaths among the most vulnerable elderly, those residing in nursing homes, account for nearly one-third of all U.S. COVID-related deaths (AARP Public Policy Institute 2021).

CIRCUMSTANCES THAT PROMOTE PANDEMICS

Several conditions or circumstances are known to promote pandemics and thus are important to identify and recognize because they point to ways to mitigate and/or prevent spread of the infection. One of the most important is whether a population was previously exposed to the infectious agent and thus developed immunity. When communities are newly exposed to an infectious agent, whole populations may be decimated. In these cases, the most effective management strategy is to develop a method to rapidly identify the infectious agent and then conduct contact tracing and quarantine.

Often, the mode of transmission of the infectious agent can affect conditions that promote spread. For example, infections that are transmitted through aerosol droplets spread more easily in crowded indoor conditions. Thus, crowded workplaces, schools, nursing homes or congregate living facilities, and social gatherings become high-risk locations.

Poor hygiene, lack of running water, and inadequately treated water and sewage all contribute to the spread of several pandemic agents. These features, in addition to other environmental conditions, such as higher-than-average temperatures and excessive rainfall, have been associated with increased risk of cholera (Jutla et al. 2013). Trade; population growth; and travel by merchants, military, crusaders, and groups from smallpox-endemic areas to previously nonexposed areas spread smallpox and have led to severe epidemics (Centers for Disease Control and Prevention 2021c). European colonization and the African slave trade similarly led to massive deaths among the Indigenous peoples of the Americas. The expansion of ease of travel today (via airlines, rail, and cruise ships) has contributed to the spread of the coronavirus.

More recently, human-made environmental changes such as logging, roadbuilding, and rapid urbanization with associated population growth have exposed people to close contact with previously more remote animal species, increasing the risk of zoonotic transmission. According to one research team, of 335 diseases that emerged between 1960 and 2004, 60% came from nonhuman animals (Vidal 2020). Ebola, hantavirus, rabies, Lyme disease, Middle East respiratory syndrome (MERS), and, most recently, COVID-19 are among the diseases that may have been introduced in this manner.

PANDEMICS AND OLDER ADULTS: VULNERABILITIES AND PREVENTION STRATEGIES

Why Seniors Are More Vulnerable

As people age, changes in the immune system increase vulnerability to infectious agents (Weyand and Goronzy 2016). The immune system is slower to respond, increasing the risk of becoming ill after exposure to an infectious agent. The immunity from vaccines may not be as complete or last as long. Recent studies have also found immunological sex differences (Márquez et al. 2020). The X chromosome has a high density of immune-related genes, and because women have two of these chromosomes, they mount stronger innate and adaptive immune responses (Schurz et al. 2019). With age, men show more decline in several aspects of immune response, which may partially explain the increased mortality among older men.

Older adults are more likely to have specific comorbidities that can increase risk for worse medical outcomes once they are infected. Seniors are also at greater risk for having cancer or other conditions (such as diabetes mellitus) that can lead to becoming immunocompromised, and they are more likely to be taking medications that further suppress immune function. The COVID-19 virus uses angiotensin converting enzyme 2 (ACE2) for entry into the host cell (Li et al. 2003). Men have higher plasma ACE2 levels than do women, and in men with heart failure, plasma levels of ACE2 are even higher than normal (Griffith et al. 2020). This difference may further explain the higher rates of morbidity and mortality among men.

Seniors may reside in communal settings, increasing their exposure to other people who may be infected. Some seniors live in multigenerational households, again increasing exposure risk. Last, as seen during the COVID-19 pandemic, when the health care system becomes overwhelmed and resources such as ventilators are scarce, age limits and life expectancy may be used as criteria influencing decisions about the distribution of resources (May and Aulisio 2020). Older people, simply as a result of their age and/or comorbidities, would thus be more vulnerable to being denied the resource.

Prevention Strategies

Public Health Interventions

Several public health interventions are used to control the spread of disease and curb the effects of global pandemics. One of the earliest of these interventions is the quarantine, which was widely used during the Black Death in the 1300s. Infected individuals were taken to fields outside town to either die or recover (Jewell 1857). Later that century, laws were passed establishing a *trentino*, or 30-day period (Sehdev 2002; Stuard 1992) to isolate the ill. This isolation period was extended to 40 days, giving rise to the term *quarantine*, derived from the Italian word *quaranta*, meaning 40.

Early forms of contact tracing, identifying and collecting information from those who were in contact with infected persons, were also used during the Black Death. Infected individuals were locked in their homes with the rest of their family, an identifying cross was painted on the door, and a watchman was stationed outside the home to make sure no one came out before the appointed time. Contact tracing has been used to manage other outbreaks, including smallpox, yellow fever, and syphilis (Cohn and O'Brien 2020).

In 1854, the spread of cholera was determined to occur through contaminated water (Tulchinsky 2018). This finding eventually led to cities in Europe and the United States making improvements to their sanitation systems during the nineteenth century. Hand hygiene through handwashing and use of alcohol-based sanitizers is important in reducing the spread of gastrointestinal, respiratory, skin, and eye infections (Centers for Disease Control and Prevention 2020c) and has been effective during the current COVID-19 pandemic. More recently, face masks and coverings and physical distancing have played a critical role in reducing spread of illnesses that spread through respiratory transmission (Centers for Disease Control and Prevention 2021d).

Vaccinations

Vaccines are a powerful public health intervention. One of the first documented uses of vaccination occurred in the year 1000 A.D. in Asia. People would scratch matter from a smallpox sore onto the arm of a healthy individual in order to build resistance against the disease (American Medical Association 1913). In 1796, the founder of modern vaccinology, Edward Jenner, inoculated an 8-year-old boy with fluid from a blister of a woman with cowpox. Jenner was able to demonstrate that the boy subsequently developed immunity to smallpox (Willis 1997). Since that time, scientists have developed vaccines that have controlled at least 12 major infectious diseases, including influenza, diphtheria, measles, mumps, poliomyelitis, rubella, and typhoid. The technology has advanced to the current use of live attenuated, inactivated, subunit, recombinant, polysaccharide, conjugate, and toxoid vaccines (National Institute of Allergies and Infectious Disease 2019). During the present-day pandemic, two vaccines have been developed using a new strategy, messenger RNA (mRNA), that causes cells to make a protein that then triggers an immune response (Centers for Disease Control and Prevention 2020f). That response produces antibodies that prevent morbidity and mortality among persons exposed to the virus.

Vaccines have been lifesaving, but dating back to just before the turn of this century, an anti-vaccination movement has gained momentum. It seems to have begun as a result of a now-debunked study linking the measles-mumps-rubella vaccine with irritable bowel syndrome and autism (Callender 2016). With the growth in internet use, a great deal of misinformation is furthering vaccine hesitancy, thus delaying the use of vaccines despite their availability. This hesitancy can relate to oneself but may extend to one's children (MacDonald and SAGE Working Group on Vaccine Hesitancy 2015). Factors that contribute to hesitancy include mandates to be vaccinated to attend school, adverse effects from vaccines, a lack of knowledge about vaccine-preventable diseases, and mistrust in corporations and public health agencies (Salmon et al. 2015).

Medical Care

In 1900, the average life expectancy in the United States was 47 years for whites and 33 years for Blacks (Centers for Disease Control and Prevention 2010). Pneumonia, influenza, tuberculosis, gastrointestinal infections, and diphtheria accounted for 34% of all deaths that year (Schanzenbach et al. 2016). The death rates from infectious disease declined dramatically over the course of the twentieth century, increasing life expectancy by 29.2 years (Hoyert et al. 1999). In addition to public health measures to control the spread of disease during pandemics and vaccines to promote immunity, modern therapeutics also have had a place in reducing the rates of morbidity and mortality associated with pandemics.

Ventilators provide mechanical ventilation to those who are unable to fully oxygenate their lungs (U.S. Food and Drug Administration 2020) and, as we have seen during the COVID-19 pandemic, have become a critical and highly used resource. Other lifesaving therapeutics in severe illness include dialysis for renal failure, organ transplantation for liver failure, and intravenous hydration and pressors for septic shock (Pollard et al. 2015). Twentieth-century advancements in medications, including antibiotics, antifungals, and antiviral medications, have also been proven to mitigate disease burden (Drexler and Institute of Medicine 2010).

LONGER-TERM SEQUELAE

Many people who survive infectious diseases that cause pandemics ultimately recover and regain their health. Some individuals, however, continue to experience longer-term medical consequences (see Table 2–1 for a summary). Smallpox often left its survivors with severe scarring and blindness. Long-term pulmonary disability, psychological impairment, and lower quality of life have been reported to persist up to 2 years after severe epidemic influenza illness (Chen et al. 2017; Luyt et al. 2012). Individuals who had polio as a child could develop post-polio syndrome

30–40 years later in life (National Institute of Neurological Disorders and Stroke 2020). Effective HIV treatments have significantly reduced AIDS and mortality. However, some conditions and chronic inflammation, which can promote certain diseases, are more common in persons with long-standing HIV infection, including cardiovascular and pulmonary disease, lymphoma, and type 2 diabetes (hyperglycemic hyperosmolar syndrome) (U.S. Department of Health and Human Services 2021). HIV-associated neurocognitive dysfunction, a spectrum of neurocognitive impairment, can affect 15%–55% of people with HIV, even among those treated with combination antiretroviral treatment (Saylor et al. 2016). Symptoms can include deficits in attention, language, motor skills, and memory and depression or psychological distress.

Although information is evolving, COVID-19 seems to be associated with longer-term sequelae as well, even among those who experienced mild acute illness (Centers for Disease Control and Prevention 2020d). These persistent symptoms may be sequelae of organ damage following the acute illness, a persistent hyperinflammatory state, ongoing viral activity, or an inadequate antibody response. The most commonly reported symptoms include fatigue, dyspnea, arthralgia, cough, and chest pain. Other symptoms include headache, fever, palpitations, myalgias, and neuropsychiatric symptoms, including cognitive impairment, depression, and new-onset psychosis. A recent multicountry study found that patients with a newly named syndrome, "long COVID," report prolonged multisystem disease and disability. Most had not been able to resume previous work at 6 months, and many were not recovered by 7 months (Davis et al. 2020). Hypotheses to explain these findings include inability to fully clear the virus, continuing low-level inflammation, and persistent immune dysfunction (Nalbandian et al. 2021). Anecdotally, some persons are reporting improvement in these symptoms following COVID-19 vaccination. At the time of this writing, the National Institutes of Health had launched a new initiative to identify the causes and, eventually, means of prevention and treatment of long COVID.

ECONOMIC CONSIDERATIONS

Given their worldwide scale and reach, pandemics exert large influences on the global population. Although some diseases such as the bubonic plague and influenza affect individuals who contract them similarly across society, others may have a disproportionate impact on specific groups and populations. Moreover, pandemics exert both direct and indirect effects on a population—effects that range from morbidity and mortality to economic disruption, population shifts over time, and exacerbation of existing social inequities.

Economists have examined the historical effects of pandemic disease on the larger economy. Pandemics such as the bubonic plague weakened feudalism, an economic and labor system in which the majority of individuals were obligated by law to work for wealthy, landed elites. Moreover, the resulting decline in the marriage rate and the growing burden of disease retarded economic growth (Bell and Lewis 2004). As the pandemic led to increased deaths, surviving workers were able to capitalize on the increased demand for their labor, laying the foundation for modern market-driven economic structures (Bell et al. 2020). Epidemics that disproportionately affect the adult population cause a contraction of the workforce in the short term. When the disease impacts child morbidity and mortality, the pandemic may also constrain birth rates and the size and strength of the workforce in the long term. Thus, the direct effects of a decreased workforce, income loss, and contraction of a society's gross domestic product may also have indirect effects on the future strength of the population in the long term (Bell and Lewis 2004; Ceylan et al. 2020). Last, whether through public health measures such as quarantine and isolation or the direct impacts on the workforce, repeated exposure to epidemic and pandemic diseases over time may significantly weaken a society's economic viability by limiting the development of social and economic structures that sustain economic growth (Bell and Lewis 2004; Charters and McKay 2020).

In general, epidemics have historically had greater impacts on individuals who are socially and economically marginalized (Substance Abuse and Mental Health Services Administration 2017). These effects may stem from decreased access to medical and public health resources or the detrimental impact on individuals who may be more susceptible to severe disease. According to public health scholars, social causes exert such a significant influence on health and disease that they may be considered fundamental causes of disease because decreased access to social resources is strongly associated with lower life expectancy, higher infant mortality rates, higher rates of chronic disease and mental illness, and racial disparities in health (Link and Phelan 1995). As one study demonstrated, regions with predominantly Black and Latinx populations had disproportionately higher rates of COVID-19 cases and deaths (Khanijahani 2021). Thus, understanding social factors as fundamental causes of disease largely predicts, for example, the disproportionate burden of COVID-19 morbidity and mortality on Black individuals and other marginalized populations, many of whom have higher rates of high-risk preexisting chronic disease and are more likely to work in occupations with higher risks of exposure (Khanijahani 2021; Link and Phelan 1995; Valles 2020).

Older and lower-income adults are more likely to experience adverse economic consequences related to disease. In addition to living expenses and costs of medications and supplemental insurance premiums, many older working adults may experience decreases in their available income. Larger impacts of pandemics on the economy may affect pensions, retirement funds, and other state and federal assistance programs, with many elderly individuals less likely to have adequate resources and opportunities to counter such economic losses (Li and Mutchler 2020). In the case of the COVID-19 pandemic, lengthy hospitalizations have become common, with many survivors requiring extended acute care hospitalizations, subacute rehabilitation, and other assisted living arrangements. The lengths of such hospitalizations may exceed those covered under existing insurance plans, exposing older, lower-income, and racial and ethnic minority individuals to significant out-of-pocket costs (Patient Access Network Foundation 2020; Schoen et al. 2017).

SUMMARY

Although pandemics have been present throughout human history, recent circumstances of globalization, ease of travel, and incursion into wild spaces have increased the opportunities for a pandemic to occur. Older adults, for many reasons, are not only more physically vulnerable to morbidity and mortality that result from pandemics but also more vulnerable to a wide array of economic consequences. Public health efforts, vaccines, and modern therapeutics can mitigate much of the impact, but by the time an infectious agent has spread to a pandemic, coordinated efforts are needed.

KEY POINTS

- Pandemics have occurred throughout the history of humankind. Certain circumstances can promote the spread of infectious illness, and depending on these circumstances, certain population groups are vulnerable to greater morbidity and mortality and may develop long-term sequelae.

- Efforts to mitigate the impact of pandemics include public health initiatives, vaccines, and modern therapeutics.

- Older and lower-income adults are more likely to experience adverse economic consequences related to disease, which can include higher living expenses, higher costs of medications and supplemental insurance premiums, and job loss.

QUESTIONS FOR REVIEW

1. Which of the following pandemics showed a W-shaped death-by-age curve?

    A. Smallpox
    B. Bubonic plague
    C. HIV/AIDS
    D. Measles
    E. 1918 influenza

Answer: E.

2. Which of the following phenomena constitute a pattern of processes that shape a society's responses to many epidemics and pandemics over time?

    A. The degree of economic devastation of the pandemic
    B. Globalization accounting for the movement of people, goods, and services
    C. Scapegoating of cultures, groups, and populations
    D. A and B
    E. B and C
    F. A, B, and C

Answer: F.

3. Which of the following is not a type of vaccine?

    A. Conjugate
    B. Inactivated
    C. Polysaccharide
    D. Multivariant
    E. Toxoid

Answer: D.

ADDITIONAL RESOURCES

Madhav N, Oppenheim B, Gallivan M, et al: Pandemics: risks, impacts, and mitigation, in Disease Control Priorities: Improving Health and Reducing Poverty, 3rd Edition. Edited by Jamison DT, Gelband H, Horton S, et al. Washington, DC, World Bank Group, 2017. Available at: www.ncbi.nlm.nih.gov/books/NBK525302. Accessed June 25, 2021.

Tomes N: The Gospel of Germs: Men, Women, and the Microbe in American Life. Cambridge, MA, Harvard University Press, 2002

Porter R: The Greatest Benefit to Mankind. New York, WW Norton, 1998

Robert Wood Johnson Foundation: The five deadliest outbreaks and pandemics in history. Princeton, NJ, Robert Wood Johnson Foundation, 2013. Available at: www.rwjf.org/en/blog/2013/12/the_five_deadliesto.html. Accessed February 27, 2021.

Rosenberg CE: Explaining Epidemics and Other Studies in the History of Medicine. Cambridge, UK, Cambridge University Press, 2008

Zaresfsky M: 3 ways physicians can help combat COVID-19 vaccine hesitancy. Chicago, IL, American Medical Association, January 6, 2021. Available at: www.ama-assn.org/delivering-care/public-health/3-ways-physicians-can-help-combat-covid-19-vaccine-hesitancy. Accessed February 27, 2021.

REFERENCES

AARP Public Policy Institute: AARP nursing home COVID-19 dashboard. Washington, DC, AARP Public Policy Institute, June 10, 2021. Available at: www.aarp.org/ppi/issues/caregiving/info-2020/nursing-home-covid-dashboard.html. Accessed June 26, 2021.

Ali M, Lopez AL, You YA, et al: The global burden of cholera. Bull World Health Organ 90(3):209–218A, 2012 22461716

American Lung Association: Trends in tuberculosis morbidity and mortality. Chicago, IL, American Lung Association, April 2013. Available at www.lung.org/getmedia/a72117a1-6c17-4415-a3dd-1c2bb7cfe2a1/tb-trend-report.pdf. Accessed June 24, 2021.

American Medical Association: The History of Inoculation and Vaccination for the Prevention and Treatment of Disease. Lecture Memoranda. AMA Meeting, Minneapolis. London, Burroughs Wellcome, 1913

Bailey M: Demographic decline in late medieval England: some thoughts on recent research. Economic History Review 49(1):1–19, 1996

Bell AR, Prescott A, Lacey H: What can the Black Death tell us about the global economic consequences of a pandemic? The Conversation, March 2020. Available at: https://theconversation.com/what-can-the-black-death-tell-us-about-the-global-economic-consequences-of-a-pandemic-132793. Accessed June 28, 2021.

Bell C, Lewis M: The economic implications of epidemics old and new. World Econ 5(4):137–174, 2004

Callender D: Vaccine hesitancy: more than a movement. Hum Vaccin Immunother 12(9):2464–2468, 2016 27159558

Centers for Disease Control and Prevention: Table 22: Life expectancy at birth, at 65 years of age, and at 75 years of age, by race and sex: United States, selected years 1900–2007. Atlanta, GA, Centers for Disease Control and Prevention, 2010. Available at: www.cdc.gov/nchs/data/hus/2010/022.pdf. Accessed June 28, 2021.

Centers for Disease Control and Prevention: Smallpox: clinical disease. Atlanta, GA, Centers for Disease Control and Prevention, December 5, 2016. Available at: www.cdc.gov/smallpox/clinicians/clinical-disease.html. Accessed December 1, 2021.

Centers for Disease Control and Prevention: Yellow fever. Atlanta, GA, Centers for Disease Control and Prevention, September 14, 2018. Available at: www.cdc.gov/globalhealth/newsroom/topics/yellowfever/index.html. Accessed June 24, 2021.

Centers for Disease Control and Prevention: Cholera—Vibrio cholerae infection. Atlanta, GA, Centers for Disease Control and Prevention, October 2, 2020a. Available at: www.cdc.gov/cholera/infection-sources.html. Accessed June 28, 2021.

Centers for Disease Control and Prevention: Diphtheria. Atlanta, GA, Centers for Disease Control and Prevention, December 2020b. Available at: www.cdc.gov/vaccines/pubs/pinkbook/dip.html. Accessed June 24, 2021.

Centers for Disease Control and Prevention: Hand hygiene recommendations. Atlanta, GA, Centers for Disease Control and Prevention, May 17, 2020c. Available at: www.cdc.gov/coronavirus/2019-ncov/hcp/hand-hygiene.html. Accessed June 28, 2021.

Centers for Disease Control and Prevention: Late sequelae of COVID-19. Atlanta, GA, Centers for Disease Control and Prevention, April 8, 2020d. Available at: www.cdc.gov/coronavirus/2019-ncov/hcp/clinical-care/late-sequelae.html. Accessed June 28, 2021.

Centers for Disease Control and Prevention: Tuberculosis. Atlanta, GA, Centers for Disease Control and Prevention, April 6, 2020e. Available at: www.cdc.gov/globalhealth/newsroom/topics/tb/index.html. Accessed June 24, 2021.

Centers for Disease Control and Prevention: Understanding mRNA COVID-19 vaccines. Atlanta, GA, Centers for Disease Control and Prevention, 2020f. Available at: www.cdc.gov/coronavirus/2019-ncov/vaccines/different-vaccines/mrna.html. Accessed June 28, 2021.

Centers for Disease Control and Prevention: Influenza (flu): flu symptoms & complications. Atlanta, GA, Centers for Disease Control and Prevention, September 21, 2021a. Available at: www.cdc.gov/flu/symptoms/symptoms.htm. Accessed December 1, 2021.

Centers for Disease Control and Prevention: Influenza (flu): burden of flu. Atlanta, GA, Centers for Disease Control and Prevention, October 4, 2021b. Available at: www.cdc.gov/flu/about/burden/index.html. Accessed December 1, 2021.

Centers for Disease Control and Prevention: Smallpox: history of smallpox. Atlanta, GA, Centers for Disease Control and Prevention, February 20, 2021c. Available at: www.cdc.gov/smallpox/history/history.html. Accessed January 31, 2021.

Centers for Disease Control and Prevention: Guidance for wearing masks. Atlanta, GA, Centers for Disease Control and Prevention, 2021d. Available at: www.cdc.gov/coronavirus/2019-ncov/prevent-getting-sick/cloth-face-cover-guidance.html. Accessed June 28, 2021.

Ceylan RF, Ozkan B, Mulazimogullari E: Historical evidence for economic effects of COVID-19. Eur J Health Econ 21(6):817–823, 2020 32500243

Charters E, McKay RA: The history of science and medicine in the context of COVID-19. Centaurus 62(2):223–233, 2020

Chen J, Wu J, Hao S, et al: Long term outcomes in survivors of epidemic Influenza A (H7N9) virus infection. Sci Rep 7(1):17275, 2017

Cohn S, O'Brien M: How physicians used contact tracing 500 years ago to control the bubonic plague. The Conversation, June 3, 2020. Available at: https://theconversation.com/contact-tracing-how-physicians-used-it-500-years-ago-to-control-the-bubonic-plague-139248. Accessed June 25, 2021.

Cox C, Amin K: COVID-19 is the number one cause of death in the U.S. in early 2021. Peterson Center on Healthcare and KFF, February 22, 2021. Available at: www.healthsystemtracker.org/brief/covid-19-is-the-number-one-cause-of-death-in-the-u-s-in-early-2021. Accessed June 26, 2021.

Davis HE, Assaf GS, McCorkell L, et al: Characterizing long COVID in an international cohort: 7 months of symptoms and their impact. medRxiv, December 27, 2020. Available at: www.medrxiv.org/content/10.1101/2020.12.24.20248802v2.full.pdf. Accessed February 27, 2021.

DeWitte SN: Age patterns of mortality during the Black Death in London, A.D. 1349–1350. J Archaeol Sci 37(12):3394–3400, 2010 21572598

DeWitte SN: Mortality risk and survival in the aftermath of the medieval Black Death. PLoS One 9(5):e96513, 2014 24806459

DeWitte SN, Wood JW: Selectivity of black death mortality with respect to pre-existing health. Proc Natl Acad Sci USA 105(5):1436–1441, 2008 18227518

Drexler M; Institute of Medicine: What You Need to Know About Infectious Disease. IV: Prevention and Treatment. Washington, DC, National Academies Press, 2010. Available at: www.ncbi.nlm.nih.gov/books/NBK209704/. Accessed June 28, 2021.

Estivariz CF, Link-Gelles R, Shimabukuro T: Poliomyelitis. Atlanta, GA, Centers for Disease Control and Prevention, November 2020. Available at: www.cdc.gov/vaccines/pubs/pinkbook/polio.html. Accessed June 24, 2021.

Gastanaduy P, Haber P, Rota PA, et al: Measles. Atlanta, GA, Centers for Disease Control and Prevention, December 2020. Available at: www.cdc.gov/vaccines/pubs/pinkbook/meas.html. Accessed June 24, 2021.

Griffith DM, Sharma G, Holliday CS, et al: Men and COVID-19: a biopsychosocial approach to understanding sex differences in mortality and recommendations for practice and policy interventions. Atlanta, GA, Centers for Disease Control and Prevention, July 16, 2020. Available at: www.cdc.gov/pcd/issues/2020/20_0247.htm. Accessed June 26, 2021.

Grove RD, Hetzel AM: Vital statistics rates in the United States: 1940–1960. Washington, DC, U.S. Government Printing Office, 1968

Hall E: Influenza. Atlanta, GA, Centers for Disease Control and Prevention, August 18, 2021. Available at: www.cdc.gov/vaccines/pubs/pinkbook/flu.html. Accessed December 1, 2021.

Hall V, Walker WL, Lindsey NP, et al: Update: noncongenital zika virus disease cases—50 U.S. states and the District of Columbia, 2016. MMWR Morb Mortal Wkly Rep 67(9):265–269, 2018 29518067

Hoyert DL, Kochanek KD, Murphy SL: Deaths: final data for 1997. Natl Vital Stat Rep 47(19):1–104, 1999 10410536

Institute of Medicine: Ethical and Legal Considerations in Mitigating Pandemic Disease, Workshop Summary. Washington, DC, National Academies Press, 2007

Jewell W: Historical Sketches of Quarantine. Philadelphia, PA, TK & PG Collins, 1857

Johns Hopkins University and Medicine: COVID-19 dashboard. Coronavirus Resource Center, 2021. Available at: coronavirus.jhu.edu/map.html. Accessed June 24, 2021.

Jutla A, Whitcombe E, Hasan N, et al: Environmental factors influencing epidemic cholera. Am J Trop Med Hyg 89(3):597–607, 2013 23897993

Khanijahani A: Racial, ethnic, and socioeconomic disparities in confirmed COVID-19 cases and deaths in the United States: a county-level analysis as of November 2020. Ethn Health 26(1):22–35, 2021 33334160

Koch A, Brierley C, Maslin MM, et al: Earth system impacts of the European arrival and Great Dying in the Americas after 1492. Quat Sci Rev 207:13–36, 2019

Li W, Moore MJ, Vasilieva N, et al: Angiotensin-converting enzyme 2 is a functional receptor for the SARS coronavirus. Nature 426(6965):450–454, 2003 14647384

Li Y, Mutchler JE: Older adults and the economic impact of the COVID-19 pandemic. J Aging Soc Policy 32(4–5):477–487, 2020 32543304

Link BG, Phelan JC: Social conditions as fundamental causes of disease. J Health Soc Behav Spec No:80–94, 1995 7560851

Luyt CE, Combes A, Becquemin MH, et al: Long-term outcomes of pandemic 2009 influenza A(H1N1)-associated severe ARDS. Chest 142(3):583–592, 2012 22948576

MacDonald NE; SAGE Working Group on Vaccine Hesitancy: Vaccine hesitancy: definition, scope and determinants. Vaccine 33(34):4161–4164, 2015 25896383

Márquez EJ, Chung CH, Marches R, et al: Sexual-dimorphism in human immune system aging. Nat Commun 11(1):751, 2020 32029736

May T, Aulisio MP: Age, "life-cycles," and the allocation of scarce medical resources. Chest 158(5):1837–1838, 2020 32585146

Mead PS: Bacterial and mycobacterial infections: plague, in Principles and Practice of Infectious Diseases. Edited by Bennett JE, Dolin R, Blaser MJ. Philadelphia, PA, Elsevier/Saunders, 2015, pp 276–283

Munro JH: Before and after the Black Death: money, prices, and wages in fourteenth-century England. Toronto, ON, Canada, University of Toronto, 2004. Available at: www.economics.utoronto.ca/public/workingPapers/UT-ECIPA-MUNRO-04-04.pdf. Accessed June 28, 2021.

Nalbandian A, Sehgal K, Gupta A, et al: Post-acute COVID-19 syndrome. Nat Med 27(4):601–615, 2021 33753937

National Institute of Aging: Why population aging matters: a global perspective. Bethesda, MD, National Institute of Aging, March 2017. Available at: www.nia.nih.gov/sites/default/files/2017-06/WPAM.pdf. Accessed June 24, 2021.

National Institute of Allergies and Infectious Disease: Vaccine types. Bethesda, MD, National Institute of Allergies and Infectious Disease, July 1, 2019. Available at: www.niaid.nih.gov/research/vaccine-types. Accessed June 25, 2021.

National Institute of Neurological Disorders and Stroke: Post-polio syndrome fact sheet. Bethesda, MD, National Institute of Neurological Disorders and Stroke, 2020. Available at: www.ninds.nih.gov/disorders/patient-caregiver-education/fact-sheets/post-polio-syndrome-fact-sheet. Accessed January 31, 2021.

National Organization for Rare Disorders: Cholera. Danbury, CT, National Organization for Rare Diseases, 2009. Available at: https:// rarediseases.org/rare-diseases/cholera. Accessed January 30, 2021.

NDTV: Heartbreaking photo shows US doctor comforting elderly Covid patient. NDTV, December 1, 2020. Available at: www.ndtv.com/world-news/heartbreaking-photo-shows-us-doctor-joseph-varon-comforting-elderly-covid-19-patient-2332355. Accessed June 24, 2021.

Ochmann S, Roser M: Smallpox. Our World in Data, 2018. Available at: https:// ourworldindata.org/smallpox. Accessed January 31, 2021.

Patient Access Network Foundation: COVID-19: the impact on Medicare beneficiaries. Washington, DC, Patient Access Network Foundation, May 2020. Available at: www.panfoundation.org/app/uploads/2020/05/COVID-19-Brief.pdf. Accessed June 25, 2021.

Pollard S, Edwin SB, Alaniz C: Vasopressor and inotropic management of patients with septic shock. P T 40(7):438–450, 2015 26185405

Salmon DA, Dudley MZ, Glanz JM, et al: Vaccine hesitancy: causes, consequences, and a call to action. Am J Prev Med 49(6)(suppl 4):S391–S398, 2015 26337116

Saylor D, Dickens AM, Sacktor N, et al: HIV-associated neurocognitive disorder—pathogenesis and prospects for treatment. Nature Rev Neurol 12(4):234–248, 2016 26965674

Schanzenbach DW, Nunn R, Bauer L: The changing landscape of American life expectancy. Washington, DC, Hamilton Project, June 2016. Available at: www.hamiltonproject.org/assets/files/changing_landscape_american_life_expectancy.pdf. Accessed February 27, 2021.

Schoen C, Davis K, Willink A: Medicare beneficiaries' high out-of-pocket costs: cost burdens by income and health status. New York, Commonwealth Fund, Issue Briefs, May 12, 2017. Available at: www.commonwealthfund.org/publications/issue-briefs/2017/may/medicare-out-of-pocket-cost-burdens. Accessed June 25, 2021.

Schurz H, Salie M, Tromp G, et al: The X chromosome and sex-specific effects in infectious disease susceptibility. Hum Genomics 13(1):2, 2019 30621780

Sehdev PS: The origin of quarantine. Clin Infect Dis 35(9):1071–1072, 2002 12398064

Simonsen L, Clarke MJ, Schonberger LB, et al Pandemic versus epidemic influenza mortality: a pattern of changing age distribution. J Infect Dis 178(1):53–60, 1998 9652423

Stuard SM: A State of Deference: Ragusa/Dubrovnik in the Medieval Centuries. Philadelphia, University of Pennsylvania Press, 1992

Substance Abuse and Mental Health Services Administration: Greater impact: how disasters affect people of low socioeconomic status. Rockville, MD, Substance Abuse and Mental Health Services Administration, July 2017. Available at: www.samhsa.gov/sites/default/files/dtac/srb-low-ses_2.pdf. Accessed February 27, 2021.

Tanne JH: Measles cases and deaths are increasing worldwide, warn health agencies. BMJ 371:m4450, 2020 33199396

Taubenberger JK, Kash JC, Morens DM: 1918 influenza: the mother of all pandemics. Atlanta, GA, Centers for Disease Control and Prevention, 2006. Available at: wwwnc.cdc.gov/eid/article/12/1/05-0979_article. Accessed June 25, 2021.

Tozay S, Fischer WA, Wohl DA, et al: Long-term complications of Ebola virus disease: prevalence and predictors of major symptoms and the role of inflammation. Clin Infect Dis 71(7):1749–1755, 2020 31693114

Tulchinsky TH: John Snow, cholera, the Broad Street pump; waterborne diseases then and now. Case Studies in Public Health, March 30:77–99, 2018.

U.S. Census Bureau: Older people projected to outnumber children for the first time in U.S. history. Washington, DC, U.S. Census Bureau, March 13, 2018. Available at: www.census.gov/newsroom/press-releases/2018/cb18-41-population-projections.html. Accessed June 24, 2021.

U.S. Department of Health and Human Services: HIV basics—overview: data and trends. U.S. Washington, DC, Department of Health and Human Services, November 25, 2020. Available at: www.hiv.gov/hiv-basics/overview/data-and-trends/global-statistics. Accessed June 24, 2021.

U.S. Department of Health and Human Services. Aging with HIV. Washington, DC, U.S. Department of Health and Human Services, May 17, 2021. Available at: www.hiv.gov/hiv-basics/living-well-with-hiv/taking-care-of-yourself/aging-with-hiv. Accessed December 3, 2021.

U.S. Food and Drug Administration: Fact sheet for healthcare providers: emergency use of ventilators during the COVID-19 pandemic. Silver Spring, MD, U.S. Food and Drug Administration, March 24, 2020. Available at: www.fda.gov/media/136424/download. Accessed November 30, 2021.

Valles SA: The predictable inequities of COVID-19 in the US: fundamental causes and broken institutions. Kennedy Inst Ethics J 30:191–214, 2020

Viboud C, Simonsen L, Fuentes R, et al: Global mortality impact of the 1957–1959 influenza pandemic. J Infect Dis 213(5):738–745, 2016 26908781

Vidal J: Destroyed habitat creates the perfect condition for coronavirus to emerge. Scientific American, March 18, 2020. Available at: www.scientific american.com/article/destroyed-habitat-creates-the-perfect-conditions-for-coronavirus-to-emerge. Accessed June 26, 2021.

Weyand CM, Goronzy JJ: Aging of the immune system. Mechanisms and therapeutic targets. Ann Am Thorac Soc 13(5)(suppl 5):S422–S428, 2016 28005419

Willis NJ: Edward Jenner and the eradication of smallpox. Scott Med J 42(4):118–121, 1997 9507590

World Health Organization: Global Influenza Strategy 2019–2030. Geneva, World Health Organization, 2019. Available at: www.who.int/influenza/Global_Influenza_Strategy_2019_2030_Summary_English.pdf?ua=1. Accessed December 1, 2021.

World Health Organization: Plague, in WHO Report on Global Surveillance of Epidemic-Prone Infectious Diseases. Geneva, World Health Organization, 2000. Available at: www.who.int/csr/resources/publications/surveillance/plague.pdf. Accessed June 24, 2021.

World Health Organization: Consensus document on the epidemiology of severe acute respiratory syndrome (SARS). Geneva, World Health Organization, 2003. Available at: www.who.int/csr/sars/en/WHOconsensus.pdf. Accessed June 24, 2021.

World Health Organization: Ebola virus disease. Geneva, World Health Organization, 2021a. Available at: www.who.int/news-room/fact-sheets/detail/ebola-virus-disease. Accessed June 24, 2021.

World Health Organization: Smallpox. Geneva, World Health Organization, 2021b. Available at: www.who.int/health-topics/smallpox#tab=tab_1. Accessed June 24, 2021.

Wu H, Tsien J (directors): 76 Days [documentary film]. New York, MTV Documentary Films, 2020

Zhang P, Li J, Liu H, et al: Long-term bone and lung consequences associated with hospital-acquired severe acute respiratory syndrome: a 15-year follow-up from a prospective cohort study. Bone Res 8(8):8, 2020 32128276

EMERGENCY PSYCHIATRIC CARE FOR OLDER ADULTS DURING THE COVID-19 PANDEMIC

Workflow, Common Presentations, and Overall Trends

Dwight Kemp, M.D., M.S.

Neha N. Sharma, M.D.

Alan Akira, M.D.

Eitan Z. Kimchi, M.D.

In this chapter we explore emergency psychiatric care for older adults during the coronavirus SARS-CoV-2 disease (COVID-19) pandemic. The emergency department (ED) is the first stop for many patients with psychiatric presentations. During the pandemic, overall rates of ED visits for psychiatric chief complaints decreased; conversely, unique challenges with workflow and dispositions increased. Inpatient psychiatric units began to require COVID-19 testing as part of their medical clearance. Patients testing positive for COVID-19 who required psychiatric admission were challenging to place. Partial hospitalization, intensive outpatient programs, and substance use disorder (SUD) treatment programs temporarily closed or converted to only virtual meetings. This presented a hardship to individuals benefiting from the milieu component of these programs and those unable to access technology. There was a lack of resources for safe quarantine locations for the homeless population. Data regarding rates of ED presentations for depression, anxiety, and suicide among older populations have been conflicting and limited. Overall, there has been no clear increase in these rates, possibly because of a lack of data examining longer-term effects of the pandemic on elder mental health or because of greater resilience to overcoming hardships in this population compared with younger age groups. Rates of substance use among the elderly population increased overall and should not be overlooked because of related detrimental morbidity and mortality. New cases of COVID-19-related psychosis have been negligible among the elderly population. Delirium was noted as a possible first presentation of COVID-19 infection among older adults and was often missed in the ED because of insufficient screening. Overall, among the vulnerable older adult population, the pandemic contributed to unexpected presentations of common psychiatric illnesses and uncovered barriers to care and dispositions from the ED.

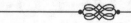

Vignette

Mr. Q is a 73-year-old man with a past medical history significant for hypertension, diabetes, and coronary artery disease and a past psychiatric history of unipolar melancholic depression in remission for 2 years. Mr. Q was transported to the ED via ambulance because of new-onset visual hallucinations. The patient was listed on the ED tracking board as a "Psych Eval." In the ED, the patient's only complaints were fatigue and poor appetite. He denied depressive symptoms, manic symptoms, other psychotic symptoms, fever, chills, cough, muscle aches, or loss of taste or smell. Mr. Q's vital signs were notable for mildly elevated blood pressure and tachycardia. He was afebrile, was breathing comfortably on room air, and had good oxygen saturation rates. His cardiac and pulmonary exam were unremarkable. The ED attending physician consulted psychiatry. The consultant interviewed Mr. Q via video telemedicine. Mr. Q appeared internally stimulated and distressed over visual hallucinations of insects crawling up and down the wall. He was oriented to person and place but not time. The consultant then obtained collateral information over the phone from Mr. Q's daughter, who reported that her father's presentation represented an acute change from baseline. Mr. Q's laboratory results revealed new abnormalities, including a leukocytosis of 14, thrombocytosis of 498, C-reactive protein of 85, lactate dehydrogenase of 293, and D-dimer of 1600. His chest X-ray showed no focal consolidations. A rapid screen for SARS-CoV-2 was positive. The emergency physician and psychiatrist diagnosed Mr. Q with delirium, and he was admitted to the general medical floor. Mr. Q had a prolonged hospital course complicated by increasing oxygen demand, agitated delirium requiring neuroleptics and physical restraint, and intensive care unit transfer for mechanical ventilation.

Between 2015 and 2050, the percentage of individuals older than 60 years is projected to grow from 12% to 22% of the population globally (World Health Organization 2021a). Fifteen percent of older adults have a mental disorder (World Health Organization 2021a).

The ED is often the gateway for psychiatric care. Patients with serious mental illness or SUDs use the ED significantly more than do patients without these conditions. In one study looking at ED visits throughout the state of North Carolina by patients with mental health disorders, the authors found that over a 3-year period, adults older than age 65 years accounted for one-quarter of all mental health disorder ED visits (Hakenewerth et al. 2015).

Emergency psychiatric care for older adults is often neglected in the literature. We must consider potential barriers to care for this population. In this chapter, we discuss how the COVID-19 pandemic affected ED utilization, considerations for disposition, and the prevalence and outcomes of common psychiatric diagnoses. We discuss how the COVID-19 pandemic put further strain on a system already stretched thin, with barriers to care that specifically affect the elderly population and lessons learned that should be incorporated into clinical decision-making and practice.

EMERGENCY DEPARTMENT VISITS

The ED is a common site for managing patients of all ages with psychiatric disorders, including older adults (Bessey et al. 2018; Theriault et al. 2020). With the first baby boomers turning 65 years old in 2011, EDs have seen a significant influx of older adults presenting with psychiatric complaints. According to the National Hospital Ambulatory Medical Care Survey, the number of ED visits by adults 65 years and older for psychiatric and substance use conditions increased by 109% between 2011 and 2016 (Theriault et al. 2020).

At the height of the COVID-19 pandemic (March 1 to April 30, 2020), ED volumes decreased across the United States because of sheltering in place and fears of infection, while hospital admissions directly corresponded with local COVID-19 cases (Giannouchos et al. 2021; Jeffery et al. 2020). Concomitantly, patients were less likely to have access to outpatient mental health care services or to be able to contact their mental health provider than they were before COVID-19 (Ferrando et al. 2021) as a direct consequence of fettering state and federal legislation (e.g., licensure and reimbursement) that predated the pandemic. The U.S.

health care system was ill-equipped early in the pandemic to manage health care remotely in accordance with emerging pandemic mitigation guidelines.

Limited data on clinical characteristics (e.g., symptoms, severity, and diagnoses) of emergency psychiatric presentations during COVID-19 are available. One study at a suburban Academic Medical Center in New York State reported no change in the volume of emergency psychiatric evaluations compared with pre-COVID levels (Ferrando et al. 2021). Twenty-seven percent of patients had moderate to severe COVID-19-related stress directly related to their symptoms, severity of illness, and diagnoses. This included worries that they or their family members might contract COVID-19 and stress related to quarantine, loss of job, diminished finances, and COVID-19-related deaths (Ferrando et al. 2021). However, these data are based on all adults and do not specifically address patients 65 years and older.

EMERGENCY DEPARTMENT PROTOCOLS, WORKFLOW, AND DISPOSITION

Disposition is an important part of the emergency psychiatric workflow. Prior to the COVID-19 pandemic, common dispositions for patients presenting to the ED with psychiatric emergencies included admission to an inpatient psychiatric unit, referral to outpatient psychiatric services, referral to an intensive outpatient or partial hospitalization program, and referral to SUD services. The workflow and disposition options for patients with psychiatric presentations were affected by the COVID-19 pandemic.

Initially passed in 1986, the Emergency Medical Treatment and Labor Act (EMTALA) is a federal law guaranteeing patients' access to emergency medical care. Hospitals with EDs are obligated to medically treat and stabilize patients seeking emergent care to the extent of their ability. EMTALA imposes several legal obligations on hospitals, one of which is to perform a medical screening examination. In 2020, addenda to EMTALA permitted the use of telemedicine to perform medical screening examinations (Brown 2021). Growing empirical evidence demonstrates that using telemedicine to treat psychiatric conditions reduces length of stay, increases cost-effectiveness, and improves satisfaction of patients and staff (Reinhardt et al. 2019). Use of telemedicine during the

COVID-19 pandemic also helped conserve personal protective equipment and reduce individual exposure to COVID-19 (Heslin et al. 2020). Telemedicine may continue to shape psychiatric care in the emergency setting in the near future.

For a variety of reasons, during the COVID-19 pandemic, many inpatient psychiatric units began to limit admissions to only patients testing negative for COVID-19. Some inpatient units do not have the ability to manage patients who need to be on contact or droplet precautions. Some staff felt uncomfortable about providing patients with masks on inpatient units (which would be necessary were a patient to test positive for COVID-19) out of fear that patients might use the string of the mask to harm themselves or others. For safety reasons, many inpatient psychiatric units are unable to administer intravenous medications or oxygen via nasal cannula to patients.

EDs started to incorporate COVID-19 screens into their routine medical workup of psychiatric patients slated for inpatient psychiatric admission, regardless of whether the patient had any signs or symptoms of COVID-19 infection. ED providers were faced with the challenge of determining how to adequately disposition patients who required an inpatient psychiatric level of care but also tested positive for COVID-19. Many of these patients were admitted to general medical units where they could be isolated. Often, these units lacked group therapy and other programs found on inpatient psychiatric units. These patients missed out on the therapeutic benefit of the milieu. In response, some institutions such as the University of Rochester Medical Center and Johns Hopkins Hospital built inpatient psychiatric units that could accommodate COVID-19-positive patients who were asymptomatic and/or demonstrated only mild symptoms (Augenstein et al. 2020).

The options for partial hospitalization and intensive outpatient programming for individuals testing positive for COVID-19 were reduced as well. As the pandemic ensued, many of these programs transitioned over to telemedicine, and some programs limited their availability or discontinued their services altogether. Telemedicine presented a unique challenge to the elderly population. One study suggested that the readiness of older adults to use telehealth services was much lower than that of younger cohorts (Lam et al. 2020). These observations are important because they raise the question of how feasible telepsychiatry outpatient follow-up may be for patients being discharged from the ED.

SUDs are becoming more prevalent among the elderly population (Yarnell et al. 2020). SUD treatment facilities, an important resource and common disposition for patients with a SUD being discharged from the ED, were also affected by the COVID-19 pandemic. Some residential and nonresidential treatment facilities temporarily closed, and others reduced their patient capacity. Because of safety precautions and limited staff, many SUD programs stopped seeing patients in person and offered only telehealth appointments. In one study, patients with SUDs attending residential facilities experienced delays in treatment initiation and received fewer services during their treatment (Pagano et al. 2021). Their retention rate in the treatment program was lower, and they experienced economic and psychosocial barriers when reentering the community. Patients with SUDs also noted technical and interpersonal challenges associated with telemedicine visits (Pagano et al. 2021).

Certain populations of patients, including homeless adults, patients with psychiatric disorders (Taquet et al. 2021), and patients with SUDs, may have been disproportionately affected by the COVID-19 pandemic. It is estimated that one-fourth to one-third of homeless individuals have a serious mental illness (Sullivan et al. 2000). Additionally, homeless individuals are more likely to use the hospital than outpatient settings for mental health treatment (North and Smith 1993). This is particularly important because older adults are comprising a growing number of the homeless population. Because of the increased prevalence of medical comorbidities among homeless adults, homeless adults who are older than age 50 years are considered *older* (Cohen 1999). Approximately half of single homeless adults are now age 50 years or older. During the COVID-19 pandemic, EDs faced ethical and logistical challenges surrounding where to discharge homeless individuals who tested positive for COVID-19 but did not require inpatient hospitalization. Some cities and states set up COVID-19 quarantine centers to help prevent the spread of infection. Others used hotels to isolate and quarantine homeless individuals who tested positive or were presumed to be positive (Fuchs et al. 2021).

SUICIDE

Suicide remains among the top 10 leading causes of death in the United States (Kochanek et al. 2020). Suicide rates among the elderly are higher than those among the general population (World Health Organization 2021b). This increase is often attributed to a multitude of risk factors, including living alone, loneliness, social isolation, underlying psychiatric disorders, and chronic health problems (Druss 2020; Sheffler et al. 2021). Epidemics of the past (e.g., the severe acute respiratory syndrome [SARS] outbreak of 2003 and the 1918 influenza pandemic) have previously been associated with a rise in underlying mental health issues (e.g., depression, PTSD) and increased suicide rates (Cheung et al. 2008; Zalsman et al. 2020). Some individuals presumed the COVID-19 pandemic would similarly be associated with increased rates of suicidal ideation and suicide attempts among older adults (Sheffler et al. 2021).

Interestingly, the limited amount of data surrounding suicidal ideation and suicide attempts among the elderly population during the COVID-19 pandemic have been conflicting. Zalsman et al. (2020) described a possible lag period that might explain conflicting findings in the current literature. Specifically, during a pandemic, short-term suicide rates may decrease initially or remain unchanged: "At times of external danger and when people are just busy surviving, they may focus less on distress and internal pain" (Zalsman et al. 2020, p. 478). Hamm et al. (2020) found that on a semistructured interview administered to 73 older adults (mean age 69) with preexisting major depressive disorder, anxiety, and suicidal ideation, symptom scores did not differ over the first 3 months of the pandemic. In Italy, there were at least five cases of COVID-19-related suicide (Wand et al. 2020). A study comparing psychiatric emergencies in the New York City area during the height of the COVID-19 pandemic versus the time before COVID-19 found no significant changes in presentations related to suicide or suicide attempts among the elderly or overall (Ferrando et al. 2021). Unchanged rates of suicide or suicide attempts in the elderly population could be accounted for by the lack of longer-term data following the pandemic. Perhaps as more data are collected, the longer-term effects of social isolation and quarantine on this high-risk population will come to light.

An alternative to consider is that older adults may be more resilient than younger age groups. Resilience has been defined as the "psychosocial and biological variables that decrease risk of onset or relapse, decrease illness severity, or increase probability or speed of recovery" (Laird et al. 2019, p. 1). Older adults may be more resilient for a variety of reasons. One such reason is that older age might be protective because of the presence of wisdom (Vahia et al. 2020). Vahia and colleagues defined wisdom as a personality trait that includes empathy, compassion, and emotional regulation. They noted that in prior studies, wisdom has been found to be inversely associated with loneliness. Older adults might also benefit from having a smaller concentration of high-quality relationships rather than numerous friendships that might be disproportionately affected by social isolation. That said, Vahia and colleagues noted that older adults with dementia, minority status, and low income might be more affected by COVID-19-related changes. Further investigation around older age and resiliency is warranted (Vahia et al. 2020).

The interpersonal theory of suicide postulates that *thwarted belongingness* (loneliness and loss of social support) and *perceived burdensomeness* (the feeling of being a burden) produce the desire to die from suicide, but the capability to act out on these thoughts is related to lived experiences and genetics (Sheffler et al. 2021). Thwarted belongingness is a key risk factor for suicide in older adults (Draper 2014). Perceived burdensomeness is seen among individuals with a variety of chronic health conditions. Thwarted belongingness and perceived burdensomeness tend to be heightened during global pandemics, which can lead to further deterioration in mental health among the elderly population. Patients who isolate because of quarantine or sheltering in place are particularly at risk of both loneliness and feeling like a burden, therefore increasing the risk of suicide.

DEPRESSION, ANXIETY, AND PTSD

Depression is one of the most common psychiatric disorders among people who die from suicide (Hawton et al. 2013). Late-life depression increases this risk of suicide and continues to significantly affect quality and quantity of life in older adults (Stone et al. 2021).

It is possible that the same risk factors discussed in the "Suicide" section regarding suicide among the elderly population during COVID-19 (i.e., social isolation, quarantine, chronic medical conditions, feeling like a burden) may also affect rates of depression in this population during a global pandemic. This is illustrated by the SARS pandemic in 2003, during which rates of depression and PTSD were found to increase overall (Hawryluck et al. 2004; Lee et al. 2006). Brooks et al. (2020) described the multiple psychological sequelae of quarantining that could contribute to these increased rates. They include increased rates of fear, nervousness, sadness, and acute stress disorder. Brooks et al. further described stressors of fear of infection, frustration, boredom, and inadequate basic supplies that could further contribute to the psychological burden experienced by individuals.

Data regarding rates of depression during the pandemic, however, have been conflicting. The Centers for Disease Control and Prevention conducted representative panel surveys in adults older than age 18 years in the summer of 2020 to assess for changes in mental health, substance use, and suicidal ideation during the COVID-19 pandemic. Their results showed that although overall rates of anxiety and depression were higher when compared with a similar time frame in 2019, the largest prevalence was in the 25- to 44-year-old age group (Czeisler et al. 2020, 2021). However, Ettman et al. (2020), through population-based surveys conducted earlier in the pandemic (i.e., March through April 2020) and before (2017–2018), found that depressive symptoms were higher across age groups (including in the older than 60 years age group). In their study of older adults with preexisting diagnoses of major depressive disorder, Hamm et al. (2020) used data from the Patient Health Questionnaire-9 and Patient-Reported Outcomes Measurement Information System Anxiety scales and found no differences in scores related to depression and anxiety compared with prepandemic scores.

ED psychiatric visits overall were found to decrease but remained consistent for percentages related to depression and suicide (Ferrando et al. 2021). Overall, the decrease in general ED psychiatry visits could be explained by lag theory regarding a delay or decrease in patients seeking psychiatric care during the pandemic (Zalsman et al. 2020). However, while the percentage of visits related to depression remained consistent, patients evaluated during COVID-19 were more likely to have anxiety regarding a COVID-19-related stressor (i.e., contracting COVID, stress of quarantine, financial constraints) (Ferrando et al. 2021).

PSYCHOSIS

Although most of the literature surrounding mental health during the COVID-19 pandemic has focused on depression, anxiety, and PTSD, it is important to comment on psychosis, particularly within the elderly population. The older population at baseline is at increased risk for developing psychosis, for which there could be numerous underlying causes. As discussed by Targum (2001), these causes include delirium, late-life schizophrenia, delusional disorder, mood disorders with psychosis, major neurocognitive disorder with psychosis, illicit substance use, medication-induced psychosis, and psychosis secondary to medical or neurological causes.

Also well studied is the link between past viral pandemics and epidemics and psychosis. In a comprehensive review, Brown et al. (2020) linked various pandemics and epidemics, for example, SARS, Middle East respiratory syndrome (MERS), Ebola, H1N1, and COVID-19, with psychosis. Case reports as early as 1889, 1918, and 1957 and as recent as 2009 have linked influenza with psychosis—sequelae including acute psychosis, delirium, major neurocognitive disorder with psychosis, and mood disorders with psychosis (Kepinska et al. 2020). In Brown et al.'s review, the most common cause of psychosis during these pandemics was steroid-induced psychosis, also possibly related to psychosocial distress or biological mechanism. Overall, Brown et al. found that the number of new cases was small enough to be attributable to typical variation alone. Furthermore, there was no clear link between pandemics and psychosis, particularly among older adults.

DELIRIUM

In a meta-analysis assessing the psychiatric and neuropsychiatric presentations associated with outbreaks caused by coronaviruses (e.g., SARS, MERS, COVID-19), Rogers et al. (2020) found that a significant proportion of patients experienced delirium during their acute phase of illness. Delirium is characterized by the acute onset of global brain dysfunction with deficits in attention, awareness, and cognition and with altered levels of consciousness (Thom et al. 2019). These deficits fluctuate in severity over time and are the direct pathophysiological consequence of an underlying medical condition or toxic exposure (Thom et al. 2019).

Risk factors for delirium with coronavirus disease include preexisting major neurocognitive disorder (a fivefold increase), severe medical illness, older age, sensory impairments, polypharmacy (especially hypnotics such as benzodiazepines, opioids, and anticholinergic medication), and male sex (Thom et al. 2019). Older age (75 years and older), medical comorbidities, and frailty increase not only the risk for more severe illness from COVID-19 infection but also the risk of atypical presentation of COVID-19 infection, such as delirium (Emmerton and Abdelhafiz 2020). Delirium is often the primary or sole symptom among adults 65 years and older (Cipriani et al. 2020; Kennedy et al. 2020). In a multisite cohort study of 817 COVID-19-positive older patients (mean age 77.7 years), Kennedy et al. (2020) found that 28% of patients presented to the ED delirious. Among those with delirium, 37% lacked typical COVID-19 symptoms such as fever and shortness of breath.

Individuals who are intoxicated or withdrawing from substances of abuse can also present with delirium. There are anecdotal reports in the literature of individuals presenting to the ED during COVID-19 experiencing severe delirium related to alcohol misuse and requiring emergent medical intervention (Brooks 2020). The severity of the delirium has been attributed to a variety of factors, including the lack of access to alcohol (precipitating alcohol withdrawal), consumption of unconventional sources of alcohol (e.g., hand sanitizer), and nutritional depletion (Brooks 2020). Clinicians should maintain a high index of suspicion for substance misuse as a potential precipitating factor for delirium in patients presenting to the ED.

In the ED, up to 75% of cases of delirium are overlooked when a validated screening tool is not used (Grossmann et al. 2014; Kennedy et al. 2020). Because delirium can be the first manifestation of COVID-19 infections, validated screening tools for delirium may play an important role in detecting infection (Cipriani et al. 2020; Kennedy et al. 2020). One such tool commonly used in the ED is the 4 As Test (4AT)., The 4AT comprises four items: Alertness, Abbreviated Mental Test, Attention, and Acute change or fluctuating course. The test takes about 2 minutes and does not require any special training to perform (Emmerton and Abdelhafiz 2020). It is well validated and shows good diagnostic accuracy among individuals 65 years and older in various care settings, including the ED, with a pooled sensitivity of 0.88 (95% CI 0.80–0.93) and specificity of 0.88 (95% CI 0.82–0.92) (Emmerton and Abdelhafiz 2020).

After determining and treating the underlying medical conditions or toxic exposures that contribute to delirium, nonpharmacological management is the mainstay in managing delirium and preventing further occurrences. This includes frequently reorienting patients, regulating their sleep-wake cycle, mobilizing them early in their treatment, and optimizing their vision, hearing, nutrition, and hydration (Radhakrishnan et al. 2021; Thom et al. 2019). Reconciling medication lists and avoiding medications likely to potentiate delirium are also key. In the ED, interventions for managing delirium are often pharmacological, including targeting agitation and other behavioral disturbances that either pose a threat to the patient or staff or interfere with medical care. In a narrative review of the literature and clinical experience, Baller and colleagues (2020) suggested a possible framework and algorithm for the pharmacological management of delirium in COVID-19 patients. In the absence of absolute contraindications to any specific class of medications, they recommended preferentially using low-potency antipsychotics and α_2 agonists to manage behavioral disturbances associated with COVID-19 infection.

SUBSTANCE MISUSE AND SUBSTANCE USE DISORDERS

Substance use–related visits to EDs are common among older adults (Bessey et al. 2018). However, SUDs are frequently overlooked in this population (Bessey et al. 2018). Historically, older adults have not reported high rates of substance use, but that is changing with the aging baby boomer generation (Han and Moore 2018). Estimates of the number of adults 50 years and older with a SUD were as high as 5.7 million in 2020 (Seim et al. 2020). The COVID-19 pandemic posed profound challenges for older adults, especially those with a SUD. Loss of loved ones, fewer social supports, and isolation through lockdowns and sheltering in place, coupled with disruption to health care, social services, and community programs, increased older adults' vulnerability to psychological distress (Satre et al. 2020). Distress increases vulnerability to addiction, and some individuals are particularly at risk of substance misuse (e.g., from genetic disposition) (Sinha 2009). According to the *Morbidity and Mortality Weekly Report*, an estimated 3% of older adults started using or increased their use of substances to cope with pandemic-related stress or emotions during the early months of the COVID-19 pandemic (Czeisler et al. 2020).

Alcohol, opioids, and hypnotics such as benzodiazepines are leading causes of substance misuse and use disorders among older adults (Seim et al. 2020). Alcohol is the most frequently used substance among older adults (Seim et al. 2020). According to the 2013–2014 National Survey on Drug Use and Health, the prevalence of alcohol use among adults 50 years and older that year was 62.1%. Rates of binge drinking were 21.5% and 9.1% among older men and women, respectively. Rates of alcohol use disorder were estimated at 5.1% and 2.4% among older men and women, respectively (Han and Moore 2018).

In the United States, alcohol sales increased by 55% during the early phase of the COVID-19 pandemic (Associated Press 2020). Increased use of alcohol could lead to a higher prevalence of alcohol use disorder (Edelman et al. 2019). Vulnerabilities related to advanced age, including diminished liver function, decreased total body water, and neuronal sensitivity to alcohol, put older adults who consume alcohol unhealthily at increased risk of severe medical, functional, and psychiatric problems requiring emergency medical and psychiatric care (Han and Moore 2018; Satre et al. 2020). The National Institutes of Health guidelines recommend that adults 65 years and older who are healthy and do not take medications consume no more than seven drinks per week and no more than three drinks per day (Han and Moore 2018). Although data are currently limited on the impact of the pandemic on alcohol-related ED visits, there are anecdotal reports in the literature of adults presenting to the ED with atypical, severe cases of delirium requiring emergent medical attention related to alcohol misuse (e.g., consuming uncongenial sources of alcohol such as hand sanitizer), withdrawal, and related nutritional depletion (Brooks 2020). Delirium and falls are the two most common sequelae of alcohol use leading to hospital admission from the ED (Bessey et al. 2018). Further, regular alcohol consumption is associated with immune impairment that increases susceptibility to pneumonia and, potentially, to COVID-19 infection (Mallet et al. 2021; Simou et al. 2018). Additionally, unhealthy alcohol use is associated with depression, anxiety, and chronic pain (Mallet et al. 2021). Some data suggest that older adults with or without comorbid depression who misuse alcohol are at increased risk of suicide (Blow et al. 2004).

The benzodiazepine prescription rate is higher among older adults than in any other age group (Seim et al. 2020). Research on disaster situations suggests that benzodiazepine prescriptions may have increased during the COVID-19 pandemic and may have contributed to increased risk of dependence and misuse among older adults (Satre et al. 2020). Among older adults, misuse of benzodiazepines has severe emergent consequences, including delirium, falls, aspiration, respiratory failure, car accidents, suicide risk, and death (Seim et al. 2020).

Opioids and other psychoactive prescription drug misuse among older adults is not uncommon and significantly affects morbidity, mortality, and health care utilization. Older patients are more likely to be prescribed opioids than are the younger population (Satre et al. 2020). Prepandemic, ED visits for prescription drug misuse increased dramatically (Han and Moore 2018). The most recent U.S. health care cost and utilization project data from 2018 indicated that between 2010 and 2015, opioid-related ED visits for patients 65 years and older increased by about 75%, whereas non-opioid-related ED visits in the same population increased by only 17% Seim et al. 2020. Furthermore, opioid-related hospitalizations increased by 35%, whereas non-opioid-related hospital admissions decreased by 17% (Seim et al. 2020). Older adults with opioid use disorder frequently have mental and physical health problems. Those with comorbid opioid use disorder and mental health conditions have increased vulnerability to poor health and psychological distress (Mallet et al. 2021; Satre et al. 2020). For instance, individuals prescribed opioids, particularly at high doses, are at increased risk of developing community-acquired pneumonia (Edelman et al. 2019), which may increase the individual's susceptibility to contracting COVID-19. Opioid misuse also increases the risk for delirium and respiratory failure, particularly when opioids are combined with hypnotics such as benzodiazepines (Seim et al. 2020).

In the early months of the COVID-19 pandemic, the largely marginalized population of older adults recovering from SUDs experienced significant psychosocial stressors, including detrimental isolation from vital supports of recovery communities, economic downturn, disruption of health care resources (e.g., medication-assisted treatment), and housing and food insecurity. These stressors exposed this vulnerable population to significantly increased risk of relapse, overdose, and other potentially devastating health and mental health consequences (Alexander et al. 2020). See "Additional Resources" section for information on substance misuse and substance use screening and treatment.

SUMMARY

Within the elderly population, patients with serious mental illness, SUDs, and homelessness are disproportionately affected by the scarce treatment resources available to them. The COVID-19 pandemic exacerbated these disparities. Patients presenting to the ED with psychiatric complaints experienced new challenges to common dispositions. The literature from past pandemics demonstrated increased rates of depression, anxiety, and PTSD. The same has been postulated during the COVID-19 pandemic, particularly among the elderly population, given their risk factors of underlying psychiatric illness, chronic medical conditions, social isolation, and loneliness. However, there have been conflicting data surrounding rates of depression, anxiety, and suicide among the elderly population during the COVID-19 pandemic, and there have been no clear or consistent increased rates. However, with lag theory, it is possible that as patients' acute medical needs are addressed, their underlying psychiatric illnesses will come to light. We suggest more long-term monitoring to address the psychological effects that come with quarantine, most importantly social isolation and loneliness.

The reader should keep in mind that patients older than age 65 with infections commonly present with atypical symptoms, including delirium. Hospitals should consider adding mental status changes as part of screening criteria. Health care providers and caregivers should be educated about atypical presentations of COVID-19 and other infections. We recommend using validated screening tools to identify and treat delirium in the ED setting. Providers should be familiar with methods to prevent, detect, and manage delirium to improve long-term outcomes.

We highlighted that SUDs are frequently overlooked among the elderly population but are common causes of significant health and mental health morbidity and mortality. Prescription drug misuse substantially increases morbidity and mortality among the elderly population.

Finally, although the COVID-19 pandemic put into glaring focus the disparities that exist in health care and how disparities in health care can be exacerbated, it nonetheless has led to innovative forms of clinical practice. Specifically, telepsychiatry expanded opportunities to evaluate and treat patients in the emergency setting. Further measures are needed to improve and support patients' access to all forms of dispositions from the ED, including inpatient, outpatient, and partial hospitalization and SUD treatment.

KEY POINTS

- The COVID-19 pandemic exacerbated the scarcity of access to treatment resources, widening the disparity gap for older adults with serious mental illness, substance use disorders, and homelessness and for other vulnerable, marginalized, and underserved groups.

- Contrary to what has been postulated from historic epidemiological data looking at prior pandemics, the COVID-19 pandemic has not led to clear or consistent increases in the rates of depression, anxiety, and suicide among the elderly. Further studies and long-term monitoring are recommended.

- As with other infections, COVID-19 commonly manifests with atypical symptoms such as delirium among adults older than 65. Validated screening tools for delirium and continuing education on delirium prevention, detection, and management are recommended to improve long-term outcomes.

- Substance misuse increased during the pandemic. Nonetheless, substance misuse and substance use disorders remain frequently overlooked among older adults. The Substance Abuse and Mental Health Services Administration provides resources for screening, brief intervention, and referral to treatment.

- The unfortunate devastation of the COVID-19 pandemic has led to innovative forms of clinical practice, including the rapid expansion of telepsychiatry in the emergency setting and beyond. The elderly population, however, may struggle to implement these innovative techniques.

QUESTIONS FOR REVIEW

1. Among the elderly population, loneliness, loss of social support, and chronic medical conditions are postulated to increase the risk of which of the following during a pandemic?

    A. Psychosis
    B. Agitation
    C. Suicide

Answer: C.

2. Conflicting data about rates of depression among the elderly population during the COVID-19 pandemic can be explained by which theory?

    A. Interpersonal theory of suicide
    B. Lag theory
    C. Thwarted belongingness

Answer: B.

3. What subpopulation among older adults is more likely to experience barriers to care?

    A. Homeless individuals
    B. Individuals with substance use disorders
    C. Both A and B

Answer: C.

ADDITIONAL RESOURCES

For a comprehensive, pre-COVID-19 overview of emergency psychiatric care for the older adults, we recommend Bessey et al.'s (2018) article "Behavioral Health Needs of Older Adults in the Emergency Department." The Substance Abuse and Mental Health Services Administration provides resources for screening, brief intervention, and referral to treatment (also known as SBIRT). The goal of SBIRT is to effectively deliver treatment early to individuals who have, or are at risk of developing, a SUD (Substance Abuse and Mental Health Services Administration 2017).

REFERENCES

Alexander GC, Stoller KB, Haffajee RL, et al: An epidemic in the midst of a pandemic: opioid use disorder and COVID-19. Ann Intern Med 173(1):57–58, 2020 32240283

Associated Press: Booze buying surges; senators push airlines for cash refunds. Associated Press, March 31, 2020. Available at: https://apnews.com/article/virus-outbreak-financial-markets-mi-state-wire-detroit-michigan-c407ecb931c6c528b4cceb0ecc216f0c. Accessed February 2, 2021.

Augenstein TM, Pigeon WR, DiGiovanni SK, et al: Creating a novel inpatient psychiatric unit with integrated medical support for patients with COVID-19. NEJM Catal 1(4):8, 2020

Baller EB, Hogan CS, Fusunyan MA, et al: Neurocovid: pharmacological recommendations for delirium associated with COVID-19. Psychosomatics 61(6):585–596, 2020 32828569

Bessey LJ, Radue RM, Chapman EN, et al: Behavioral health needs of older adults in the emergency department. Clin Geriatr Med 34(3):469–489, 2018 30031428

Blow FC, Brockmann LM, Barry KL: Role of alcohol in late-life suicide. Alcohol Clin Exp Res 28(5)(suppl):48S–56S, 2004 15166636

Brooks SK, Webster RK, Smith LE, et al: The psychological impact of quarantine and how to reduce it: rapid review of the evidence. Lancet 1395(10227):912–920, 2020 32112714

Brooks V: COVID-19's effects on emergency psychiatry. Current Psychiatry 19(7):33–36, 38–39, 2020

Brown E, Gray R, Lo Monaco S, et al: The potential impact of COVID-19 on psychosis: a rapid review of contemporary epidemic and pandemic research. Schizophr Res 222:79–87, 2020 32389615

Brown HL: Emergency care EMTALA alterations during the COVID-19 pandemic in the United States. J Emerg Nurs 47(2):321–325, 2021 33388166

Cheung YT, Chau PH, Yip PS: A revisit on older adults suicides and severe acute respiratory syndrome (SARS) epidemic in Hong Kong. Int J Geriatr Psychiatry 23(12):1231–1238, 2008 18500689

Cipriani G, Danti S, Nuti A, et al: A complication of coronavirus disease 2019: delirium. Acta Neurol Belg 120(4):927–932, 2020 32524537

Cohen CI: Aging and homelessness. Gerontologist 39(1):5–14, 1999 10028766

Czeisler MÉ, Lane RI, Petrosky E, et al: Mental health, substance use, and suicidal ideation during the COVID-19 pandemic—United States, June 24–30, 2020. MMWR Morb Mortal Wkly Rep 69(32):1049–1057, 2020 32790653

Czeisler MÉ, Lane RI, Wiley JF, et al: Follow-up survey of US adult reports of mental health, substance use, and suicidal ideation during the COVID-19 pandemic, September 2020. JAMA Netw Open 4(2):e2037665, 2021 33606030

Draper BM: Suicidal behaviour and suicide prevention in later life. Maturitas 79(2):179–183, 2014 24786686

Druss BG: Addressing the COVID-19 pandemic in populations with serious mental illness. JAMA Psychiatry 77(9):891–892, 2020 32242888

Edelman EJ, Gordon KS, Crothers K, et al: Association of prescribed opioids with increased risk of community-acquired pneumonia among patients with and without HIV. JAMA Intern Med 179(3):297–304, 2019 30615036

Emmerton D, Abdelhafiz A: Delirium in older people with COVID-19: clinical scenario and literature review. SN Compr Clin Med 2:1790–1797, 2020

Ettman CK, Abdalla SM, Cohen GH, et al: Prevalence of depression symptoms in US adults before and during the COVID-19 pandemic. JAMA Netw Open 3(9):e2019686, 2020 32876685

Ferrando SJ, Klepacz L, Lynch S, et al: Psychiatric emergencies during the height of the COVID-19 pandemic in the suburban New York City area. J Psychiatr Res 136:552–559, 2021 33158555

Fuchs JD, Carter HC, Evans J, et al: Assessment of a hotel-based COVID-19 isolation and quarantine strategy for persons experiencing homelessness. JAMA Netw Open 4(3):e210490, 2021 33651111

Giannouchos TV, Biskupiak J, Moss MJ, et al: Trends in outpatient emergency department visits during the COVID-19 pandemic at a large, urban, academic hospital system. Am J Emerg Med 40:20–26, 2021 33338676

Grossmann FF, Hasemann W, Graber A, et al: Screening, detection and management of delirium in the emergency department—a pilot study on the feasibility of a new algorithm for use in older emergency department patients: the modified Confusion Assessment Method for the Emergency Department (mCAM-ED). Scand J Trauma Resusc Emerg Med 22:19, 2014 24625212

Hakenewerth AM, Tintinalli JE, Waller AE, et al: Emergency department visits by older adults with mental illness in North Carolina. West J Emerg Med 16(7):1142–1145, 2015 26759669

Hamm ME, Brown PJ, Karp JF, et al: Experiences of American older adults with pre-existing depression during the beginnings of the COVID-19 pandemic: a multicity, mixed-methods study. Am J Geriatr Psychiatry 28(9):924–932, 2020 32682619

Han BH, Moore AA: Prevention and screening of unhealthy substance use by older adults. Clin Geriatr Med 34(1):117–129, 2018 29129212

Hawryluck L, Gold WL, Robinson S, et al: SARS control and psychological effects of quarantine, Toronto, Canada. Emerg Infect Dis 10(7):1206–1212, 2004 15324539

Hawton K, Saunders K, Topiwala A, et al: Psychiatric disorders in patients presenting to hospital following self-harm: a systematic review. J Affect Disord 151(3):821–830, 2013 24091302

Heslin SM, Nappi M, Kelly G, et al: Rapid creation of an emergency department telehealth program during the COVID-19 pandemic. J Telemed Telecare Sept 1, 2020 32873137 Epub ahead of print

Jeffery MM, D'Onofrio G, Paek H, et al: Trends in emergency department visits and hospital admissions in health care systems in 5 states in the first months of the COVID-19 pandemic in the US. JAMA Intern Med 180(10):1328–1333, 2020 32744612

Kennedy M, Helfand BKI, Gou RY, et al: Delirium in older patients with COVID-19 presenting to the emergency department. JAMA Netw Open 3(11):e2029540, 2020 33211114

Kepinska AP, Iyegbe CO, Vernon AC, et al: Schizophrenia and influenza at the centenary of the 1918–1919 Spanish influenza pandemic: mechanisms of psychosis risk. Front Psychiatry 11(72):72, 2020 32174851

Kochanek KD, Xu J, Arias E: Mortality in the United States, 2019. NCHS Data Brief (395):1–8, 2020 33395387

Laird KT, Krause B, Funes C, et al: Psychobiological factors of resilience and depression in late life. Transl Psychiatry 9(1):88, 2019 30765686

Lam K, Lu AD, Shi Y, et al: Assessing telemedicine unreadiness among older adults in the United States during the COVID-19 pandemic. JAMA Intern Med 180(10):1389–1391, 2020 32744593

Lee TM, Chi I, Chung LW, et al: Ageing and psychological response during the post-SARS period. Aging Ment Health 10(3):303–311, 2006 16777659

Mallet J, Dubertret C, Le Strat Y: Addictions in the COVID-19 era: current evidence, future perspectives a comprehensive review. Prog Neuropsychopharmacol Biol Psychiatry 106:110070, 2021 32800868

North CS, Smith EM: A systematic study of mental health services utilization by homeless men and women. Soc Psychiatry Psychiatr Epidemiol 28(2):77–83, 1993 8511667

Pagano A, Hosakote S, Kapiteni K, et al: Impacts of COVID-19 on residential treatment programs for substance use disorder. J Subst Abuse Treat 123:108255, 2021 33375986

Radhakrishnan NS, Mufti M, Ortiz D, et al: Implementing delirium prevention in the era of COVID-19. J Alzheimers Dis 79(1):31–36, 2021 33252073

Reinhardt I, Gouzoulis-Mayfrank E, Zielasek J: Use of telepsychiatry in emergency and crisis intervention: current evidence. Curr Psychiatry Rep 21(8):63, 2019 31263972

Rogers JP, Chesney E, Oliver D, et al: Psychiatric and neuropsychiatric presentations associated with severe coronavirus infections: a systematic review and meta-analysis with comparison to the COVID-19 pandemic. Lancet Psychiatry 7(7):611–627, 2020 32437679

Satre DD, Hirschtritt ME, Silverberg MJ, et al: Addressing problems with alcohol and other substances among older adults during the COVID-19 pandemic. Am J Geriatr Psychiatry 28(7):780–783, 2020 32359882

Seim L, Vijapura P, Pagali S, et al: Common substance use disorders in older adults. Hosp Pract (1995) 48 (suppl 1):48–55, 2020 32073917

Sheffler JL, Joiner TE, Sachs-Ericsson NJ: The interpersonal and psychological impacts of COVID-19 on risk for late-life suicide. Gerontologist 61(1):23–29, 2021 32959869

Simou E, Britton J, Leonardi-Bee J: Alcohol and the risk of pneumonia: a systematic review and meta-analysis. BMJ Open 8(8):e022344, 2018 30135186

Sinha R: Modeling stress and drug craving in the laboratory: implications for addiction treatment development. Addict Biol 14(1):84–98, 2009 18945295

Stone DM, Jones CM, Mack KA: Changes in suicide rates—United States, 2018–2019. MMWR Morb Mortal Wkly Rep 70(8):261–268, 2021 33630824

Substance Abuse and Mental Health Services Administration: Screening, Brief Intervention, and Referral to Treatment (SBIRT). Rockville, MD, Substance Abuse and Mental Health Services Administration, September 15, 2017. Available at: www.samhsa.gov/sbirt. Accessed March 10, 2021.

Sullivan G, Burnam A, Koegel P, et al: Quality of life of homeless persons with mental illness: results from the course-of-homelessness study. Psychiatr Serv 51(9):1135–1141, 2000 10970916

Taquet M, Luciano S, Geddes JR, et al: Bidirectional associations between COVID-19 and psychiatric disorder: retrospective cohort studies of 62 354 COVID-19 cases in the USA. Lancet Psychiatry 8(2):130–140, 2021 33181098

Targum SD: Treating psychotic symptoms in elderly patients. Prim Care Companion J Clin Psychiatry 3(4):156–163, 2001 15014599

Theriault KM, Rosenheck RA, Rhee TG: Increasing emergency department visits for mental health conditions in the United States. J Clin Psychiatry 81(5):20m13241, 2020 32726001

Thom RP, Levy-Carrick NC, Bui M, et al: Delirium. Am J Psychiatry 176(10):785–793, 2019 31569986

Vahia IV, Jeste DV, Reynolds CF III: Older adults and the mental health effects of COVID-19. JAMA 324(22):2253–2254, 2020 33216114

Wand APF, Zhong B-L, Chiu HFK, et al: COVID-19: the implications for suicide in older adults. Int Psychogeriatr 32(10):1225–1230, 2020 32349837

World Health Organization: Ageing and Health. Geneva, World Health Organization, 2021a. Available at: www.who.int/news-room/fact-sheets/detail/ageing-and-health#:~:text=Between%202015%20and%202050%2C%20the,%2D%20and%20middle%2Dincome%20countries. Accessed November 1, 2021.

World Health Organization: Suicide data. World Health Organization, 2021b. Available at: www.who.int/teams/mental-health-and-substance-use/suicide-data. Accessed June 28, 2021.

Yarnell S, Li L, MacGrory B, et al: Substance use disorders in later life: a review and synthesis of the literature of an emerging public health concern. Am J Geriatr Psychiatry 28(2):226–236, 2020 31340887

Zalsman G, Stanley B, Szanto K, et al: Suicide in the time of COVID-19: review and recommendations. Arch Suicide Res 24(4):477–482, 2020 33200946

CHAPTER 4

INPATIENT GERIATRIC PSYCHIATRY DURING A GLOBAL PANDEMIC

Antoinette M. Valenti, M.D.
Ebony Dix, M.D.
Col. (Ret.) Elspeth Cameron Ritchie, M.D., M.P.H.

People infected with coronavirus SARS-CoV-2 disease (COVID-19) can present with mild symptoms typically seen with the common cold or flu, or they may present with severe symptoms leading to pneumonia, myocardial injury, renal failure, and even death. Patients with poor mental health are at high risk for contracting COVID-19 (Yao et al. 2020). Age and medical comorbidities increase the risk of severe illness and mortality due to COVID-19 (Wu and McGoogan 2020). Older adults with severe mental illness are more susceptible to delirium, which may be the only presenting feature of infection with COVID-19 despite a negative polymerase chain reaction (PCR) test. The case presented in this chapter illustrates the difficulty in diagnosing atypical presentations of COVID-19 in older adults with underlying severe mental illness as well as some of the many challenges associated with isolating patients while providing inpatient psychiatric care. This case also demonstrates an area of opportunity for developing models of care within the inpatient psychiatric setting during a global pandemic.

Vignette

On March 19, 2020, 8 days after the World Health Organization declared COVID-19 a global pandemic, Mr. G, a 70-year-old African American man with schizophrenia, end-stage renal disease on hemodialysis, hypertension, diabetes mellitus, hepatitis C, and latent tuberculosis was referred from his assisted living facility to the emergency department for evaluation of disorganized, bizarre, and aggressive behaviors. Mr. G's chief complaint was lethargy. He had received his long-acting depot neuroleptic shot 3 days prior to admission after several months of noncompliance.

On admission to the hospital inpatient psychiatry unit, Mr. G's outpatient medications were reinitiated, and his latent tuberculosis treatment was continued. Five days later, he complained of weakness and fell. At the time of his fall, he had altered mental status. The rapid response team was called and found that Mr. G was hypoglycemic and remained hypoglycemic after drinking several servings of juice. He was transferred to inpatient medicine for altered mental status in the setting of hypoglycemia.

On transfer to the hospital's inpatient medicine unit, a chest X-ray demonstrated a new right lower lobe opacity, and a computed tomography (CT) scan of Mr. G's chest confirmed right lower lobe consolidation and a long-standing pleural effusion. Treatment for aspiration pneumonia was initiated, and Mr. G continued hemodialysis and treatment for his latent tuberculosis. A PCR test for COVID-19 was performed, and the results were negative. While on the medicine service, Mr. G had episodes of disruptive and violent behaviors, including throwing feces at staff and pouring water on the floor. He received several doses of emergency medications for his agitation. Psychiatry was consulted after he attempted to wrap an overhead cord around his neck and to use the end of a power cord to puncture his left upper extremity fistula. It was determined that Mr. G's aggressive and unsafe behaviors would be better managed on the hospital's inpatient psychiatry unit, and he was transferred.

On the psychiatry unit, Mr. G continued to be agitated and psychotic, with disorganized thoughts and hallucinations. He had another unwitnessed fall, hitting his head. He showed no focal neurological deficits on examination, and a head computed tomography (CT) scan showed no acute findings. He was placed on 1:1 observation for fall prevention. Over the next 2 days, Mr. G fluctuated between somnolence, normal arousal, and increased agitation. His presentation was consistent with hyperactive delirium superimposed on his underlying psychotic disorder. The medicine service was consulted for his waxing and waning presentation, and adjustments were made in his medications to reduce sedation. However, Mr. G continued to have bouts of physical aggressiveness with staff and disruptive behaviors, such as exposing himself. He began to refuse dialysis. The renal consulting team, which had been following him closely, determined that he did not need emergent dialysis.

Mr. G remained somnolent, and on the following day he was noted to have agonal breathing and a drop in hemoglobin concentration. That same day, his roommate tested positive for COVID-19 and was transferred to the medicine unit for isolation. This prompted ordering a repeat PCR COVID-19 test for Mr. G. This time his test was positive, and he was transferred to the inpatient medicine service for isolation. Shortly after transfer, he developed fever and worsening oxygen saturation. Two days later he had a witnessed aspiration event, for which he was started on a new course of antibiotic treatment. His oxygen requirements increased, his mental status declined further, and he was transferred to the medical intensive care unit (ICU). A repeat CT scan of his head was unremarkable. Three days later, he was determined to require intubation to protect his airway as well as central line placement. Within minutes, Mr. G developed bradycardia, followed by pulseless electrical activity and full cardiac arrest. Resuscitation efforts were unsuccessful. The cause of death was determined to be complications of COVID-19, manifested initially by delirium alone.

Given that Mr. G tested positive after having interacted with his COVID-19-positive roommate, there was concern about a COVID-19 outbreak on the inpatient psychiatry unit. All inpatients were tested, and two more asymptomatic patients tested positive and were immediately placed in isolation. This prompted vigorous attempts to contain the virus on the psychiatry unit. The unit was closed to new admissions, and discharges were held. Staff and patients were provided with masks to wear except when eating or sleeping. Patients were asked to eat in their rooms rather than in the dining room. Groups were conducted in small numbers with patients spaced 6 feet apart. All patients were tested every 2 days.

Despite these efforts, patients continued to test positive, and two other patients were transferred to medicine for treatment. Given the failed efforts to contain the virus, the decision was made to require two consecutive negative COVID-19 tests before discharging patients and to close the unit to admissions until infection control protocols could be reviewed and refined. A group of subject matter experts recommended screening and COVID-19 testing prior to admission, single-room occupancy throughout admission, and more frequent cleaning of common areas, in addition to the use of face coverings and limiting the numbers assembled for groups and dining, allowing adequate spacing among patients. Moreover, the no-visitation policy already in place was continued. With these additional measures in place, the unit was safely reopened to admissions.

The case vignette illustrates the multitude of challenges involved in identifying and treating older adults with chronic mental illness infected with COVID-19 on an inpatient psychiatric unit. Older adults with chronic mental illness are among those at highest risk for contracting COVID-19 and suffering severe clinical outcomes (Yao et al. 2020). In this chapter we expand on three critically important areas highlighted in the vignette that represent opportunities for ongoing examination, research, and development in the arena of inpatient geriatric psychiatry. First, we review the diagnostic complexity that exists in detecting and treating older adults infected with COVID-19. Those infected may be difficult to identify because of the heterogeneity of symptoms, ranging from mild to severe and overlapping with other conditions. Furthermore, a negative PCR test for COVID-19 may be falsely reassuring either because of an inadequate sample collection or because the predictive value of the test may vary from time of exposure and symptom onset (Kucirka et al. 2020). Next, we evaluate some of the unique challenges in the management and prevention of a COVID-19 outbreak on an inpatient geriatric psychiatry unit. Several structural, environmental, and patient-specific factors must be considered, given the congregate care setting of a psychiatric unit. Additional attention is required to address workforce-related issues to safely deliver clinical care (Cheung et al. 2020). Mitigation strategies and innovative service delivery practices became essential for adapting to the new landscape of inpatient psychiatry during the COVID-19 pandemic. Last, we conclude with a discussion of some examples of models of care that have been developed at various institutions across the country to care for psychiatric inpatients during the pandemic.

LESSONS FROM THE CASE VIGNETTE

Diagnostic Complexity

Epidemiological findings indicate that the COVID-19 pandemic had a disproportionately high impact on morbidity and mortality in older adults (D'Adamo et al. 2020) and patients with severe mental disorders (Li et al. 2020a). Patients with schizophrenia are at higher risk of infection secondary to underlying medical comorbidities and difficulty following social distancing instructions. Despite the recognition that patients with severe mental disorders such as schizophrenia are especially vulnerable, diagnosis of COVID-19 in those with atypical presentations can be missed because the primary psychiatric disorder may also present with confusion, agitation, and bizarre behaviors.

Although initial descriptions of COVID-19 focused on respiratory and gastrointestinal symptoms, there is a growing body of evidence for neuropsychiatric manifestations such as headache, anosmia, ageusia, paresthesias, encephalitis, and encephalopathy (Lechien et al. 2020; Mao et al. 2020). Altered mental status is seen in up to 70% of patients with COVID-19, including those without the usual COVID-19 symptoms (Chen et al. 2020; Mao et al. 2020; O'Hanlon and Inouye 2020). In some cases, such as with Mr. G in the vignette, delirium may be the only presenting symptom, and therefore, the recognition of delirium can be instrumental in identifying otherwise asymptomatic patients (Alkeridy et al. 2020).

Moreover, neuropsychiatric symptoms seem to be associated with more severe disease (Mao et al. 2020). A study of 707 patients in Brazil verified delirium as an independent predictor of in-hospital death in adults ≥50 years old with COVID-19 (Garcez et al. 2020). Although altered mental status and/or confusion was not initially known to be a symptom associated with COVID-19, the World Health Organization now recognizes it as a presenting feature of COVID-19 infection in the absence of respiratory symptoms (World Health Organization 2021). Interestingly, delirium associated with COVID-19 appears to be most often of the hyperactive subtype, with one study demonstrating up to 86.6% of individuals with COVID-19 having presented with a hyperactive delirium (Beach et al. 2020; Helms et al. 2020).

Delirium not only is a presenting symptom for COVID-19 but also affects the course of illness. Patients with COVID-19 delirium are known to have an increased length of hospital stay, more ICU admissions (Chachkhiani et al. 2020; Khan et al. 2020), increased use of and longer duration on ventilators (Garcez et al. 2020; Helms et al. 2020), and increased mortality (Chachkhiani et al. 2020; Vena et al. 2020). Therefore, early recognition is critical for both treatment and isolation from others.

It is not surprising that delirium may be the presenting symptom for COVID-19. Coronaviruses are avidly neurotropic (Desforges et al. 2014; Wu et al. 2020). The neuroinvasive capacity of coronaviruses allows them to breach the CNS via the olfactory nerve or through blood circulation. After invading the CNS, they may increase demyelination, interleukin release, and the permeability of the blood-brain barrier, thereby causing direct damage to the brain (Wu et al. 2020). These types of neuroinflammatory pathways are known to contribute to the development of delirium (Fong et al. 2015; Maldonado 2018; van Munster et al. 2009).

Mr. G, the patient in the vignette, presented in March 2020, well before it was recognized that delirium could be the sole presenting symptom for COVID-19. Such knowledge perhaps could have led to an earlier diagnosis, raising the index of suspicion for COVID-19 in the setting of symptoms (e.g., agitation) that were readily seen simply as manifestations of an underlying psychotic disorder.

Mr. G initially presented for care because of an acute exacerbation of his schizophrenia. A PCR COVID-19 test 1 week after his admission was negative, suggesting that his change in mental status at the time of admission was most likely secondary to an exacerbation of his schizophrenia; however, one cannot exclude the possibility of a false-negative test (Kucirka et al. 2020). Midway through Mr. G's 28-day hospitalization, there was concern for delirium after a fall in which he also hit his head. It is unknown whether the fall caused his altered mental status or his altered mental status led to the fall. Nonetheless, his delirium preceded his rather acute decline in respiratory status. Even after careful review and discussion of his hospital course, it was difficult to determine when his agitation was no longer solely secondary to his psychotic illness but also a manifestation of hyperactive delirium. At the time of Mr. G's COVID-19 diagnosis, his presentation was most consistent with hyperactive delirium superimposed on an exacerbation of his schizophrenia.

Several factors contributed to the delay in the diagnosis of Mr. G's hyperactive delirium, which in turn delayed his diagnosis of COVID-19. First, his initial presentation was characterized by disorganization, hallucinations, and agitation, all of which can be seen in a relapse of schizophrenia precipitated by medication nonadherence as well as in hyperactive delirium. Second, as noted above, at that time it was not known that delirium could be the sole presenting symptom of COVID-19; if that fact had been known, it might have led to earlier ordering of the PCR test for COVID-19 and his more timely isolation from other patients, decreasing viral transmission on the unit. Third, Mr. G's disruptive behaviors were life-threatening, and therefore, safety and determining which unit would best manage his behaviors became the focus of treatment, distracting attention from other considerations. Finally, some of the protective measures that were put in place, such as social isolation, restrictions on visitors, and reduced staff care time with patients due to infection risk became barriers to early detection and prevention of delirium.

Challenges of the Inpatient Psychiatric Setting

Up to this point, we have described a case vignette from the early days of the COVID-19 pandemic, when so much was unknown. The case illustrates the considerable challenges associated with evaluating, diagnosing, and treating patients needing hospitalization for acute psychiatric illness. It also demonstrates that as experience with the pandemic grew, it became increasingly evident that there was substantial risk of contagion on an inpatient psychiatric unit. Early on, nursing homes had borne the brunt of the COVID-19 pandemic, with nearly one-third of COVID-19-related fatalities nationwide (Chidambaram et al. 2020). However, COVID-19 spread rapidly in residential settings, including psychiatric hospitals (Callaghan et al. 2020; Kimball et al. 2020; Mosites et al. 2020; Wallace et al. 2020). The first known COVID-19 outbreak in a U.S. inpatient geriatric psychiatry unit occurred soon after March 11, 2020, in King County, Washington, and highlighted the need for protocols to contain such an outbreak (Corcorran et al. 2021). There were outbreaks of COVID-19 in facilities around the country, leading to the closure of inpatient units and, in some instances, the opening up of COVID-19-positive psychiatric units.

The landscape of knowledge related to COVID-19 changed rapidly. Thus, hospitals across the country adapted their care delivery models under the guidance of the Centers for Disease Control and Prevention and local health department policies. Unlike medical and surgical floors, the physical structure and design of inpatient and residential psychiatric care settings present unique infection prevention challenges. Patients are not confined to their rooms, typically have roommates, use communal bathrooms, eat in a dining room, and are encouraged to participate in groups throughout the day. This use of shared space requires the development of special safety and screening protocols that ensure the safety of patients and staff while allowing effective treatment to take place.

As soon as COVID-19 tests were widely available, many institutions began testing patients in the emergency department prior to admission to psychiatry. The dilemma that arose was where to send patients needing inpatient psychiatric care who either tested positive and were asymptomatic or tested positive and had symptoms that required medical treatment.

Models of Care

Some institutions created inpatient psychiatric units specifically designed for COVID-19-positive patients with minimal or no symptoms. Early examples were described in publications from Johns Hopkins (Angelino et al. 2020) and the University of California, Los Angeles (UCLA; Cheung et al. 2020), and a later example was discussed in a publication from Yale (Li et al. 2021).

Given that congregating in close quarters is a risk factor for this patient population, Johns Hopkins developed an effective approach to create an inpatient unit where the delivery of psychiatric care posed minimal risk to patients and staff for transmission. First, they instituted comprehensive screening of patients prior to an admission so that positive cases could be identified and treated to avoid exposing other hospitalized patients. Screening included questions about recent contacts and travel as well as temperature checks. It was important to keep in mind that patients could convert to a positive status after admission. Therefore, once a patient was admitted to an inpatient unit, precautions were taken to promptly identify fever and other symptoms that might have developed so isolation could begin. The practice of daily screening questions and temperature checks was implemented, and frequent handwashing and the use of face coverings was frequently reinforced.

Dining and group experiences were done in shifts to accommodate smaller groups and ensure adequate spacing of patients during these activities. All rooms were converted to single occupancy. Johns Hopkins also took steps to decrease the risk of introducing COVID-19 to the unit, reducing access for nonessential personnel and visitors. The use of videoconferencing for such visits was encouraged. It was recognized that telehealth faces unique challenges in the inpatient setting, particularly if a patient is grossly disorganized, violent, and/or not redirectable. Despite these challenges, there was merit in using this form of communication for nonessential in-person consultations, allowing family visitation and trainees to participate in care. This type of social connectedness used for family visitation often was instrumental in detecting and preventing altered mental status. Videoconferencing also allowed for better communication without the use of personal protective equipment (PPE), which can impair conversation during important nonpharmacological interventions for altered mental status such as orientation.

At other institutions, the culmination of such challenges eventually led to the development of a COVID-19-positive psychiatric unit. It became essential to develop a protocol and design for a psychiatric unit for patients who tested positive and were asymptomatic because in many instances there were simply not enough resources on an internal medicine unit to house patients only for quarantine purposes. During the first couple months of the pandemic, colleagues from UCLA and Yale published a collaborative piece in which they identified eight critical concepts to carefully consider when developing a psychiatric COVID-19-positive unit, including the establishment of clear guidelines for the following: 1) criteria for admission and discharge; 2) social-distancing, isolation, and PPE requirements; 3) medical comanagement and/or consultation; 4) code blue protocol; 5) staffing and workflow; 6) restraint and agitation management; 7) discharge and follow-up planning; and 8) patients' rights (Cheung et al. 2020). Some of the specifics within these categories are given in Table 4–1.

According to the Cheung et al. (2020) guidelines, at institutions without a COVID-19-positive unit, patients testing positive are admitted to a medical unit, regardless of symptom status, and placed in a single negative pressure room and followed by the psychiatry consultation service. Patients in isolation might need a sitter, who is required to wear full PPE for the duration of their shift, unless the room is constructed in

---

Table 4–1. Guidelines for minimizing COVID-19 infection on a psychiatric inpatient unit

---

Screening patients prior to admission or transfer to an inpatient psychiatry unit

• Ask questions about symptoms, recent travel, and close contact with people who have tested positive for COVID-19

• Check temperature

• Test for COVID-19

Preventing transmission among patients throughout an inpatient psychiatry unit

• Ask daily screening questions about symptoms

• Perform at least daily temperature checks

• Promote frequent handwashing

• Require single-room occupancy

• Increase the frequency of cleaning

• Require wireless surgical masks or face coverings for all staff and patients[a]

• Eat in shifts with patients 6 feet apart

• Limit groups to small numbers with patients 6 feet apart

• Educate and offer vaccination

Limiting the introduction of COVID-19 to an inpatient psychiatry unit by others

• Ask screening questions and check temperature of staff at beginning of shifts

• Offer family visitation via videoconferencing

• Perform consultations/admission interview by telehealth

• Allow trainees to participate in care by telehealth

Discharge planning

• Educate and offer vaccination if not yet vaccinated

• Explain follow-up care and discharge to residential setting if continued self-quarantine is necessary

---

[a]Surgical masks have a wire to conform to the nasal bridge; removal of the wire is recommended on an inpatient psychiatry unit for safety reasons.

a way that enables a sitter to remain outside the room and monitor the patient through a window. The psychiatry consultation team following the patient may be unable to evaluate patients in person because of their isolation status. Providing recommendations based on chart review or using telehealth technology if available may limit the team's ability to accurately assess for tremor, gait abnormalities, and abnormalities in muscle tone and reflexes.

Patients with acute behavioral disturbances that warrant restraint use require the presence of several staff members dressed in the appropriate PPE to manage the patient. Most institutions refer to Centers for Disease Control and Prevention guidelines for the duration of isolation and contact precautions for these patients to determine when they can be safely admitted to an inpatient psychiatric unit. However, admission to inpatient psychiatry presents a separate set of challenges.

On the inpatient psychiatric unit, infection prevention measures are strictly enforced because of the communal living environment and lack of single-occupancy rooms. Patients are required to wear a mask at all times except during meals and when sleeping. Mask wearing can be problematic because in some cases the metal clip inside the mask will have to be removed until a more suitable mask can be provided. Many patients cannot or will not tolerate the mask. Frequent handwashing and use of hand sanitizer is encouraged, and many patients need constant reminders about this. Patients are educated on how to properly cough or sneeze into their elbow. Common rooms for meals and group therapy have capacity limits to allow for social distancing. Signs are put up to serve as reminders to patients about hygiene, masks, and social distancing.

Patients are monitored multiple times per day for symptoms suggestive of COVID-19, which include fever, anosmia, and gastrointestinal problems. An algorithm to determine when to test a patient and a protocol for safely isolating and managing symptomatic patients, also known as persons under investigation, have been developed. One way to test patients safely is to designate an isolation room where one or more symptomatic patients can be roomed and tested. One nurse is identified to interact with the persons under investigation and is provided with an N95 mask, gown, gloves, and face shield. One staff member is assigned to sit outside the isolation room to redirect patients to remain in the room if needed and to safeguard PPE supplies outside the room reserved for an emergency staff assist. The nurse is designated to care for patients until the test results come back or the shift ends. Results are typically returned within a few hours, and if positive, the patient is transferred to medicine and the rest of the ward is tested.

Although practices are evolving over time, usually, the ward is closed to new admissions and all remaining patients are tested, and once all tests return negative, the unit is deep cleaned and reopened for admissions. In the instance of a cluster of COVID-19 cases, some wards change from double-room occupancy to single-room occupancy. When a patient tests positive, staff are advised to get tested only if certain criteria are met according to their local and institutional infection prevention guidelines. Visitor restrictions on the inpatient units parallel those on the regular hospital floors. During one of the many ebbs and flows in COVID-19 case rates, hospital administration decided that visitors could be permitted on a limited basis; however, shortly after a patient tested positive on one of the inpatient wards, the visitor restriction was reimposed.

Other clinical operations on inpatient units have been significantly impacted. A protocol was developed to address physical holds and restraints to ensure that all staff required for the event have the appropriate training and access to PPE. Social distancing is not always possible when patients require assistance with activities of daily living. If consultation from a medical or surgical subspecialist is needed, it is often conducted via chart review and over the phone with the provider rather than in person. Some consultants are able to use video telehealth technology to interview the patient, but this limits their ability to conduct a physical exam. Legal hearings and proceedings are all done over the phone or with videoconferencing technology, but many patients with psychosis, sensory impairment, or cognitive disorders cannot or will not participate in these meetings.

COVID-19 changed the landscape of how providers interface with patients. Both parties must manage their own anxieties about possibly becoming infected with the virus. Patients might worry about their risk of getting sick from a provider or staff member or just by virtue of being in the hospital. Providers must be diligent about self-monitoring for symptoms throughout the day, and some have adopted the practice of wearing scrubs and changing out of contaminated clothing prior to returning home. In some settings, staff developed staggered work schedules, in which they alternate between being on-site seeing patients and being off-site seeing patients using video telemedicine technology. This schedule enables the development of a contingency plan if a staff member becomes exposed or sick and needs to quarantine, but this is a challenge for many patients. Some patients are unable or unwilling to interact with providers using telehealth technology, and with face-to-face interactions, PPE makes it more difficult to pick up facial expressions and nonverbal cues.

Working remotely creates both challenges and opportunities for many inpatient providers not only in delivering patient care but also in maintaining contact with other staff members. Many team huddles and meetings have been moved to videoconferencing platforms because of social distancing practices. Although initially isolating, videoconferencing has opened up lines of communication for inpatient care teams to more easily engage in interdisciplinary collaboration of care.

Finally, discharge planning requires special consideration, particularly for older adults going to assisted living facilities, skilled nursing facilities, or group homes with shared dining and social spaces, both of which are known major risk factors for the transmission of COVID-19. As of this writing, vaccination against COVID-19 has become more and more widespread, increasing confidence in the safety of these dispositions. However, vaccine acceptance is not universal among patients (and staff), and even when patients are able to receive their first injection in the hospital, it is not always easy to ensure that the second injection and any boosters, if necessary, will be administered at the appropriate time. There have been many variants of the COVID-19 virus, some more infectious than others. At the time of publication, the delta variant has been the most infectious strain. Vaccination is recommended and encouraged because it is the best protection against severe illness, hospitalization, and death.

SUMMARY

In summary, COVID-19 has proven to be novel not only for its virulence but also for its ability to alter the landscape of clinical psychiatry. During the course of the pandemic, we have learned many lessons about how to deliver care to our patients, especially those who are at highest risk of severe illness and complications from COVID-19. Increased awareness and diagnostic vigilance have enabled us to better detect and manage emerging cases. We have gained a better understanding of the neurobiological mechanisms by which COVID-19 acts in patients presenting with atypical features and neuropsychiatric manifestations, particularly in older adults with medical and psychiatric comorbidities. Through collaborative efforts across nationwide health systems and the implementation of structured protocols, models of care delivery have been developed to safely meet the inpatient psychiatric needs of this vulnerable population. Innovations in telehealth technology have given rise to a hybrid workforce capable of providing multidisciplinary care in the inpatient psychiatric setting.

However, the protocols for COVID-19 will remain in flux to accommodate the advances in our understanding of the virus and its sequelae. Revisions will be required to ensure adherence to institutional, local, and federal public health guidelines. Some of the evolving policies will include universal screening and testing of patients, adjustments to visitor policies, PPE guidance for patients and staff, and management of asymptomatic COVID-19-positive patients who require an inpatient level of psychiatric care.

KEY POINTS

- COVID-19 directly affects the CNS, and delirium is commonly seen in hospitalized patients and may be the only presenting symptom.

- Both elderly people and those with severe mental illness are more susceptible to delirium, and therefore, clinicians must remain vigilant for this syndrome as an atypical presentation of COVID-19 in this patient population.

- Providing safe and effective inpatient mental health care while trying to contain and prevent the spread of a highly contagious respiratory virus is a challenge but can be executed in a variety of ways with careful planning and multiple precautions in place.

QUESTIONS FOR REVIEW

1. Hospitalized patients with delirium and COVID-19 are noted to have which of the following?

    A. Increased length of hospital stay
    B. Increased admissions to the ICU
    C. Increased ventilator utilization
    D. All of the above

Answer: D.

2. Which is true of delirium in COVID-19 patients?

    A. It is more likely to be hypoactive.
    B. It may be the only presenting symptom of COVID-19.
    C. It indicates a favorable prognosis.
    D. It is independently associated with in-hospital death in adults 50 years and older.
    E. B and D

Answer: E.

3. Which is *not* true of telepsychiatry and videoconferencing use?

    A. These modalities are used equally in inpatient and outpatient psychiatry settings.

    B. These modalities are a good way to keep trainees engaged in patient care while not exposing patients to more in-person staff than is absolutely necessary.

    C. These modalities are a great way for patients and families to maintain contact and "visit" while patients are hospitalized.

    D. These modalities can limit nonessential in-person interactions with patients and staff.

Answer: A.

REFERENCES

Alkeridy WA, Almaghlouth I, Alrashed R, et al: A unique presentation of delirium in a patient with otherwise asymptomatic COVID-19. J Am Geriatr Soc 68(7):1382–1384, 2020 32383778

Angelino AF, Lyketsos CG, Ahmed MS, et al: Design and implementation of a regional inpatient psychiatry unit for patients who are positive for asymptomatic SARS-CoV-2. Psychosomatics 61(6):662–671, 2020 32800571

Beach SR, Praschan NC, Hogan C, et al: Delirium in COVID-19: a case series and exploration of potential mechanisms for central nervous system involvement. Gen Hosp Psychiatry 65:47–53, 2020 32470824

Callaghan AW, Chard AN, Arnold P, et al: Screening for SARS-CoV-2 infection within a psychiatric hospital and considerations for limiting transmission within residential psychiatric facilities—Wyoming, 2020. MMWR Morb Mortal Wkly Rep 69(26):825–829, 2020 32614815

Chachkhiani D, Soliman MY, Barua D, et al: Neurological complications in a predominantly African American sample of COVID-19 predict worse outcomes during hospitalization. Clin Neurol Neurosurg 197:106173, 2020 32877769

Chen T, Wu D, Chen H, et al: Clinical characteristics of 113 deceased patients with coronavirus disease 2019: retrospective study. BMJ 368:m1091, 2020 32217556

Cheung EH, Strouse TB, Li L: Planning for a psychiatric COVID-19-positive unit. Medscape, May 17, 2020. Available at: www.medscape.com/viewarticle/930659. Accessed June 29, 2021.

Chidambaram P, Garfield R, Neuman T: COVID-19 has claimed the lives of 100,000 long-term care residents and staff. KFF, November 25, 2020. Available at: www.kff.org/policy-watch/covid-19-has-claimed-the-lives-of-100000-long-term-care-residents-and-staff/. Accessed June 29, 2021.

Corcorran MA, Olin S, Rani G, et al: Prolonged persistence of PCR-detectable virus during an outbreak of SARS-CoV-2 in an inpatient geriatric psychiatry unit in King County, Washington. Am J Infect Control 49(3):293–298, 2021 32827597

D'Adamo H, Yoshikawa T, Ouslander JG: Coronavirus disease 2019 in geriatrics and long-term care: the ABCDs of COVID-19. J Am Geriatr Soc 68(5):912–917, 2020 32212386

Desforges M, Le Coupanec A, Brison E, et al: Neuroinvasive and neurotropic human respiratory coronaviruses: potential neurovirulent agents in humans. Adv Exp Med Biol 807:75–96, 2014 24619619

Fong TG, Davis D, Growdon ME, et al: The interface between delirium and dementia in elderly adults. Lancet Neurol 14(8):823–832, 2015 26139023

Garcez FB, Aliberti MJR, Poco PCE, et al: Delirium and adverse outcomes in hospitalized patients with COVID-19. J Am Geriatr Soc 68(11):2440–2446, 2020 32835425

Helms J, Kremer S, Merdji H, et al: Delirium and encephalopathy in severe COVID-19: a cohort analysis of ICU patients. Crit Care 24(1):491, 2020 32771053

Khan SH, Lindroth H, Perkins AJ, et al: Delirium incidence, duration, and severity in critically ill patients with coronavirus disease 2019. Crit Care Explor 2(12):e0290, 2020 33251519

Kimball A, Hatfield KM, Arons M, et al: Asymptomatic and presymptomatic SARS-CoV-2 infections in residents of a long-term care skilled nursing facility—King County, Washington, March 2020. MMWR Morb Mortal Wkly Rep 69(13):377–381, 2020 32240128

Kucirka LM, Lauer SA, Laeyendecker O, et al: Variation in false-negative rate of reverse transcriptase polymerase chain reaction-based SARS-CoV-2 tests by time since exposure. Ann Intern Med 173(4):262–267, 2020 32422057

Lechien JR, Chiesa-Estomba CM, De Siati DR, et al: Olfactory and gustatory dysfunctions as a clinical presentation of mild-to-moderate forms of the coronavirus disease (COVID-19): a multicenter European study. Eur Arch Otorhinolaryngol 277(8):2251–2261, 2020 32253535

Li L, Li F, Fortunati F, Krystal JH: Association of a prior psychiatric diagnosis with mortality among hospitalized patients with coronavirus disease 2019 (COVID-19) infection. JAMA Netw Open 3(9):e2023282, 2020a 32997123

Li L, Stanley R, Fortunati F: Emerging need and early experiences with a COVID-specific psychiatric unit. Psychiatr Serv 71(8):873, 2020b 32741335

Li L, Roberts SC, Kulp W, et al: Epidemiology, infection prevention, testing data, and clinical outcomes of COVID-19 on five inpatient psychiatric units in a large academic medical center. Psychiatry Res 298:113776, 2021 33571800

Maldonado JR: Delirium pathophysiology: an updated hypothesis of the etiology of acute brain failure. Int J Geriatr Psychiatry 33(11):1428–1457, 2018 29278283

Mao L, Jin H, Wang M, et al: Neurologic manifestations of hospitalized patients with coronavirus disease 2019 in Wuhan, China. JAMA Neurol 77(6):683–690, 2020 32275288

Mosites E, Parker EM, Clarke KEN, et al: Assessment of SARS-CoV-2 infection prevalence in homeless shelters—four U.S. cities, March 27–April 15, 2020. MMWR Morb Mortal Wkly Rep 69(17):521–522, 2020 32352957

O'Hanlon S, Inouye SK: Delirium: a missing piece in the COVID-19 pandemic puzzle. Age Ageing 49(4):497–498, 2020 32374367

van Munster BC, Korse CM, de Rooij SE, et al: Markers of cerebral damage during delirium in elderly patients with hip fracture. BMC Neurol 9(1):21, 2009 19473521

Vena A, Giacobbe DR, Di Biagio A, et al: Clinical characteristics, management and in-hospital mortality of patients with coronavirus disease 2019 in Genoa, Italy. Clin Microbiol Infect 26(11):1537–1544, 2020 32810610

Wallace M, Hagan L, Curran KG, et al: COVID-19 in correctional and detention facilities—United States, February–April 2020. MMWR Morb Mortal Wkly Rep 69(19):587–590, 2020 32407300

World Health Organization: COVID-19 clinical management: living guidance, 25 January 2021. Geneva, Switzerland, World Health Organization, 2021. Available at: https://apps.who.int/iris/handle/10665/338882. Accessed June 29, 2021.

Wu Y, Xu X, Chen Z, et al: Nervous system involvement after infection with COVID-19 and other coronaviruses. Brain Behav Immun 87:18–22, 2020 32240762

Wu Z, McGoogan JM: Characteristics of and important lessons from the coronavirus disease 2019 (COVID-19) outbreak in China: summary of a report of 72314 cases from the Chinese Center for Disease Control and Prevention. JAMA 323(13):1239–1242, 2020 32091533

Yao H, Chen JH, Xu YF: Patients with mental health disorders in the COVID-19 epidemic. Lancet Psychiatry 7(4):e21, 2020 32199510

GERIATRIC MENTAL HEALTH CARE

Lessons From a Pandemic

Marc Agronin, M.D., DFAPA, DFAAGP

> Nursing home residents aren't getting half of our resources or half of our attention, yet they account for roughly half the deaths.
> —David Grabowski (Godfrey 2020)

Nursing homes have been hot spots of both cases and mortality during the coronavirus SARS-CoV-2 disease (COVID-19) pandemic. The confluence of older, medically compromised residents in congregate living with frequent contact with outside workers and visitors has created a particular vulnerability to infectious spread in these long-term care settings. At the same time, the well-recognized neuropsychiatric effects of COVID-19 infection have hit nursing home residents hard, especially those who already have significant baseline impairment. Nursing home staff as frontline health care workers have faced enormous stress during the pandemic. Residents have suffered from prolonged social isolation. Fortunately, there have been numerous approaches to mitigating these stresses and many lessons learned that can be applied to future infectious outbreaks.

Vignette

An 82-year-old nursing home resident with Parkinson's disease was noted to have a fever and cough. A COVID-19 nasal swab test came back positive. Over several days he was noted to be stiffer with slower movements, despite his usual anti-Parkinson's regimen. On day 7 he was noted to be more confused and weak. He was hospitalized and found to be delirious and dehydrated. Even after recovery from acute symptoms of COVID-19, he was unable to walk and had increased neurocognitive impairment. Aggressive physical rehabilitation led to improved mobility over several months and modest improvement in cognition, but he did not return to his previous cognitive and functional baseline.

Throughout 2020, nursing homes and other long-term care settings emerged early on as significant COVID-19 pandemic hot spots. In fact, by June 2020 nearly one-third of all deaths in the United States from the novel coronavirus were seen in nursing homes (Paulin 2020). Data from the Centers for Disease Control and Prevention (2021) indicate that as of late March 2021 there were 644,247 confirmed cases of COVID-19 in U.S. nursing homes and 131,386 deaths, representing nearly 25% of all COVID-19 deaths in the United States. California, Texas, and Pennsylvania account for approximately 23% of all cases and one in five deaths in nursing homes. The weekly number of both cases ($N=33,595$) and deaths ($N=6,007$) peaked in nursing homes the week of December 20, 2020. Staff have also been hit hard, with 558,659 confirmed cases and 1,632 deaths (Centers for Disease Control and Prevention 2021).

The prevalence of COVID-19 in the surrounding community is consistently associated with COVID-19 cases and/or deaths in nursing homes (Gorges and Konetzka 2020). But additional factors contribute to the heightened risk of infectious spread in general within a nursing home and the much higher risk of mortality. Most residents are old, ill, and frail and are often immunocompromised (Eveleth 2020). They live in close quarters with roommates and have congregate dining and social and recreational activities and are cared for by staff who live in the community (many with young children), may take public transportation to work, and then come into the facility and circulate among the residents. Among staff, there is the potential for lack of adequate personal protective equipment (PPE) and training, coupled with, in some instances, relatively lax approaches to infection control. Finally, these residents are frequently exposed to multiple family members from the community who may visit every day.

To mitigate these risks early on in the pandemic, the Department of Veterans Affairs (VA) nursing homes as well as most other long-term care facilities instituted multiple interventions (Psevdos et al. 2021). Among the strategies implemented were the following:

- Screening residents and staff for COVID-19 symptoms
- Limiting new admissions
- Implementing a 14-day observation period for residents returning to the facility from acute care
- Restriction of visitations except for compassionate situations (such as a terminally ill individual)
- Infection control education for both residents and staff
- Promoting consistent staffing
- Promoting use of telehealth for consultations and clinic visits outside the facility
- Establishment of cohorted COVID-19 units within the nursing home to facilitate isolation of asymptomatic positive cases

As a result, the VA reported much lower COVID-19 rates and related mortality (Spotswood 2020). As of February 2021, the reported infection rate at VA facilities was 5.47 per 100 residents, and the mortality rate was less than 0.5% (Kime 2021). Rates of success with similar measures to mitigate infectious spread in private long-term care facilities and assisted care facilities varied on the basis of the degree of implementation. To aid in these efforts, the Centers for Medicare and Medicaid Services (2020) provided guidelines for nursing homes in spring 2020, covering everything from screening to visitation and proper use of PPE. Many states adopted the Centers for Medicare and Medicaid Services guidelines, but there was great variability in how states chose to gather and report nursing home cases and deaths as well as impose restrictions on visitation. Regulations across states for reporting cases and deaths and restricting visitation were generally less consistently applied to assisted living facilities (True et al. 2020).

HOW DOES COVID-19 AFFECT THE BRAIN?

The significant morbidity and mortality in older medically and psychiatrically compromised nursing home residents stem not only from the preeminent pulmonary symptoms of COVID-19 infection but also from the common neurological and neuropsychiatric complications. Coronaviruses—especially COVID-19—are neuroinvasive and may directly enter the CNS through the olfactory bulb (Desforges et al. 2019). Acute infection affects the brain through hypoxia, glial cell activation, and cytokinemia. Its damage to brain tissue has been seen in autopsies with cerebral edema and neuronal degeneration and demyelination (Wu et al. 2020). In addition, COVID-19 infection can damage the endothelial lining of the blood-brain barrier and also bind to angiotensin converting enzyme 2 receptors, which in turn can increase blood pressure and the risk of hemorrhagic stroke.

More than one-third of COVID-19 patients develop a variety of neurological symptoms or neuropsychiatric disorders, especially those with more severe infections, with even higher rates of more than 40% in those who require hospitalization or time in an intensive care unit (Taquet et al. 2021; Wu et al. 2020). The most common acute neurological symptoms include loss of smell and taste, headache, and "brain fog." More concerning symptoms include peripheral neuropathy, delirium, stroke, encephalitis, neurocognitive impairment, psychosis, and mood disturbances (Mao et al. 2020). Older individuals with multiple comorbidities and preexisting neurological and psychiatric conditions are at particular risk. In one study of COVID-19 patients in Wuhan, China, nearly 37% had neurological symptoms, including headaches, paresthesias, stroke, and encephalopathy. Data from 125 case reports (median age=71) of neurological and neuropsychiatric complications in a U.K. surveillance study from April 2020 showed cerebrovascular events in 62% of the sample, of whom 74% had ischemic stroke, 12% had intracerebral hemorrhage, and 1% had CNS vasculitis. Of concern was that 18% of the sample were younger than 60 years old (Varatharaj et al. 2020). In this same sample, acute mental status changes were seen in 31%, of whom 23% had encephalopathy and 18% had encephalitis. Psychiatric diagnoses were seen in 59% of the sample, of whom 43% had psychosis, 26% had neurocognitive changes, and 17% had mood disorders. Of this group, 50% were younger than 60 years old (Varatharaj et al. 2020). A much larger sample of COVID-19 patients indicated that anxiety disorders were the most common neuropsychiatric diagnosis, seen in 17.39% of individuals, followed by mood disorders (13.66%), substance use (6.58%), and psychotic disorders (1.4%) (Taquet et al. 2021).

These data point to several key lessons that can be applied to nursing home residents. First, mental health issues must be treated as both acute and long-lasting sequelae of COVID-19 infection (Rogers et al. 2020). Clinicians should look for key indicators of infection, including changes in energy, alertness, concentration, orientation, sleep, and appetite. COVID-19 testing is appropriate for any patient with suspected infection who exhibits neurological changes, regardless of whether there are respiratory symptoms or classic symptoms of fever and cough. Patients need aggressive identification and treatment of neurocognitive changes, delirium, psychosis, and mood and anxiety disorders. Older individuals, especially those with frailty and dementia, need to be physically mobilized as soon as possible to reduce deconditioning, build confidence, and promote engagement with others.

COVID-19 IMPACT ON LIFE IN LONG-TERM CARE

By necessity, nursing home residents were largely confined to their rooms for nearly the entire first 6–8 months of the COVID-19 pandemic—and longer in many facilities—with limited movement and social interactions that continued for more than a year. Initial restrictions included no congregate dining or activities, no in-person family visits, limited access to medical and mental health services, and lack of access to therapeutic activities and services. Residents experienced a general lack of exercise, sunlight, and social interactions. Even when staff began to facilitate video chats with family, it was a passive and frustrating experience for many residents who were not tech savvy or even those who were tech capable and were totally reliant on staff and family availability.

The consequences of restrictions to room, activity, and social interactions were largely ignored during the early part of the pandemic because nursing home staff were focused on dealing with the imminent danger of infection spreading throughout the facility. However, social isolation was a well-recognized problem even before the pandemic, affecting 25% of older adults and higher percentages of nursing home residents, and it has adverse effects on well-being, physical health, and mental health (National Academies of Sciences, Engineering, and Medicine 2020). During the pandemic, residents spent large amounts of time alone, without family contact and familiar faces, seeing and wearing masks, and listening to the news or hearing about losses. Staff were often unrecognizable with extensive PPE that covered their faces, heads, and bodies. Residents with little to no understanding of the pandemic could become anxious and confused by seeing people wandering around them with full PPE garb. In some individuals, these experiences led to profound social isolation, boredom, sadness and grief, fear and anxiety, confusion, relapse of mental health conditions, or even failure to thrive (Agronin 2021). Sadly, for many residents this social isolation was not a new experience, but it certainly was more severe than before.

Even when restrictions began to be lifted, life in nursing homes was far from normal well after a year into the pandemic. Uncertainty remained as to when life would return to prepandemic normality and whether long-standing new infection control procedures would remain in place. Fortunately, the implementation of COVID-19 vaccinations for both nursing home residents and staff in December 2020 and January 2021 had a relatively rapid and positive impact on reducing infections in facilities (Mor et al. 2021). In one study of VA Community Living Centers, there was a 75% drop in COVID-19 positive tests among all residents 4 weeks after vaccination (Rudolph et al. 2021). However, despite the relative safety and success of vaccination in nursing homes, including data showing COVID-19 cases decreasing by 83% among nursing home staff, many frontline nurses and certified nursing assistants chose not to get vaccinated because of various fears and concerns, many of which were based on rumors and myths, often promulgated by social media (Bailey and Dubnow 2021). The gaps in vaccination rates became even more problematic when the COVID-19 delta variant began surging in 2021, affecting both unvaccinated and a percentage of fully vaccinated individuals.

ENGAGEMENT STRATEGIES

Given the potentially devastating effects of both COVID-19 infection itself and social isolation on neuropsychiatric function, many facilities employed several strategies to better engage and mobilize residents, and these strategies can be applied to ongoing or future infectious outbreaks and other similar circumstances. First, staff have to become like family members during acute lockdowns in order to maintain some consistent and supportive contacts. To facilitate this familiarity with staff required to wear masks and other PPE, both identifying name tags and photos can be worn over facial or bodily coverings. Important clinical assessments and appointments can be carried out through telehealth platforms, especially for individuals confined to highly restrictive COVID-19 units. Family video chats can be facilitated by nursing, social work, mental health, and therapeutic programming staff on a regular basis. Activities such as music therapy at the door can be brought to the residents' rooms, and fun snacks and meals can be delivered to the room. Activities can be conducted via video or closed-circuit TV if available, and drive-through family visits using masks and social distancing (or even protective see-through barriers in some instances) can help residents maintain contact in a safe manner. Once visitation is liberalized, visits can be held outdoors with small numbers of visitors, family education about proper infection control procedures, and use of appropriate PPE.

During pandemics, special attention needs to be given to the differences in communication styles among people from different generations, cultures, and walks of life. Although there are common concerns among everyone, differences in style and outlook may amplify some of the divergent ways in which these fears and stresses are expressed, and the same words or expressions may be verbalized and interpreted with different emphases and meanings (Agronin 2020). Under stress, individuals tend to speak *to* and not *with* each other. At the same time, older individuals can demonstrate incredible psychological resilience during a pandemic, including emergent strengths of wisdom, purpose, positivity, and creativity that can help them and those around them (Agronin 2018). Recommended strategies to better engage with older nursing home residents and help them identify and amplify these strengths include asking questions about their past and present perspectives and being patient and empathic while listening intently to what they have to say. These approaches can begin to break down the social isolation that is so pervasive during quarantines.

THE STRESS OF BEING A FRONTLINE CAREGIVER

Nursing home staff in all areas, from clinical roles to housekeeping, security, maintenance, and administration, have all played frontline roles during the COVID-19 pandemic and, as a result, have faced enormous stress from actual and feared infectious exposure at work. They also face financial loss if they miss extended work time when sick. Clinical staff face the unique stress of having to wear extensive PPE throughout their workday, which can include in totality both a restrictive N95 mask and a surgical or cloth mask covering it, face shield, head covering, one to two layers of gloves, gown or jumpsuit, and shoe covers. This PPE is burdensome to put on and change and, when worn all day, can increase body heat and sweating and promote dehydration and fatigue. Staff who provide bedside care, especially in COVID-19 units, face the additional stress of potential infectious exposure with every resident contact. Many of these staff then return home, where they care for their families, who themselves may have infectious exposure. In addition, many have their own medical risk factors for COVID-19 such as obesity, hypertension, and diabetes.

Data from studying frontline caregivers in other pandemics have shown increased risk for acute stress reactions and PTSD and increased risk for anxiety, panic attacks, depression, and suicide (Morganstein 2020; World Health Organization 2020). A North American support team of psychiatrists and other mental health professionals who provided telephone and video contacts with Chinese heath care workers found several stages of emotional change: bewilderment, shock, anger, anxiety, burnout, and desperation. The best time to intervene was during stages of anger and anxiety, with time-limited, professional therapeutic tools (Cheng 2020).

STRATEGIES TO HELP FRONTLINE STAFF

One study that interviewed nursing assistants during the pandemic identified several key sources of organizational empowerment that helped to mitigate psychological stress, including providing key information, resources, various forms of support, and opportunities to innovate in providing care (Travers et al. 2020). In terms of information, staff education must be deliberate and repetitive in terms of infection control procedures, including the proper use of PPE, and attuned to multilingual and multicultural staff differences. It should also include information on stress identification and reduction, with a focus on deep breathing, hydration, taking breaks, and sleep hygiene. Supportive resources include on-site counseling and referrals to employee assistance programs or other professional mental health services and a confidential mental health hotline. A key source of support can come through daily staff huddles with safe social gathering to provide updates, reassurance, inspiration, education, and opportunities to vent and ask questions (Morganstein 2020). Some of these meetings should include interactions with staff from human resources and administration. These meetings will enable staff to brainstorm on ways to actively help themselves and their residents and promote creativity and innovation in care.

One helpful term that can be used to promote stress reduction is the use of "emotional PPE," which refers to strategies to self-identify and manage emotional and mental stress and related symptoms. This may include several components:

- Emotional "pulse taking" by asking yourself regularly "How am I feeling right now?"
- Prestress and poststress surveillance and reduction techniques such as deep-breathing relaxation and mindfulness strategies
- Support groups and individual counseling on anxiety, depression, grief, and acute and posttraumatic stress reactions
- Encouraging, supporting, and inspiring these behaviors on a daily basis

In addition, it is important to recognize and reward staff as health care heroes and use this recognition to encourage caring behaviors and support for one another. These approaches help to build morale, reduce staff burnout and turnover, and channel staff in need to available resources.

It is imperative for leadership in these settings to engage these strategies and maintain them over time, even in the postpandemic period. Finally, there are many individuals who want to help, from family members and local businesses to volunteers and civic and religious groups. The key is to find them and engage them.

COVID-19 AND NEW MODELS OF LONG-TERM CARE

COVID-19 has demonstrated that during a pandemic, large institutional care settings with shared rooms and communal areas lead to less than optimal care and prove fatal in far too many cases. This outcome suggests that alternative models merit consideration. A recent study found that those nursing homes with low registered nurse and total staffing levels had a higher probability of having residents with COVID-19 (Harrington et al. 2020). Several investigators and professional organizations have recommended establishing minimum staffing standards at both the federal and state levels as a preventive intervention to better contain COVID-19 (Figueroa et al. 2020; Gorges and Konetzka 2020).

Alternative models of long-term care have also been proposed. One such alternative, The Green House Project, has received a great deal of attention and review (Zimmerman et al. 2016). Each Green House is designed with private bedrooms that surround a center of life in the home, an area for cooking, dining, and social activities. The cottages have adjoining external patios or balconies. The workforce consists of a small group of universal workers, licensed as certified nursing assistants, who work in just one home and get to know the 10–12 residents well. This structure reduces the numbers of external and stranger interactions and allows the home to feel more personal and humanistic. A comparison analysis found that residents of Green House homes spent less time hospitalized than did residents in several hundred traditional nursing homes. Most recently, a University of North Carolina study found that COVID-19 incidence and mortality rates were lower among Green House and small facilities when compared with those from more traditional nursing homes (Zimmerman et al. 2021).

SUMMARY

The COVID-19 pandemic has had a catastrophic impact on nursing homes and other long-term care settings, with a steep and stressful learning curve. We know that the neuropsychiatric effects of COVID-19 infection are common and can persist for months and that early and aggressive intervention is needed and must breach the barriers to care. Even though we must keep residents safe during infectious outbreaks, staying isolated in one's room is lonely and stressful, but there are creative ways to engage individuals. This pandemic has presented an opportunity to consider promising and alternative models of long-term care. Frontline caregivers have been true heroes during this pandemic, facing daily stress that can be overwhelming. We have learned that there are effective ways to support them over time.

KEY POINTS

- Nursing homes and other long-term care settings have been epicenters of COVID-19 infections and deaths.

- Neuropsychiatric symptoms are frequent associated symptoms and postinfectious sequelae of COVID-19 infection.

- In addition to high rates of infection and morbidity due to COVID-19, long-term care residents have suffered significantly from social isolation, with resultant increases in psychiatric symptoms.

- Long-term care staff have faced significant stresses during the COVID-19 pandemic, which warrant prompt mental health interventions.

QUESTIONS FOR REVIEW

1. Nursing home deaths have comprised what percentage of total U.S. deaths from COVID-19?

    A. 5%
    B. 10%
    C. 25%
    D. 50%

Answer: C.

2. According to one study, the most common neuropsychiatric disorder associated with COVID-19 infection was which of the following?

   A. Psychotic disorders
   B. Anxiety disorders
   C. Mood disorders
   D. Alzheimer's disease

Answer: B.

3. One of the most devastating aspects of life for nursing home residents during the COVID-19 pandemic has been which of the following?

   A. Worsening glucose levels
   B. Hip fractures
   C. Arrhythmias
   D. Social isolation

Answer: D.

ADDITIONAL RESOURCES

Centers for Disease Control and Prevention: COVID-19 nursing home data. Atlanta, GA, Centers for Disease Control and Prevention, March 21, 2021. Available at: https://data.cms.gov/stories/s/bkwz-xpvg. Accessed April 7, 2021.

National Academies of Sciences, Engineering, and Medicine: Social Isolation and Loneliness in Older Adults: Opportunities for the Health Care System. Washington, DC, National Academies Press, 2020.

National Center for PTSD: Provider Self-Care Toolkit. Washington DC, U.S. Department of Veterans Affairs. Available at: www.ptsd.va.gov/professional/treat/care/toolkits/provider. Accessed April 27, 2021.

World Health Organization: Mental health and psychosocial considerations during the COVID-19 outbreak. Geneva, Switzerland, World Health Organization, March 18, 2020. Available at: www.who.int/docs/default-source/coronaviruse/mental-health-considerations.pdf?sfvrsn=6d3578af_10. Accessed April 27, 2021.

REFERENCES

Agronin ME: The End of Old Age: Living a Longer, More Purposeful Life. New York, Hachette, 2018

Agronin ME: Why it's so hard to talk to your parents about the coronavirus—and vice versa. The Wall Street Journal, April 22, 2020. Available at: www.wsj.com/articles/why-its-so-hard-to-talk-to-your-parents-about-the-coronavirus-and-vice-versa-11587236112. Accessed April 27, 2021.

Agronin ME: What COVID-19 taught us about the high cost of isolation. The Wall Street Journal, April 12, 2021. Available at: www.wsj.com/articles/covid-19-isolation-11618005941. Accessed April 27, 2021.

Bailey M, Dubnow S: Covid cases plummet 83% among nursing home staffers despite vaccine hesitancy. KHN, March 15, 2021. Available at: http://khn.org/news/article/covid-cases-plummet-among-nursing-home-staffers-despite-vaccine-hesitancy. Accessed April 27, 2021.

Centers for Disease Control and Prevention: COVID-19 nursing home data. Atlanta, GA, Centers for Disease Control and Prevention, 2021. Available at: https://data.cms.gov/stories/s/bkwz-xpvg. Accessed April 27, 2021.

Centers for Medicare and Medicaid Services: COVID-19 long-term care facility guidance. Baltimore, MD, Centers for Medicare and Medicaid Services, April 2, 2020. Available at: www.cms.gov/files/document/4220-covid-19-long-term-care-facility-guidance.pdf. Accessed April 27, 2021.

Cheng P: Supporting frontline health care professionals: lessons from Wuhan experience. Psychiatric News, April 9, 2020. Available at: psychnews.psychiatryonline.org/doi/10.1176/appi.pn.2020.4b34. Accessed June 29, 2021.

Desforges M, Le Coupanec A, Dubeau P, et al: Human coronaviruses and other respiratory viruses: underestimated opportunistic pathogens of the central nervous system? Viruses 12(1):1–28, 2019 31861926

Eveleth R: It's time for an end-of-life discussion about nursing homes. Wired, June 26, 2020. Available at: www.wired.com/story/its-time-for-an-end-of-life-discussion-about-nursing-homes. Accessed April 27, 2021.

Figueroa JF, Wadhera RK, Papanicolas I, et al: Association of nursing home ratings on health inspections, quality of care, and nurse staffing with COVID-19 cases. JAMA 324(11):1103–1105, 2020 32790822

Godfrey E: The coronavirus is especially deadly in nursing homes. The Atlantic, April 29, 2020. Available at: www.theatlantic.com/politics/archive/2020/04/coronavirus-especially-deadly-nursing-homes/610855. Accessed June 29, 2021.

Gorges RJ, Konetzka RT: Staffing levels and COVID-19 cases and outbreaks in U.S. nursing homes. J Am Geriatr Soc 68(11):2462–2466, 2020 32770832

Harrington C, Ross L, Chapman S, et al: Nurse staffing and coronavirus infections in California nursing homes. Policy Polit Nurs Pract 21(3):174–186, 2020 32635838

Kime P: COVID-19 death rate at VA nursing homes is 13 times lower than national average. Military.com, February 10, 2021. Available at: www.military.com/daily-news/2021/02/10/covid-19-death-rate-va-nursing-homes-13-times-lower-national-average.html. Accessed June 29, 2021.

Mao L, Jin H, Wang M, et al: Neurologic manifestations of hospitalized patients with coronavirus disease 2019 in Wuhan, China. JAMA Neurol 77(6):683–690, 2020 32275288

Mor V, Gutman R, Yang X, et al: Short-term impact of nursing home SARS-CoV-2 vaccinations on new infections, hospitalizations, and deaths. J Am Geriatr Soc Apr 16, 2021 33861873 Epub ahead of print

Morganstein J: Coronavirus and mental health: taking care of ourselves during infectious disease outbreaks. American Psychiatric Association, February 19, 2020. Available at: www.psychiatry.org/news-room/apa-blogs/apa-blog/2020/02/coronavirus-and-mental-health-taking-care-of-ourselves-during-infectious-disease-outbreaks. Accessed April 27, 2021.

National Academies of Sciences, Engineering, and Medicine: Social Isolation and Loneliness in Older Adults: Opportunities for the Health Care System. Washington, DC, National Academies Press, 2020

Paulin E: How to track COVID-19 nursing home cases and deaths in your state. What states are reporting and how to find it. Washington, DC, AARP, June 11, 2020. Available at: www.aarp.org/caregiving/health/info-2020/coronavirus-nursing-home-cases-deaths.html. Accessed April 27, 2021.

Psevdos G, Papamanoli A, Barrett N, et al: Halting a SARS-CoV-2 outbreak in a US Veterans Affairs nursing home. Am J Infect Control 49(1):115–119, 2021 33157181

Rogers JP, Chesney E, Oliver D, et al: Psychiatric and neuropsychiatric presentations associated with severe coronavirus infections: a systematic review and meta-analysis with comparison to the COVID-19 pandemic. Lancet Psychiatry 7(7):611–627, 2020 32437679

Rudolph JL, Hartronft S, McConeghy K, et al: Proportion of SARS-CoV-2 positive tests and vaccination in Veterans Affairs Community Living Centers. J Am Geriatr Soc Apr 16, 2021 33861871 Epub ahead of print

Spotswood S: VA touts lower CLC COVID-19 rates vs. community nursing homes. U.S. Medicine, July 9, 2020. Available at: www.usmedicine.com/late-breaking-news/va-touts-lower-clc-covid-19-rates-vs-community-nursing-homes. Accessed April 15, 2021.

Taquet M, Geddes JR, Husain M, et al: 6-month neurological and psychiatric outcomes in 236 379 survivors of COVID-19: a retrospective cohort study using electronic health records. Lancet Psychiatry 8(5):416–427, 2021 33836148

Travers JL, Schroeder K, Norful AA, et al: The influence of empowered work environments on the psychological experiences of nursing assistants during COVID-19: a qualitative study. BMC Nurs 19:98, 2020 33082713

True S, Ochieng N, Cubanski J, et al: Under the radar: states vary in regulating and reporting COVID-19 in assisted living facilities. KFF, June 16, 2020. Available at: www.kff.org/coronavirus-covid-19/issue-brief/under-the-radar-states-vary-in-regulating-and-reporting-covid-19-in-assisted-living-facilities/. Accessed April 27, 2021.

Varatharaj A, Thomas N, Ellul MA, et al: Neurological and neuropsychiatric complications of COVID-19 in 153 patients: a UK-wide surveillance study. Lancet Psychiatry 7(10):875–882, 2020 32593341

World Health Organization: Mental health and psychosocial considerations during the COVID-19 outbreak. Geneva, World Health Organization, March 18, 2020. Available at: www.who.int/docs/default-source/coronaviruse/mental-health-considerations.pdf?sfvrsn=6d3578af_10. Accessed April 27, 2021.

Wu Y, Xu X, Chen Z, et al: Nervous system involvement after infection with COVID-19 and other coronaviruses. Brain Behav Immun 87:18–22, 2020 32240762

Zimmerman S, Bowers BJ, Cohen LW, et al: New evidence on the Green House model of nursing home care: synthesis of findings and implications for policy, practice, and research. Health Serv Res 51(suppl 1):475–496, 2016 26708381
Zimmerman S, Dumond-Stryker C, Tandan M, et al: Nontraditional small house nursing homes have fewer COVID-19 cases and death. J Am Med Dir Assoc 22(3):489–493, 2021 33516670

CHAPTER 6

DEMENTIA CARE AND THE COVID-19 PANDEMIC

Mari Umpierre, Ph.D., LCSW
Shehan Chin, LMSW
Karla Steinberg, LMSW
Micheline Dugué, M.D.

About 5.8 million adults in the United States live with dementia. Many are cared for at home by family or informal caregivers. In March 2020, when New York City became the epicenter of the coronavirus SARS-CoV-2 disease (COVID-19) pandemic in the United States, the dementia care service landscape changed dramatically in the city. In this chapter we describe how services were adapted to address the psychosocial care needs of this highly vulnerable group, highlighting the experiences of patients and providers in New York City.

Vignette

Mrs. M is a 71-year-old bilingual (Cantonese and English) Chinese woman who immigrated to the United States in the 1980s and is her husband's main caregiver. Mr. M is 78 years old and has moderate Alzheimer's disease. He was diagnosed at age 63 and remained stable for about 5 years. As his dementia progressed, his behavior and cognition deteriorated. About 7 years after Mr. M's initial diagnosis, Mrs. M noticed significant

changes in his day-to-day functioning, including behavioral disturbances, wandering, agitation, aggression, and oppositional style. At that
time he was referred to an adult day care program four times per week.
He adjusted well to the setting, and the family situation improved and
stabilized.

In March 2020, the adult day care center closed as a result of the
COVID-19 pandemic. With the routine change, Mr. M refused to take his
medication, which resulted in increased agitation, wandering, and overall confusion. To better manage the behavioral challenges and to minimize his agitation and confusion, Mrs. M tried reorganizing her daily
routine, but her husband's behavior and mood continued to deteriorate.

The situation led to a crisis call to her social worker. Together they
made a plan to address and cope with behavior changes that included a
telephone consultation with her husband's psychiatrist to review whether
his current medications should be modified. The plan also included
speaking with Mr. M in a calming voice, giving him space, using distractions, and exploring different strategies for him to accept taking his
medication regularly.

In January 2021, the approximate number of people in the United
States living with dementia was a staggering 5.8 million (www.alz.org).
Although there are many potential causes of dementia, the most common is Alzheimer's disease. Using 2010 census data, prevalence projections indicate that by the year 2050, 13.8 million adults are expected to
be living with Alzheimer's disease, although it should be noted that the
only definitive diagnosis for Alzheimer's disease is through examining
the brain postmortem (Rocca et al. 2011). One in ten adults 65 years and
older has Alzheimer's disease (Hebert et al. 2013). Among all races,
women are nearly two times more likely than men to be affected by Alzheimer's disease (Matthews et al. 2019). Per the Centers for Disease Control and Prevention (2018), the cases of Alzheimer's disease and other
dementias broken down by race are as follows:

> Among people ages 65 and older, African Americans have the highest prev-
> alence of Alzheimer's disease and related dementias (13.8 percent), fol-
> lowed by Hispanics (12.2 percent), and non-Hispanic whites (10.3 percent),
> American Indian and Alaska Natives (9.1 percent), and Asian and Pacific
> Islanders (8.4 percent).
>
> By 2060, the researchers estimate there will be 3.2 million Hispanics
> and 2.2 million African Americans with Alzheimer's disease and related
> dementias. The increases are a result of fewer people dying from other
> chronic diseases and surviving into older adulthood when the risk for
> Alzheimer's disease and related dementias increases.

As the number of dementia patients grows exponentially, so does
the need for medical and psychosocial care services to meet their needs,

the needs of their family members, and those of their informal and formal caregivers (over)burdened by caring for this population.

MEDICAL AND BEHAVIORAL COMORBIDITIES

Medical comorbidities are known to affect the course of dementia (Poblador-Plou et al. 2014) and lead to increased morbidity and mortality (Marengoni et al. 2009). Seniors with dementia have an average of four medical comorbidities compared with two in those who do not have dementia. These common comorbidities, such as hypertension and diabetes, are typically addressed in the primary care setting. Visual, orodental, and genitourinary problems can further complicate dementia (Martín-García et al. 2013). Critical medical problems such as heart failure, and now COVID-19, can overshadow the diagnosis and treatment of dementia. Seniors with dementia have half the long-term survival after hospitalization of those without dementia (Sampson et al. 2013). Seniors with dementia and COVID-19 have a 6-month mortality of 20.99% and hospitalization risks of 59.26% (Wang et al. 2021).

The cost of care for comorbidities increases in the context of dementia, with higher inpatient and skilled nursing facility utilization (Hill et al. 2002). Costs for patients with early-stage Alzheimer's disease and comorbid diseases treated with cognitive enhancers were lower than for patients not receiving therapy. Better management of advancing cognitive decline and behavioral and psychological symptoms of dementia (BPSD) could reduce the cost of care for comorbid illnesses.

BPSD are present in 90% of people with dementia (Davies et al. 2018). Agitation and aggression, along with sleep disturbance, make it difficult for them to remain home even with caregivers and are often the reason for institutionalization. Available medication management with the cognitive enhancement that has the strongest randomized clinical trial evidence includes acetylcholinesterase inhibitors (donepezil, galantamine, rivastigmine) to optimize memory and cognitive functioning (Howard et al. 2012) and N-methyl-D-aspartate receptor antagonists (memantine) to manage cognitive decline with disease progression (Grossberg et al. 2009). There are currently no FDA-approved medications for the treatment of BPSD. However, clinical trials have used several agents for symptomatic management. The American Psychiatric Association has published guidelines on the use of antipsychotics to treat agitation or psychosis in dementia (American Psychiatric Association 2016). Additional guidelines offer recommendations for depression and apathy (Rabins et al. 2017).

PATIENT-FOCUSED DEMENTIA CARE SERVICES

Specialized service programs to address patient care needs throughout the mild, moderate, and/or severe stages of the disease are designed to provide socialization and care to the patient and respite for the caregiver. Being engaged and active maximizes the dementia patient's overall well-being and may decrease the incidence of behavioral disturbances and other psychological symptoms. Thus, patient-focused dementia care services and programs are likely to be beneficial.

At the beginning of the COVID-19 pandemic, the dementia care service landscape changed dramatically. Day programs, senior centers, and many nonresidential care settings that catered to older adults for daily services essentially shut their doors. The impact was felt deeply among patients and families. Many organizations moved to an online model, but for many people with dementia the transition was not an easy one. Access to computers, tablets, and internet services is uneven among the elderly (Barbosa Neves et al. 2019; Martins Van Jaarsveld 2020).

In New York City, the epicenter of the health crisis in the early months of the pandemic, a few in-person services continued to be offered at no cost. One such program was a respite program, the COVID 19 Community Relief Program, offered by Renewal Care, a licensed home care services agency. This program offered free in-home services (companion care or home health aide) for no fewer than 60 hours total, from mid- to late May through July 1, with the possibility of continuing services either paid privately or funded through grant extension. It addressed the needs of patients in the moderate to severe stages of Alzheimer's disease.

The Riverstone program (see "Additional Resources" at the end of the chapter), a day treatment program, stopped providing traditional in-person services and transformed into a virtual program delivering care (over the telephone and/or via the online Zoom platform). Mirroring the linguistic and cultural context of the Manhattan community where the organization is located, services to patients and to their caregivers continued to be provided in English and Spanish.

New York City–based programs such as Arts & Minds (see "Additional Resources") focus on serving the individual *behind* the illness, and, like many other services, transitioned to virtual modalities. Arts & Minds participants engage in virtual museum visits with a trained museum educator who guides and enriches participants' experience of viewing the artworks. The visit concludes with an interactive discussion that fosters reflection and self-expression among patients with dementia and their caregivers. When visits are conducted in person, participants also engage in art-making activities. This component of the experience is not part of the virtual program.

In general, patients in the mild stages of neurocognitive disease are able to function independently and engage in social interactions with peers and family. For these patients, The Memory Tree has been a valuable resource, both before and during the pandemic. Designed to meet the specific needs of those navigating the mild stages of Alzheimer's disease and related dementias, it provides socialization activities, enrichment, and support. Shortly after the onset of the pandemic, The Memory Tree transitioned from in-person programs in several locations throughout the city to virtual programs and services over the phone and via Zoom.

FAMILY AND INFORMAL CAREGIVING

A diagnosis of dementia is not synonymous with global incapacity. In the early stages of the disease, patients are able to maintain autonomy and independence in their day-to-day life. Family members or loved ones may provide support, collaboration, and care as part of their routine family responsibilities. At this stage family members do not always self-identify as caregivers (Eifert et al. 2015). Caregiving tasks and responsibilities increase in complexity as the disease progresses (Adams 2006). When family caregivers are well supported (e.g., have informational, emotional, and instrumental resources), balancing the demands of the role is less taxing, leads to the provision of higher-quality family care for the dementia patient (Mayo et al. 2000), and minimizes perceptions of stress. When family caregivers lack support and resources, it is the opposite—they experience greater financial, physical, and psychosocial costs that can ultimately compromise the quality of care they are able to provide (Zarit and Whitlatch 1992).

The transition from being a loved one to embarking on the dementia caregiving career may be experienced as burdensome (Adams 2006). Caregiver burden, as defined by Zarit and colleagues (1985), is the extent to which caregivers perceive the adverse effect that caregiving has on their emotional, social, financial, and physical functioning (Zarit et al. 1985). Additionally, dementia caregivers in stressful circumstances tend to develop role overload (Savla et al. 2021), which may lead to depression and anxiety (Clyburn et al. 2000). Nevertheless, family caregivers underutilize psychosocial care and support to address their own self-care and psychological needs (Adams 2006; Wald et al. 2003). Although many caregivers perceive caregiving throughout the disease as a family duty, it can also be rewarding, reaffirm family ties, and honor the relationship between the patient and caregiver (Tarlow et al. 2004).

As would be expected during the COVID-19 pandemic, caregiving was perceived by many as stressful, taxing, and burdensome (Cohen et al. 2020). Caregivers in urban and rural settings endured the loss of formal social services and partially or completely lost informal sources of support, including help from family, friends, and/or neighbors. Social distancing disrupted everyday routines for dementia patients (Lai et al. 2020) and decreased access to services and overall support, leaving dementia caregivers at risk of experiencing role overload, loneliness, isolation (), and caregiver burden.

In cities such as New York, family members who had not lived together for decades were suddenly roommates or apartment mates again. Many parents went to live with their adult children or extended family members. In some instances, family members came to live with the patient with dementia. Some were not aware of their loved one's cognitive decline and discovered serious changes during the lockdown.

CAREGIVER-FOCUSED SERVICES DURING THE PANDEMIC

As illustrated in the vignette, many patients experienced distress, agitation, wandering, overall confusion, and behavioral challenges that negatively affected their own and their caregiver's well-being (Cohen et al. 2020; Carpinelli Mazzi et al. 2020). In Italy, Carpinelli Mazzi et al. (2020) explored the effects of COVID-19 lockdown measures on the psychological outcomes of dementia caregivers and found that the disruptions caused by stay-at-home orders negatively affected the behavior and mood of patients as well as the caregiver's overall psychological well-being. In Argentina, Cohen et al. (2020) studied caregiver stress among dementia caregivers during COVID-19 and found similar results.

The stress of having a family member with dementia to care for, with the added stressor of the family member not understanding why his or her routine had changed during the pandemic, proved a lot to deal with for many caregivers. Psychoeducation became especially important as family members now were seeing their loved ones for longer stretches of time under higher levels of stress and without the knowledge and information needed to manage their behavioral and psychological symptoms. This change was particularly difficult in New York City, where dwellings tend to be small and can feel overcrowded.

CaringKind, an Alzheimer's disease and related dementias organization focused on helping caregivers in New York City (see "Additional Resources"), maintained its multilingual support hotline for overwhelmed family members throughout the pandemic. A much-needed service provided by CaringKind before and during lockdown is Alzheimer's disease and related dementias psychoeducation training. In these classes, family members learn about the disease, what to expect as the disease progresses, and how to communicate and interact effectively with their loved one with dementia. The trainings reinforce communication (listening *and* speaking) skills and address changes in the relationship dynamics as well as how to be prepared to accept and cope with them as they emerge.

At the Icahn School of Medicine at Mount Sinai's Alzheimer's Disease Research Center located at Mount Sinai Hospital's campus, a telephonic group that was in place before the pandemic continued to meet without interruption. As in Italy and Argentina, research partners and caregivers who participated in the New York City group reported feeling more strained, underserved, and isolated from friends and family members. During group sessions, they shared challenging experiences accessing basic needs and supplies such as food and medicines, toiletries, and products to prevent contamination (hand sanitizers and wipes) due to overall shortages in the city. Most group members were among those at the highest risk of getting the most severe forms of the disease (older than age 65 years), and all reported feeling very concerned for themselves and for their loved ones with dementia.

As the COVID-19 health crisis intensified in the city, the group provided space and time for members to share concerns, obtain support, and receive concrete advice. During the pandemic, videoconferencing technology became available at no additional cost, making it feasible to change the telephonic group to a Zoom video group. All participants were receptive to the idea of videoconferencing. The transition was successful, and the group continued to meet biweekly via Zoom. Incorporating the visual component helped to deepen the emotional connections that already existed among group members who had not had the opportunity to meet in person.

A theme frequently brought up in the group was the fear of contracting the virus and what it implied for loved ones with dementia. The same topic came up during social work check-in calls conducted as part of the Research Partners Self-Care and Support Program. This grant-funded social work service program provides support, connects participants with resources, and promotes their intentional self-care. A self-care action plan, initially prepared by the social worker and caregiver or research partner, is reexamined as the needs of the caregivers change. With this in mind, during the pandemic, the social worker reached out over the phone to all program participants. Telephone check-in appointments were established to identify concrete and support needs. To help caregivers prepare for an emergency, the self-care action plan was refined and expanded during social work telephone visits. It included a list of informal support networks (e.g., family, friends, neighbors) as well as available community resources who could be called in an emergency to take over the tasks of the primary caregiver. For example, when the social worker reached out to Mrs. M, she reported feeling very stressed for two reasons: 1) her husband's behavioral disturbances had increased, and 2) she was afraid of getting COVID-19 and not being able to care for him at home. The social worker validated Mrs. M's worries and concerns, provided support, and updated Mrs. M's self-care action plan (Table 6–1).

Research partners and caregivers who participated in telephone check-in sessions delivered by the Research Partners Self-Care and Support Program's social worker presented with similar concerns and challenges. Table 6–2 contains a list of common challenges and matching recommendations.

SUMMARY AND LESSONS LEARNED

In normal times, partnerships between medical and psychosocial care providers, caregivers, and community services are essential for providing quality dementia care. During the COVID-19 pandemic, caring for patients with dementia in the community required not only strong collaborations and strategic planning but also incorporating the use of technology. From telemedicine appointments to virtual day programs and support groups for caregivers, the pandemic spearheaded a digital revolution (Cuffaro et al. 2020) that has affected not only dementia care but all areas of society. Now, more than ever, digital literacy is a requirement for managing day-to-day life.

Table 6–1. Personalized self-care action plan for caregivers/research partners

---

Caring for yourself is one of the most important things you can do as a caregiver. This form will help you to identify your self-care practices and refine and enrich what you are already doing.

1. Please make a note of things you do to take care of yourself.

   I attend support groups and take walks outside as often as I can.

2. How often do you get a chance to engage in these activities?

   I participate in a support group every other week at Mount Sinai and every month at CaringKind.

   I take walks every day for 30 minutes.

3. What gets in the way?

   My responsibility to take care of my husband gets in the way, especially when he is in a bad or aggressive mood.

4. Make a note of possible solutions/strategies to overcome these challenges.

   When my husband is in a bad mood, I ask my son to watch him for 30 minutes so he gets distracted and I take time to destress.

   Getting my husband distracted is one way of helping him to change his mood. He is receptive to watching TV.

   I disregard what he says to me because I remember that it is his disease speaking.

   If I have to engage with him, I try changing the subject.

5. Who is or could be your "self-care buddy," someone who reminds you to take time for yourself? You may select more than one person.

   I have two very good friends who encourage me to take time for myself. We are in touch regularly. They remind me to take care of myself.

6. Take a moment to reflect on your family/social support network; make a note of who comes to mind.

   My eldest son who lives in the basement of my home will be able to help take care of my husband if I get sick with COVID-19.

   My sister-in-law calls me on the phone, and we talk; this helps me emotionally. She can't come over to help me out. We used to go grocery shopping together. I enjoyed doing this with her before the pandemic. I miss going out with her.

7. Often caregivers feel that they do not have the resources they need to take care of their loved ones. What resources/services do you already have to support you in your role?

   I used to have help at home, a private pay home health aide, but I am worried about getting infected, and I asked her not to come in for now.

Table 6–1. Personalized self-care action plan for caregivers/research partners *(continued)*

I participate in the biweekly Alzheimer's Disease Research Center research partners/caregiver group and in the CaringKind monthly group.

8. What resources/services do you need?

I need help with my husband's agitation and behavior changes.

I need help finding recreational activities for my husband, to keep him occupied.

In case I cannot go out to the grocery store, I need to find food delivery.

9. Do you have a plan to obtain them? Let us review it and refine the plan together.

Contact my husband's psychiatrist to let her know that he has become more aggressive and agitated since he does not attend the day program. Ask her to review his medication in case she can add something to help decrease his agitation.

Get in touch with the day program and see what activities they are providing to patients during the pandemic.

Help my husband participate in the virtual day program activities.

Locate and use Chinese grocery delivery services and get in touch with New York City's Grab-and-Go meals.

Keep connected with New York City's vaccine rollout news.

Access to the hardware, software, and broadband services needed for all to benefit from technology equally is a challenge on micro, mezzo, and macro levels. However, using a personalized approach, clinicians, including geriatric psychiatrists, can incorporate brief assessments of their patient's (and their patient's caregiver's) access to and comfort with the use of technology. This information can inform the preparation of treatment and care plans. Furthermore, clinicians should familiarize themselves with digital literacy capacity–building services (e.g., Senior Planet). Clinicians can recommend participation in these programs not only for patients in the early and mild stages of the disease but also for their caregivers.

Discussing digital literacy skill building will help to open conversations with caregivers about their intentional self-care. Supporting caregivers is an essential component of dementia care. With countless of in-person and Web-based programs devoted to supporting caregivers in real time and/ or on demand, strongly recommending participation in these programs can help reduce psychological burden and isolation for the caregiver, improving overall quality of life for all. Dementia services research participation can also be offered as another component of self-care for family members, as illustrated earlier, although direct benefit cannot be prom-

Table 6–2. Recommendations and actions in response to caregiver challenges

Challenge	Recommendations and actions
Fear of what will happen to a loved one if the caregiver gets sick with COVID-19	Prepare a backup plan incorporating members of the family and community resources who can take on primary caregiving responsibilities. Encourage the caregiver to actively prepare a backup plan, discussing it with family members and friends. Refer the caregiver to PSS Circle of Care for assistance with overall geriatric care management needs.
Difficulties shopping for food and necessities	Refer to Meals on Wheels.
Difficulties understanding and implementing COVID-19 prevention practices due to confusing public health messaging	Clarify Centers for Disease Control and Prevention social distancing rules and recommendations to prevent community spread and discuss ways to help the patient comply with them.
Feeling disconnected and isolated due to social distancing	Clarify the difference between social distance and physical distance. Highlight the importance of social connections and encourage the caregiver to reach out to loved ones using phone/video/mail. Create a list of people for the caregiver to stay in touch with, with the plan being to talk to at least one person from the list each day. Make a plan to check in with the caregiver every other week.
Decrease in home care hours or discontinued care	Promote self-advocacy skills and provide concrete recommendations to alleviate role overload (e.g., scheduling respite time, incorporating relaxation exercises, refining time management skills).

Table 6-2. Recommendations and actions in response to caregiver challenges *(continued)*

Challenge	Recommendations and actions
Cessation of caregiver in-person support groups	Extend invitation to join virtual or telephonic support group. Provide one-on-one social work check-ins frequently.
Temporary cessation of individual psychotherapy sessions in person combined with a transition to telehealth not being feasible for a variety of reasons, including lack of privacy in the home and discomfort with use of technology	Increase the frequency of check-ins, with calls scheduled at the caregiver's convenience for brief (15-minute) conversations. Encourage digital literacy skill building and discuss with psychotherapists the need to schedule sessions at more convenient times.
Cessation of adult day care services	Recommend virtual programs for the patient with dementia, including Alzheimer's Foundation of America Teal Room, as well as caregiver-focused services, including chair yoga provided free of charge by the same organization. Increase frequency of check-in calls to provide emotional support. Encourage connecting with adult day care centers and participating in virtual services delivered on a modified schedule.
Digital literacy knowledge gaps	Introduce the caregiver to Senior Planet and AARP.

ised form research participation. Dementia research participation can be offered as an opportunity for patients and their family caregivers to obtain support and indirect opportunities to optimize their quality of life. For example, in a qualitative study conducted by Connell et al. (2001) about caregivers' attitudes toward their family member's participation in Alzheimer's disease research, a significant finding was that all caregivers expressed a high degree of satisfaction with the social interactions, contact, and support they received from research and clinical staff. Furthermore, Connell and colleagues (2001) reported that caregivers expressed feeling that they were "not alone and had somewhere to turn for help." Physicians and especially geriatric psychiatrists are in an excellent position to educate families on the opportunities that research participation may bring for them.

Although digital technology is part of our day-to-day life, a digital divide still exists, especially in rural communities. As the COVID-19 pandemic continues, patients and families without adequate access to technology or without internet access will require traditional services, with multidisciplinary care teams adapting services and incorporating resources to deliver optimal care.

KEY POINTS

- About 5.8 million people in the United States live with dementia and, even in the moderate stages of the disease, may frequently present with behavioral disturbances.

- Because of social and physical distancing recommendations, in-person dementia care services were significantly reduced or stopped altogether during the pandemic, and as a result many persons with dementia became confused and agitated in reaction to disrupted schedules and lack of engagement. Family and informal caregivers found themselves alone and without support to care for their loved ones.

- Partnerships between medical and psychosocial care providers, caregivers, and community services are essential for providing quality dementia care in normal times. During the COVID-19 pandemic and beyond, caring for a person with dementia in the community requires strong collaborations, strategic planning, and the use of technology to meet the complex needs of this population and their family and informal caregivers.

QUESTIONS FOR REVIEW

1. When is dementia caregiving perceived as burdensome by the majority of caregivers?

    A. During the early stages of the disease
    B. During the moderate stages of the disease
    C. When they do not have the knowledge and resources to carry out their caregiving responsibilities

Answer: C.

2. Behavioral and psychological disturbances are present in what percentage of dementia patients?

    A. 50%
    B. 90%
    C. 20%

Answer: B.

3. Geriatric psychiatrists are in a unique position to do which of the following?

    A. Engage patients and their caregivers in conversations about participation in dementia research and the opportunities that it may bring.
    B. Explore dementia caregivers' access to and comfort with digital technology and use this information to inform the design of dementia patients' treatment plans.
    C. Both A and B

Answer: C.

ADDITIONAL RESOURCES

Alzconnected (free online caregiver community funded by the Alzheimer's Association): www.alzconnected.org/?_ga=2.44445412.1924198137.1572459148-779403807.1569860036

Alzheimer's Association: 1-800-272-3900, www.alz.org

Alzheimer's Foundation of America caregiving resources: https://alzfdn.org/caregiving-resource

Alzheimer's Foundation of America Teal Room: https://alzfdn.org/afa tealroom

American Psychiatric Association: The American Psychiatric Association Practice Guideline on the Use of Antipsychotics to Treat Agitation or Psychosis in Patients With Dementia. Available at: https://doi.org/10.1176/appi.books.9780890426807.

Arts & Minds: https://artsandminds.org/programs

CaringKind (information, resources, direct service to patients and to their caregivers): www.caringkindnyc.org/aboutus

Cyberseniors.com (free technology assistance for seniors): www.youtube.com/watch?v=bemDf6wuHJ0

Family Caregiver Alliance caregiver webinars, capacity-building resource: www.caregiver.org/fca-webinars

Meals on Wheels: www.mealsonwheelsamerica.org/find-meals

The Memory Tree: www.thememorytree.org

National Institute on Aging: Alzheimer's Caregiving: Caring for Yourself: www.nia.nih.gov/health/alzheimers-caregiving-caring-yourself

New York City Grab-and-Go-Meals: www.schools.nyc.gov/school-life/ food/community-meals

Papa (college students trained to be social buddies and helpers for older adults): www.joinpapa.com, www.youtube.com/watch?v=9OVyD9 InLdw

Rabins PV, Rovner, BW, Rummans, T, et al.: Practice Guideline for the Treatment of Patients With Alzheimer's Disease and Other Dementias. APA Guideline Watch, October 2014. Available at: https:// psychiatryonline.org/pb/assets/raw/sitewide/practice_guidelines/ guidelines/alzheimerwatch.pdf.

Riverstone program: www.riverstonenyc.org/memory-center-remote

Sweet Readers (young students engaging virtually in reading and other activities with patients with dementia patients): www.sweetreaders. org/about-us/people/co-founders/karen-young

REFERENCES

Adams KB: The transition to caregiving: the experience of family members embarking on the dementia caregiving career. J Gerontol Soc Work 47(3–4):3–29, 2006 17062520

American Psychiatric Association: The American Psychiatric Association Practice Guideline on the Use of Antipsychotics to Treat Agitation or Psychosis in Patients With Dementia. Arlington, VA, American Psychiatric Association, 2016

Barbosa Neves B, Franz R, Judges R, et al: Can digital technology enhance social connectedness among older adults? A feasibility study. J Appl Gerontol 38(1):49–72, 2019 29166818

Carpinelli Mazzi M, Iavarone A, Musella C, et al: Time of isolation, education and gender influence the psychological outcome during COVID-19 lockdown in caregivers of patients with dementia. Eur Geriatr Med 11(6):1095–1098, 2020 33052535

Centers for Disease Control and Prevention: U.S. burden of Alzheimer's disease, related dementias to double by 2060. Atlanta, GA, Centers for Disease Control and Prevention, 2018. Available at: www.cdc.gov/media/releases/ 2018/p0920-alzheimers-burden-double-2060.html. Accessed June 29, 2021.

Clyburn LD, Stones MJ, Hadjistavropoulos T, et al: Predicting caregiver burden and depression in Alzheimer's disease. J Gerontol B Psychol Sci Soc Sci 55(1):S2–S13, 2000 10728125

Cohen G, Russo MJ, Campos JA, et al: Living with dementia: increased level of caregiver stress in times of COVID-19. Int Psychogeriatr 32(11):1377–1381, 2020 32729446

Connell CM, Shaw BA, Holmes SB, Foster NL: Caregivers' attitudes toward their family members' participation in Alzheimer disease research: implications for recruitment and retention. Alzheimer Di Assoc Disord 15(3):137–145, 2001 11522931

Cuffaro L, Di Lorenzo F, Bonavita S, et al: Dementia care and COVID-19 pandemic: a necessary digital revolution. Neurol Sci 41(8):1977–1979, 2020 32556746

Davies SJ, Burhan AM, Kim D, et al: Sequential drug treatment algorithm for agitation and aggression in Alzheimer's and mixed dementia. J Psychopharmacol 32(5):509–523, 2018 29338602

Eifert EK, Adams R, Dudley W, et al: Family caregiver identity: a literature review. Am J Health Educ 46(6):357–367, 2015

Grossberg GT, Pejovic V, Miller ML, et al: Memantine therapy of behavioral symptoms in community-dwelling patients with moderate to severe Alzheimer's disease. Dement Geriatr Cogn Disord 27(2):164–172, 2009 19194105

Hebert LE, Weuve J, Scherr PA, et al: Alzheimer disease in the United States (2010–2050) estimated using the 2010 census. Neurology 80(19):1778–1783, 2013 23390181

Hill JW, Futterman R, Duttagupta S, et al: Alzheimer's disease and related dementias increase costs of comorbidities in managed Medicare. Neurology 58(1):62–70, 2002 11781407

Howard R, McShane R, Lindesay J, et al: Donepezil and memantine for moderate-to-severe Alzheimer's disease. N Engl J Med 366(10):893–903, 2012 22397651

Lai FHY, Yan EWH, Yu KKY, et al: The protective impact of telemedicine on persons with dementia and their caregivers during the COVID-19 pandemic. Am J Geriatr Psychiatry 28(11):1175–1184, 2020 32873496

Marengoni A, Rizzuto D, Wang HX, et al: Patterns of chronic multimorbidity in the elderly population. J Am Geriatr Soc 57(2):225–230, 2009 19207138

Martín-García S, Rodríguez-Blázquez C, Martínez-López I, et al: Comorbidity, health status, and quality of life in institutionalized older people with and without dementia. Int Psychogeriatr 25(7):1077–1084, 2013 23575107

Martins Van Jaarsveld G: The effects of COVID-19 among the elderly population: a case for closing the digital divide. Front Psychiatry 11:577427, 2020 33304283

Matthews KA, Xu W, Gaglioti AH: Racial and ethnic estimates of Alzheimer's disease and related dementias in the United States (2015–2060) in adults aged≥65 years. Alzheimers Dement 15(1):17–24, 2019 30243772

Mayo NE, Wood-Dauphinee S, Côté R, et al: There's no place like home: an evaluation of early supported discharge for stroke. Stroke 31(5):1016–1023, 2000 10797160

Poblador-Plou B, Calderón-Larrañaga A, Marta-Moreno J, et al: Comorbidity of dementia: a cross-sectional study of primary care older patients. BMC Psychiatry 14(1):84, 2014 24645776

Rabins PV, Rovner BW, Rummans T, et al: Guideline watch (October 2014): practice guideline for the treatment of patients with Alzheimer's disease and other dementias. Focus Am Psychiatr Publ 15(1):110–128, 2017 31997970

Rocca WA, Petersen RC, Knopman DS, et al: Trends in the incidence and prevalence of Alzheimer's disease, dementia, and cognitive impairment in the United States. Alzheimers Dement 7(1):80–93, 2011 21255746

Sampson EL, Leurent B, Blanchard MR, et al: Survival of people with dementia after unplanned acute hospital admission: a prospective cohort study. Int J Geriatr Psychiatry 28(10):1015–1022, 2013 23280594

Savla J, Roberto KA, Blieszner R, et al: Dementia caregiving during the "stay-at-home" phase of COVID-19 pandemic. J Gerontol B Psychol Sci Soc Sci 76(4):e241–e245, 2021 32827214

Tarlow BJ, Wisniewski SR, Belle SH, et al: Positive aspects of caregiving: contributions of the REACH project to the development of new measures for Alzheimer's caregiving. Res Aging 26(4):429–453, 2004

Wald C, Fahy M, Walker Z, Livingston G: What to tell dementia caregivers—the rule of threes. Int J Geriatr Psychiatry 18(4):313–317, 2003 12673607

Wang Q, Davis PB, Gurney ME, et al: COVID-19 and dementia: analyses of risk, disparity, and outcomes from electronic health records in the US. Alzheimers Dement Feb 9, 2021 33559975 Epub ahead of print

Zarit SH, Whitlatch CJ: Institutional placement: phases of the transition. Gerontologist 32(5):665–672, 1992 1427279

Zarit SH, Orr NK, Zarit JM: The Hidden Victims of Alzheimer's Disease: Families Under Stress. New York, New York University Press, 1985

CHAPTER 7

TELEHEALTH MODELS OF CARE FOR GERIATRIC BEHAVIORAL HEALTH DURING A PANDEMIC

Magdalena Bednarczyk, M.D.
Donald M. Hilty, M.D., M.B.A.
Shilpa Srinivasan, M.D., DFAPA, DFAAGP
Sandra Swantek, M.D., FAPA

In this chapter we provide an overview of telepsychiatry's usefulness in evaluating and treating psychiatric disorders among older adults. Although the COVID-19 pandemic led to dramatic increases in virtual modalities as a safety measure, it also demonstrated the feasibility and acceptance of use by clinicians and older adults, which will likely lead to a continuation of telepsychiatry use beyond the pandemic. We discuss the history and use of telepsychiatry, followed by a review of current models of care. We propose educational competencies supporting clinicians building a telemedicine skill set. Finally, we discuss access and policy issues amplified by economic disparities affecting access to technology.

Vignette

Mrs. S is an 81-year-old widowed woman who has been living in an assisted living facility (ALF) for 3 years. She has diabetes mellitus, diabetic peripheral neuropathy, hypertension, and major neurocognitive disorder due to Alzheimer's disease. She was referred to see a geriatric psychiatrist because of sad mood, insomnia with possible auditory hallucinations, and social withdrawal. As a result of the coronavirus SARS-CoV-2 disease (COVID-19) lockdown at the ALF, her initial psychiatric visit was virtual, and her son was able to join virtually as well.

The first appointment was fraught with multiple challenges. Technical difficulties occurred, and the absence of tech-knowledgeable staff readily available for troubleshooting led to an inadequate examination and early termination of the visit. Improved coordination with ALF staff led to several mitigation strategies, including using a fully charged tablet for the encounter (with a backup charger nearby just in case), providing a tablet stand to the patient for ease of use, and having an office setup free of visual obstructions. As additional insurance, the facility staff and the psychiatrist exchanged telephone contact information for addressing technical problems. Further, the ALF staff member, wearing a mask, was present and assisted with various physical aspects of the examination of Mrs. S, who was also wearing a mask. This visit proceeded smoothly, and the assessment was completed. Treatment recommendations were given and discussed with the patient, her son, and the ALF staff.

OVERVIEW OF TELEMEDICINE AND TELEPSYCHIATRY

Telepsychiatry, the use of technology to deliver psychiatric care at a distance, expands access for many patients, enhances patient-physician collaboration, improves health outcomes, and reduces medical costs (Chen et al. 2020). Although used interchangeably, the terms *telehealth* and *telemedicine* are not synonymous. Telehealth delivers a wide range of medical care, public health services, and education. Telemedicine focuses on exchanging medical information, diagnosis, and treatment (Office of the National Coordinator for Health Information Technology, www.healthit.gov). For our purposes, we use *telepsychiatry* and *telemedicine* interchangeably.

Telepsychiatry was first used at the Nebraska Psychiatric Institute in 1959, but a lack of evidence supporting efficacy slowed its expansion. Decades of research culminated in 2010 with the first publication of evidence-based practice guidelines (Yellowlees et al. 2010). Concerns about privacy, safety, technology limitations, reimbursement, regulatory credentialing, and education remained barriers to widespread acceptance (Bashshur and Shannon 2009).

Since then, the evidence base has grown. Patients and caregivers report satisfaction with telemedicine equal to that of in-person visits (Bishop et al. 2002; Parikh et al. 2013). Allied health professionals report high satisfaction with technology that improves access to psychiatric services. Psychiatrists have used telepsychiatry to successfully treat late-life depression, anxiety, dementia, and cognitive impairment in settings including patient homes, long-term care, inpatient facilities, outpatient facilities, and primary care (Gould and Hantke 2020; Hilty et al. 2013).

Prepandemic, 80% of all primary care telemedicine visits included mental health topics (Mehrotra et al. 2016). Meanwhile, mental health clinicians used telepsychiatry in only 1% of their encounters (Mehrotra et al. 2016). Centers for Medicare and Medicaid Services (CMS) regulations limited older adults' access to telepsychiatry in underserved rural and geographic regions (Centers for Medicare and Medicaid Services 2018).

In the decade before the COVID-19 pandemic, adults older than age 65 increasingly used the internet. Nearly two-thirds of older adults had home internet access or smartphones by 2019, which was still less than the 90% of all U.S. adults online by 2016 (Anderson and Perrin 2017; Pew Research Center 2021). Adults 80 years and older accessed telepsychiatry less often than did their younger counterparts. Compared with peers, older adults unable to make a video visit were more likely 85 years or older, male, unmarried persons of color residing in a nonmetropolitan area, with less education, lower income, and poorer self-reported health (Lam et al. 2020). About 12% of older adults using smartphones for internet access were more likely to be lower-income racial and ethnic minorities with less than a college degree (Lam et al. 2020). As age increases, internet use decreases (Swantek and Bednarczyk 2020). Whether this relation between age and internet use changes as more technology-savvy elders reach their eighth decade remains to be seen (Pew Research Center 2021). Rural elderly face additional barriers due to the lack of infrastructure needed for high-speed internet and broadband access (Tomer et al. 2020).

Telepsychiatry Expansion

Successful telepsychiatry use depends on specific variables: internet or smartphone access and technology literacy, which depends on age, education, income level, race or ethnicity, and geographic location. As the pandemic prompted stay-at-home orders, CMS lifted restrictions that previously limited telemedicine to certain rural and underserved areas. For the first time, telepsychiatry opened to all older adults living in a suburban, urban, or remote rural area.

By fall 2020, telemedicine use rapidly increased in ambulatory organizations, even as it varied across organizations and medical specialties
(Mehrotra et al. 2020). Telemedicine use increased in larger organizations, and its use in behavioral health grew, accounting for 41% of visits
(Busch et al. 2021). Age-related differences in telepsychiatry access
emerged: Younger elders familiar with smartphones and internet access
quickly adjusted to telemedicine, but adults 80 years and older struggled with multiple barriers. Clinicians relied on telephone visits for
these oldest and most vulnerable elders. An estimated 30% of telemedicine visits were audio only during the pandemic, prompting debate
over the continued reimbursement of audio-only visits after the crisis
(Uscher-Pines et al. 2021).

Statistics reported by federally qualified health centers (FQHCs)
document the magnitude and speed of telemedicine adoption. FQHCs
are outpatient health centers providing comprehensive primary care to
30 million low-income individuals, including low-income older adults
(Uscher-Pines et al. 2021). Prepandemic, FQHCs made minimal use of
behavioral health telemedicine. In March 2020, FQHCs substituted in-
person visits with telephone and video visits. There were 6.6 in-person,
18.2 telephone, and 4.0 video behavioral health visits per 1,000 patients
per month during the pandemic period, with 22.8% occurring in person, 63.3% via telephone, and 13.9% via video. Telephone visits peaked
in April 2020, comprising 71.6% of behavioral health visits (Uscher-
Pines et al. 2021). Similarly, by November 2020, the Department of Veterans Affairs reported a 1,653% increase in weekly video visits since the
beginning of the pandemic, peaking at more than 41,000 visits in a single day, of which nearly 25% were for mental health (Ferguson et al.
2021). During this time, 77.5% of veterans and almost 35% of the mental
health providers were first-time users of telemedicine video modalities
(Ferguson et al. 2021).

Telepsychiatry Requirements

Successful telemedicine use requires that patients and clinicians have
access to the internet; the skills to operate and troubleshoot equipment;
and the ability to communicate without the cues available in person.
These factors can vary dramatically depending on the individual's age,
education, income level, race or ethnicity, and geographic location.

In 2018, an estimated 38% (13 million) of all U.S. older adults could not
access a video visit (Lam et al. 2020). Only 6% (approximately 2.8 million) had a support person to help make the connection (Lam et al.
2020). Audio-only visits suffice for some older adults; however, hearing,

communication, or cognitive deficits are potential barriers for approximately 20% of older adults (Lam et al. 2020).

Robust evidence supports the use of telemedicine for older adults in many settings of care and with several psychiatric conditions, including nursing home consultation on, screening for, and diagnosis of cognitive disorders; community care for cognitive disorders; treatment of depression in integrated and collaborative care models; and psychotherapy (Choi et al. 2020; Gentry et al. 2019; Sheeran et al. 2013). As the vignette illustrated, challenges occur in assessments done by video and even more during an audio-only session. Challenges diminish with effective coordination, technological support, and collateral informants. As noted in the previous subsection, CMS temporarily eased licensing requirements during the pandemic. Whether these changes persist postpandemic remains to be seen. As a result, clinicians would benefit from understanding state practice and licensing regulations (CMS, Medicare, and Medicaid policies).

MODELS OF CARE

Telepsychiatry challenges historical assumptions about health care delivery by creating new models of care, replacing episodic in-person interactions with more easily accessed care delivered more effectively at potentially less cost while mitigating specialist shortages (Gould and Hantke 2020; Speedie et al. 2008). Three technologies form the basis of telepsychiatry: internet interventions, video telepsychiatry, and mobile applications. Combined with in-person care, these technologies help patients, families, caregivers, and primary care providers (e.g., geriatricians) (Chan et al. 2017; Hilty et al. 2021b).

Spontaneous, Synchronous, or Asynchronous Use

On a spectrum of low to high engagement and technology requirements, older adults use website information, support and chat groups, social media, resources for self-directed assessment and care, asynchronous patient-clinician communication (i.e., mobile health app, text, or email), e-consultations within the electronic health system, video, wearable sensors, and hybrid care models combining in-person visits with technology (Chan et al. 2017; Hilty et al. 2021b). Although spontaneous technology may be valuable and enjoyable, it is helpful to consider the source used (e.g., internet, social media, e-consultation, video), the user's goal or aim, and liabilities and approaches to make it meaningful and prudent. For example, easy-to-use options such as chat rooms and social media may vary in quality but offer a positive form of support for a patient, spouse, or caregiver. However, more meaningful change may require an in-depth evaluation and clinical relationship via video.

Effective Clinical Care and Health Care System Workflow

Technology may change the nature of interaction for participants and communication related to information exchange, clarity, responsiveness, and comfort (Hilty et al. 2021b). The goal of technology is to simulate real-time experiences related to feelings, perception, images, and interaction. Even low-cost telepsychiatry video systems facilitate engagement and a social presence for participants sharing a virtual space, getting to know one another, and discussing complex issues.

Creating the Synchronous Therapeutic Environment

Ultimately, the goal via any modality is to create an environment that facilitates therapeutic engagement and emotional well-being for all parties (Maheu et al. 2019). The patient's requests, needs, and preferences are the clinician's priority. *Telemedicine encounters should prioritize the longitudinal relationship between the patient and the treating health care professional. An established patient-clinician relationship diminishes concerns for inappropriate prescribing and lessens diversion risk while allowing prescribing of controlled substances via telemedicine.* Although video is well accepted, reflection can help determine whether another technology (e.g., email, text) is helpful and suitable (Hilty et al. 2021b; Maheu et al. 2019). As care changes with the addition of new technology (telephone, text messaging, app), the clinician must attend to the legal and ethical mandates surrounding the therapeutic relationship (e.g., privacy, dealing with emergencies).

Shifting Care to Asynchronous Technologies

Clinical care in person, by video, and by asynchronous technologies share things in common, but there are differences as well (Hilty et al. 2020a; Zalpuri et al. 2018). One shift is moving from structural (e.g., office visit) to functional in-time clinical care, which may affect the *therapeutic frame, communication, boundaries, and trust* (Hilty et al. 2020b). As an asynchronous technology, electronic health records (EHRs) give the health care team access to clinical notes, treatment plans, medication lists, patient medical images, and data. Although EHRs are efficient, without a physical examination, the clinician relying on EHRs accepts the inherent risk of input error guiding clinical decisions. Correspondence via technology outside the office visit creates a new sense of continuity, connection, and ease of communication that once was impossible (Hilty et al. 2020b). Another shift is in-time data collection with wearables and sensors—for heart rate, steps or activity, and other parameters in older adults—yielding more valid, reliable, and meaningful data to aid clinician decision-making (Hilty et al. 2021a). Although older adults are included infrequently in tests of wearable or interactive applications,. evidence-informed applications hold promise (Gould and Hantke 2020).

TELEMEDICINE COMPETENCIES AND ASYNCHRONOUS TECHNOLOGY COMPETENCIES

Health care reformers suggested information technology competencies in 2003 (Institute of Medicine 1996). Competency-based education focuses on clinical skill development in addition to knowledge acquisition. Competencies dovetail with lifelong learning as a part of ongoing practice, but clinicians strive for quality care for many other reasons. Clinical experience, propelled forward by COVID-19, appears to predict interest and concern level. Conservatively, clinical experience of perhaps 1–5 hours is needed to debunk preliminary questions and concerns, and a dose of 6–10 hours or more is required to gain skills (Cruz et al. 2021).

Competencies exist for video adult care (Hilty et al. 2015; Maheu et al. 2019), social media (Zalpuri et al. 2018), mobile health (Hilty et al. 2020a), wearable sensor (Hilty et al. 2021a), and asynchronous (Hilty et al. 2021b) technologies. To date, no specific telecompetencies exist for children, adolescents, families, or older adults, although these technologies have been embraced for older veterans (Armstrong et al. 2018).

Competencies for video and other technologies are organized into the six domains of the Accreditation Council for Graduate Medical Education (2017): patient care, medical knowledge, systems-based practice, professionalism, practice-based learning and improvement, and interpersonal and communication skills (Table 7–1). Some studies used subdomain headings applicable across behavioral health professions (Maheu et al. 2019) and shifted content to a three-level learner system (i.e., beginner, competent/proficient, and expert; Hilty et al. 2015) from a variety of levels reported in the literature (Accreditation Council for Graduate Medical Education 2017; Dreyfus and Dreyfus 1980).

Table 7–1. Outline of geriatric telepsychiatry competencies for patient care based on the domains of the Accreditation Council for Continuing Medical Education Framework

Area and topic	Novice or advanced beginner[a]	Competent or proficient user[b]	Expert[c]
Patient care			
History taking	Obtain standard history with geriatric and medical emphases	Contextualize history related to technology (i.e., uses, preferences) Anticipate issues for older adults	Prevent and overcome obstacles to starting and flow of care
Engagement and interpersonal skills	Develop therapeutic alliance with trust and rapport	Adjust interview to technology; replace in-person gesture (e.g., handshake) with verbal one Prevent distractions and interruptions	Provide tips to maximize engagement and avoid distractions (e.g., dress, room, technology) Research best practices
Assessment and physical examination	Be thorough Stratify risk/protective factors Learn tools (e.g., MMSE)	Assess danger risk and adjust follow-up plan as well virtually as in person Ensure full MMSE alternative or administer tools with adjustments	Synthesize information Select tools contextually (e.g., MMSE, Trails A and B, other) Teach use of distance examination vs. in person
Management and treatment planning	Outline treatment plan Learn consultation vs. management roles Follow up with others (e.g., geriatrician, PCP)	Contextualize treatment plan to patient, caregiver, setting, and care continuum Decide on consultation vs. management plan (e.g., give PCP medication instructions) Engage patient, referring doctor, and other team members	Tailor recommendations to resources, culture, and patient preference; complement local services with e-services Select supplemental technologies (e.g., email, telephone) and assess impact on the process

Table 7–1. Outline of geriatric telepsychiatry competencies for patient care based on the domains of the Accreditation Council for Continuing Medical Education Framework *(continued)*

Area and topic	Novice or advanced beginner[a]	Competent or proficient user[b]	Expert[c]
Prescribing	Inquire about past medications and medical conditions Learn prescribing process manually and by computer (in-person and/or telepsychiatric care) Prescribe within skill set/scope (e.g., adult) and seek help for other populations and/or controlled substances	Request information from distant site resources to complement history Give prescriber (e.g., PCP) a few options Plan for prescribing electronically: request patient, pharmacy, and computer connection to remote site/pharmacies Anticipate likelihood for regular vs. controlled medication and check state and federal requirements; assess alternative reasonable prescribers on the basis of their roles and scope	Diagnose common "holes" in required information and teach substitution Research, evaluate, and teach on administrative barriers and solutions (e.g., state and federal best practices) Teach legal standards and management of emergencies Research the validity of exceptions or so-called workarounds Advocate for patient care within reasonable legal/regulatory standards
Documentation	Note hard copy and/or use rudimentary EHR	Take advantage of EHR, with attention to informed consent, preferences, goals for technology, problems, and privacy	Teach standards and additional necessary information and model documentation for TP
Privacy and confidentiality	Learn in-person basic regulations	Use TP regulations and, if none, apply judgment to convert in-person ones Inform patients of common errors (e.g., mobile phone privacy limitations)	Practice within all standards and evolving telepractice movements to make recommendations to others on parameters

Table 7–1. Outline of geriatric telepsychiatry competencies for patient care based on the domains of the Accreditation Council for Continuing Medical Education Framework *(continued)*

Area and topic	Novice or advanced beginner[a]	Competent or proficient user[b]	Expert[c]
Communication			
Communication skills	Communicate clearly with patient and professionals	Amplify presence via communication (15% of appointment time): lean forward, use gestures and digital drawings, and show websites	Build technical workflow to enable devices for interaction and optimize participants' telepresence
Cultural diversity and social determinants	Consider participants' needs and preferences	Adjust to patient culture/preferences for therapeutic relationship Include caregiver and others	Teach cultural humility, formulation, and generalizations for practice
Language ability/interpreter	Use the interpreter as best as possible with supervision	Ask language preference Plan for best interpreter option (e.g., trained professionals rather than staff and family)	Consider verbal and nonverbal dimensions and teach about interpreter conflicts of interest
Systems-based practice			
Outreach to community	Participate and engage as issues arise	Identify potential resources, needs, and roles and include participants Use community-centered approach	Develop plan to assess, develop, and maintain relationships Anticipate barriers and solutions
Interprofessional education	Participate in and learn from experiences with others	Work with/lead IPE team and begin to teach within IPE framework	Problem solve with and support others Serve as resource for telemedicine data

Table 7-1. Outline of geriatric telepsychiatry competencies for patient care based on the domains of the Accreditation Council for Continuing Medical Education Framework *(continued)*

Area and topic	Novice or advanced beginner[a]	Competent or proficient user[b]	Expert[c]
Care models	Perform role assigned and grasp care provider vs. consultant role	Evaluate preliminary role vs. flexibility along a stepped continuum of roles; Adapt to collaborative, stepped care	Have facility with models of consultation and integrated, stepped, and hybrid care; Adapt practice to fit context
Rural health	Learn rural health basics related to care	Learn about rural access, epidemiology, and barriers	Teach, practice, and role model
Special populations	Adjust to a difference (e.g., medical/surgical floor, nursing home, veteran)	Recognize differences and adapt assessment and management; Adjust participants to include family members, caregivers, or nursing personnel when collecting information and adjust treatment plan	Teach and role model best practices; View population- and public health–level (e.g., underserved, culture) issues
Licensure regulations for TP and model used	Learn in-person regulations because states may differ	Be aware that in-person and TP regulations may differ and seek consultation if necessary	Research, teach, and practice within TP regulations state to state or within the federal system (e.g., veterans)

Table 7–1. Outline of geriatric telepsychiatry competencies for patient care based on the domains of the Accreditation Council for Continuing Medical Education Framework *(continued)*

Area and topic	Novice or advanced beginner[a]	Competent or proficient user[b]	Expert[c]
Professionalism			
Attitude	Learn and be open to technology Do not assume older adults do not like or will not use technology	Role model openness to technology, IPE, and care process Manage problems that arise	Apply work in human resources, business, and other fields to medicine
Integrity and ethical behavior	Demonstrate respect for others	Role model best practices when unexpected and/or untoward event occurs Maintain quality/standard of care	Teach elements of and how to build a culture related to ethical practice
Scope	Help the patient be successful and seek consultation if needed	Identify potential concerns and practice within scope(s) after assessment of pros and cons	Provide feedback on scope and boundary issues Prevent and troubleshoot problems
Practice-based learning			
Administration	Learn basics of in-person care and video care	Be aware of important differences between in-person and video care and use other technologies in care plan with purpose	Teach about practice with adjustments to video care due to clinical, legal/regulatory, and other issues

Table 7–1. Outline of geriatric telepsychiatry competencies for patient care based on the domains of the Accreditation Council for Continuing Medical Education Framework *(continued)*

Area and topic	Novice or advanced beginner[a]	Competent or proficient user[b]	Expert[c]
Safety and quality improvement	Systematically assess safety and quality of care Learn how to participate in QI processes as applicable	Identify, plan for, and manage risks Apply QI information to cases, training, and systems	Research evolving QI, medicolegal, and practice trends Adjust planning and reevaluate
Teaching and learning	Participate and contribute	Organize, contextualize, and evaluate training and identify future options	Provide context, pedagogical foundation, teaching strategies, and evaluation steps
Knowledge			
Evolution of video practice	Know relevance and history of fundamentals	Know relevance, history, and evidence base (e.g., apply guidelines)	Research evidence-based and clinical guidelines
Mobile health and other technology	Learn principles of uses in health care	Be ready to use and evaluate with purpose to achieve treatment goal	Provide practice guides, trainings, and in-time help for questions
Technology			
Adaptation to technology	Present self well with verbal and nonverbal aspects	Plan for differences, identify barriers, and put patient at ease	Identify additional ways to engage and express empathy
Remote site design	Observe	Identify problems and solutions	Preplan for iterative improvement Modify on the basis of care options

Table 7–1. Outline of geriatric telepsychiatry competencies for patient care based on the domains of the Accreditation Council for Continuing Medical Education Framework (*continued*)

Area and topic	Novice or advanced beginner[a]	Competent or proficient user[b]	Expert[c]
Technology (*continued*)			
Technology operation	Learn microphone, camera, and other basics	Operate hardware, software, and accessories and perform basic troubleshooting	Optimize components on the basis of context and manage all troubleshooting Consider clinician, plant, and other industrial psychology components

Note.   EHR = electronic health record; IPE = interprofessional education; MMSE = Mini-Mental State Examination; PCP = primary care provider; QI = quality improvement; TP = telepsychiatry.
[a]Clinician is learning clinical and technology-based skills.
[b]Clinician can apply good in-person skill to technology-based care with appreciation of context.
[c]Clinician has advanced knowledge, skill, and experience in care, research, administration, and/or policy.

For patient care history taking, a comparison of novice/advanced beginner and competent/proficient clinicians may help. A novice or advanced beginner might be fine starting the session but might not replace a handshake with other nonverbal behaviors or might not consider the omission of olfactory data (e.g., perfume, alcohol on the patient's breath). He or she might not know how to use an interpreter smoothly and efficiently at either end or by telephone. A competent or proficient clinician would open with a brief informed consent discussion and navigate from video to other technologies. A competent or proficient clinician would adjust the screen and audio during the interview, particularly if screening for movement disorders, intoxication or withdrawal, or other medical problems. A competent or proficient clinician or an expert would consider whether the technology affects the patient presentation, flow of conversation, or transference development.

Prescribing skills are a vital part of the short- and long-term treatment plan for patients when using a treatment or management model. A competent and proficient physician asks for information from the remote site before the meeting. The request includes medical history, medication, pharmacy, and other information. The clinician assesses whether the computer connects to remote sites or pharmacies and develops a plan for prescribing electronically. Clinicians concerned about substance abuse and misuse must know state and federal regulations for controlled medications. Requirements for an in-person evaluation and other matters vary by state, so clinicians may need to seek advice and document the process on a case-by-case basis (McCann et al. 2019).

REIMBURSEMENT AND POLICY

Historically, older adults confront multiple barriers to accessing health care, including lack of transportation and limited numbers of physicians accepting Medicare and Medicaid. Prepandemic, Medicare paid for telemedicine services only if the patient received the service while present in a strictly defined originating site. These medical encounters did not include reimbursed communication, counseling, management, or care coordination with nonclinical staff (Centers for Medicare and Medicaid Services 2018). Further, such uses of telemedicine, particularly audio-only health care, raise concerns for fraud, abuse, and unnecessary and lower-quality care. Although fraud is important to address, eliminating coverage for telemedicine or telephone visits would disproportionately affect underserved, elderly, and poor populations, further limiting their access to mental health care services (Uscher-Pines et al. 2021).

BEYOND THE COVID-19 PANDEMIC

As technology becomes an essential component of personal and professional life, what is needed are clearly defined policies and guidance on integrating telemedicine into the health care system. Medical societies and consumer groups are advocating for the continuation of telemedicine following the pandemic (American Medical Association 2017; Daniel et al. 2015; Krupinski and Bernard 2014; O'Connor 2020; Robeznieks 2021). The evolution of telepsychiatry care will depend on a constellation of the following variables: legislation and licensing, reimbursement, professional guidelines, health care system modifications, infrastructure, and user-friendly tools and technology.

Legislation and Professional Licensing Requirements

Before the pandemic, legal and regulatory constraints limited telemedicine implementation and wide acceptance. Although the temporary lifting of many of these hurdles allowed for broader telepsychiatry use, many of these changes could potentially influence new post-COVID-19 pandemic telemedicine regulations, including clinician licensure, prescribing, credentialing, and scopes of practice.

Reimbursement

CMS enacted changes aimed to lift previous restrictions governing the use of telemedicine during the pandemic. These changes included the following:

- Removing restrictions to the geographic location of the patient, allowing telemedicine services to be provided across state lines and in patients' homes
- Removing the requirement for established in-person patient-clinician relationships before initiation of telemedicine services
- Broadening the list of services provided by telemedicine and expanding to allow nonmedical practitioners to provide patient care via telemedicine encounters

- Allowing telephone evaluation and management services previously restricted to video or in-person encounters
- Eliminating frequency limitations for telemedicine encounters
- Providing Medicare reimbursement for telemedicine services, including psychotherapy, equal to that for in-person visits (Health Resources and Services Administration 2021)

Following resolution of the COVID-19 pandemic, Medicare could reverse many of the temporary changes that have allowed broad and rapid implementation and dissemination of telemedicine. Professional and consumer groups are actively engaged in discussion with policymakers regarding the future of telemedicine (Henry 2021). Successful large-scale utilization of telemedicine requires addressing these policy issues.

Professional Guidelines

Telemedicine visits should augment, not replace, in-person clinic visits. Specific criteria are needed to guide the appropriateness of telemedicine versus in-person visits and to allow the clinician to use professional judgment to determine whether a telemedicine visit is appropriate for the individualized needs of each patient (Daniel et al. 2015).

Health Care System Modifications: HIPAA-Compliant, User-Friendly Systems

Health care systems must invest in developing secure telemedicine platforms that ensure privacy and compliance with state and federal regulations, including the Health Insurance Portability and Accountability Act (HIPAA). User-friendly platforms for individuals with sensory impairment and those with limited technology literacy will improve patient access and the overall customer experience. Health systems and community-based practices should ensure that telemedicine does not increase health care access disparities for patients with low literacy or socioeconomic level or advanced age, further widening the digital poverty gap.

Infrastructure

Increased telemedicine use is possible only with universal internet access, regardless of race, socioeconomic level, or geographic location. Reduced-cost or free home broadband or mobile devices with data plans are essential to improving access. Several new funding streams and pilot programs are under way on emergency broadband benefits, COVID-19 telehealth programs, and improving broadband availability and quality data (Connolly et al. 2021; Federal Communications Commission 2021).

User-Friendly Tools and Technology

The creation of user-friendly technology for computer-naive and sensory-impaired persons will help increase the availability of these services for older adults who struggled to or could not use telemedicine services during the pandemic. Older adults can successfully meet with a mental health clinician regardless of technology naivete, sensory or cognitive impairment, or the patient or provider location. Additionally, specialty consultations from a geriatric psychiatrist in an office anywhere may now affect the care of older adults in more settings than previously possible.

SUMMARY

Expanded telemedicine access makes patient-centered, integrated care available to every older person regardless of race, ethnicity, education, socioeconomics, or geographic location. Universal internet and broadband service infrastructure, access to user-friendly technologies, and continuation of pandemic regulatory waivers for telemedicine would positively change older adults' lives and mental health regardless of their rural, suburban, or urban location. Addressing legal and regulatory issues limiting expanded access would remove additional barriers, as would instituting equitable reimbursement regardless of the location of the patient or clinician or whether the technology included video or used only audio. Research evaluating the successes; remaining barriers and challenges; and safety, training, and personnel needs would allow for ongoing refinement of telepsychiatry across the health care delivery landscape after the pandemic and beyond. As we look to the end of the pandemic, we enter a time of posttraumatic growth, a time of cultural adaptation and change responding to the inequities laid bare during the pandemic. It is the least that we can do in honor of the lives lost across the country.

KEY POINTS

- With adequate preparation and support, older adults can use and benefit from telepsychiatry.

- A previsit assessment can identify the chief concern and patient and staff attitudes toward telepsychiatry, along with physical considerations (e.g., sensory function, gait, balance, extrapyramidal symptoms).

- Whether the visit is the first or there are other considerations, a clinical exam may require staff assistance, particularly if the patient is cognitively impaired, delirious, combative, or sensory impaired.

- To conduct an adequate physical exam, a device that allows viewing the patient from wide-angle, close-up, and focused views allows assessment for various clinical concerns, including the presence of movement disorder or fall risk.

- Virtual visits can facilitate the inclusion of caregivers and family members. Inclusion allows the psychiatrist to observe the caregiver-patient interactions and collect collateral information.

- Ongoing clinical experience, teaching, and professional development facilitate telepsychiatry skills and attitudes, ensuring a high quality of care and improved outcomes.

QUESTIONS FOR REVIEW

1. Quality of care and good outcomes in telepsychiatry depend on which of the following?

    A. Patient access to technology
    B. Patient attitudes
    C. CMS approval of telepsychiatry
    D. HIPAA-compliant technology
    E. Clinical experience and professional development

Answer: E.

2. There is evidence supporting the use of telepsychiatry for which of the following?

    A. Palliative care
    B. Treatment of cognitive disorders
    C. Nursing home consultation
    D. Treatment of anxiety
    E. B, C, and D

Answer: E.

3. Older adults' successful telemedicine use depends on which of the following?

    A. Residence in a CMS-approved underserved area
    B. Ownership of a flip phone
    C. Neighbors
    D. Technology literacy
    E. The geriatric psychiatrist's knowledge of technology

Answer: D.

ADDITIONAL RESOURCES

American Psychiatric Association: Telepsychiatry toolkit. Washington, DC, American Psychiatric Association, 2021. Available at: www.psychiatry.org/psychiatrists/practice/telepsychiatry/toolkit. Accessed July 1, 2021.

American Telemedicine Association: Practice Guidelines for Video-Based Online Mental Health Services. Arlington, VA, American Telemedicine Association, August 13, 2009. Available at: www.americantelemed.org/resources/practice-guidelines-for-video-based-online-mental-health-services-2. Accessed July 1, 2021.

APA Committee on Telepsychiatry and APA College Mental Health Caucus: College Mental Health, Telepsychiatry: Best Practices, Policy Considerations and COVID-19. Washington, DC, American Psychiatric Association, August 2020. Available at: www.psychiatry.org/File%20Library/Psychiatrists/Practice/Telepsychiatry/APA-College-Mental-Health-Telepsychiatry-COVID-19.pdf. Accessed July 1, 2021.

Grady B, Myers KM, Nelson EL, et al: Evidence-based practice for telemental health. Telemed J E Health 17(2):131–148, 2011 21385026

Myers K, Cain S, Work Group on Quality Issues, et al: Practice parameter for telepsychiatry with children and adolescents. J Am Acad Child Adolesc Psychiatry 47(12):1468–1483, 2008 19034191

Shore JH, Yellowlees P, Caudill R, et al: Best practices in videoconferencing-based telemental health April 2018. Telemed J E Health 24(11):827–832, 2018 30358514

Parekh R: Geriatric Considerations in Telepsychiatry. Washington, DC, American Psychiatric Association, 2021. Available at: www.psychiatry.org/psychiatrists/practice/telepsychiatry/toolkit/geriatric-telepsychiatry. Accessed July 1, 2021.

Yellowlees P, Shore JH, Roberts L, et al: Practice guidelines for video-conferencing-based telemental health—October 2009. Telemed J E Health 16(10):1074–1089, 2010 21186991

REFERENCES

Accreditation Council for Graduate Medical Education: Common program requirements. Accreditation Council for Graduate Medical Education, July 1, 2017. Available at: www.acgme.org/acgmeweb/Portals/0/PFAssets/ProgramRequirements/CPRs2013.pdf. Accessed June 30, 2021.

American Medical Association: AMA telemedicine policy. American Medical Association, 2017. Available at: www.ama-assn.org/media/22056/download. Accessed June 30, 2021.

Anderson M, Perrin A: Tech adoption climbs among older adults. Washington, DC, Pew Research Center, May 2017. Available at: www.pewresearch.org/internet/2017/05/17/tech-adoption-climbs-among-older-adults. Accessed June 30, 2021.

Armstrong C, Edwards-Stewart A, Ciulla R, et al: Department of Defense Mobile Health Practice Guide, 4th Edition. Washington, DC, Defense Health Agency Connected Health, U.S. Department of Defense, 2018

Bashshur RL, Shannon GW: History of Telemedicine Evolution, Context, and Transformation. New Rochelle, NY, Mary Ann Liebert, 2009, pp 384–390

Bishop JE, O'Reilly RL, Maddox K, et al: Client satisfaction in a feasibility study comparing face-to-face interviews with telepsychiatry. J Telemed Telecare 8(4):217–221, 2002 12217104

Busch AB, Sugarman DE, Horvitz LE, et al: Telemedicine for treating mental health and substance use disorders: reflections since the pandemic. Neuropsychopharmacology 46(6):1068–1070, 2021 33479513

Centers for Medicare and Medicaid Services: Information on Medicare telemedicine. Baltimore, MD, Centers for Medicare and Medicaid Services, November 15, 2018. Available at: www.cms.gov/About-CMS/Agency-Information/OMH/Downloads/Information-on-Medicare-Telehealth-Report.pdf. Accessed July 1, 2021.

Chan S, Godwin H, Gonzalez A, et al: Review of use and integration of mobile apps into psychiatric treatments. Curr Psychiatry Rep 19(12):96, 2017 29082425

Chen JA, Chung WJ, Young SK, et al: COVID-19 and telepsychiatry: early outpatient experiences and implications for the future. Gen Hosp Psychiatry 66:89–95, 2020 32750604

Choi NG, Marti CN, Wilson NL, et al: Effect of telehealth treatment by lay counselors vs by clinicians on depressive symptoms among older adults who are homebound: a randomized clinical trial. JAMA Netw Open 3(8):e2015648, 2020 32865577

Connolly SL, Stolzmann KL, Heyworth L, et al: Rapid increase in telemental health within the Department of Veterans Affairs during the COVID-19 pandemic. Telemed J E Health 27(4):454–458, 2021 32926664

Cruz C, Orchard K, Shoemaker EZ, et al: A survey of residents/fellows, program directors, and faculty about telepsychiatry: clinical experience, interest, views, and misconceptions. J Tech Behav Sci Feb 9, 2021 33585672 Epub ahead of print

Daniel H, Sulmasy LS, Health and Public Policy Committee of the American College of Physicians: Policy recommendations to guide the use of telemedicine in primary care settings: an American College of Physicians position paper. Ann Intern Med 163(10):787–789, 2015 26344925

Dreyfus SE, Dreyfus HL: A five-stage model of the mental activities involved in directed skill acquisition. Berkeley, University of California Operations Research Center, 1980. Available at: www.researchgate.net/publication/235125013_A_Five-Stage_Model_of_the_Mental_Activities_Involved_in_Directed_Skill_Acquisition. Accessed July 1, 2021.

Federal Communications Commission: FCC reviews progress on emergency broadband benefits, COVID-19 telehealth program, and efforts to improve broadband availability data. Federal Communications Commission, February 17, 2021. Available at: www.fcc.gov/document/fcc-reviews-emergency-broadband-telehealth-broadband-data-progress. Accessed November 10, 2021.

Ferguson JM, Jacobs J, Yefimova M, et al: Virtual care expansion in the Veterans Health Administration during the COVID-19 pandemic: clinical services and patient characteristics associated with utilization. J Am Med Inform Assoc 28(3):453–462, 2021 33125032

Gentry MT, Lapid MI, Rummans TA: Geriatric telepsychiatry: systematic review and policy considerations. Am J Geriatr Psychiatry 27(2):109–127, 2019 30416025

Gould CE, Hantke NC: Promoting technology and virtual visits to improve older adult mental health in the face of COVID-19. Am J Geriatr Psychiatry 28(8):889–890, 2020 32425468

Health Resources and Services Administration: Medicare payment policies during COVID-19. Rockville, MD, Health Resources and Services Administration, January 28, 2021. Available at: https://telehealth.hhs.gov/providers/billing-and-reimbursement/medicare-payment-policies-during-covid-19/. Accessed November 10, 2021.

Henry TA: Congress must ensure telehealth access after pandemic's over. Chicago, IL, American Medical Association, March 11, 2021. Available at: www.ama-assn.org/practice-management/digital/congress-must-ensure-telehealth-access-after-pandemic-s-over. Accessed November 10, 2021.

Hilty DM, Ferrer DC, Parish MB, et al: The effectiveness of telemental health: a 2013 review. Telemed J E Health 19(6):444–454, 2013 23697504

Hilty DM, Crawford A, Teshima J, et al: A framework for telepsychiatric training and e-health: competency-based education, evaluation and implications. Int Rev Psychiatry 27(6):569–592, 2015 26540642

Hilty DM, Chan S, Torous J, et al: A framework for competencies for the use of mobile technologies in psychiatry and medicine. JMIR Mhealth Uhealth 8(2):e12229, 2020a 32130153

Hilty DM, Randhawa K, Maheu MM, et al: A review of telepresence, virtual reality, and augmented reality applied to clinical care. J Technol Behav Sci 5:178–205, 2020b

Hilty DM, Armstrong CM, Luxton DD, et al: Sensor, wearable and remote patient monitoring competencies for clinical care and training: scoping review. J Technol Behav Sci Jan 22, 2021a 33501372 Epub ahead of print

Hilty DM, Torous J, Parish MB, et al: A literature review comparing clinicians' approaches and skills to in-person, synchronous, and asynchronous care: moving toward competencies to ensure quality care. Telemed J E Health 27(4):356–373, 2021b 32412882

Institute of Medicine: Telemedicine: A Guide to Assessing Telecommunications for Health Care. Washington, DC, National Academies Press, 1996

Krupinski EA, Bernard J: Standards and guidelines in telemedicine and telehealth. Healthcare (Basel) 2(1):74–93, 2014 27429261

Lam K, Lu AD, Shi Y, Covinsky KE: Assessing telemedicine unreadiness among older adults in the United States during the COVID-19 pandemic. JAMA Intern Med 180(10):1389–1391, 2020 32744593

Maheu M, Drude K, Hertlein K, et al: An interdisciplinary framework for tele-behavioral health competencies. J Technol Behav Sci 3(2):108–140, 2019

McCann RA, Lingam HA, Felker BL, et al: Practical and regulatory considerations of teleprescribing via CVT. Curr Psychiatry Rep 21(12):122, 2019 31741088

Mehrotra A, Jena AB, Busch AB, et al: Utilization of telemedicine among rural Medicare beneficiaries. JAMA 315(18):2015–2016, 2016 27163991

Mehrotra A, Chernew M, Linetsky D, et al: The impact of the COVID-19 pandemic on outpatient care: visits return to pre-pandemic levels, but not for all providers and patients. New York, Commonwealth Fund, May 19, 2020. Available at: www.commonwealthfund.org/publications/2020/apr/impact-covid-19-outpatient-visits. Accessed July 1, 2021.

O'Connor K: Psychiatrists continue to advocate during pandemic. Psychiatric News, August 4, 2020. Available at: https://doi.org/10.1176/appi.pn.2020.8a12. Accessed July 1, 2021.

Parikh M, Grosch MC, Graham LL, et al: Consumer acceptability of brief video-conference-based neuropsychological assessment in older individuals with and without cognitive impairment. Clin Neuropsychol 27(5):808–817, 2013 23607729

Pew Research Center: Internet/broadband fact sheet. Washington, DC, Pew Research Center, April 7, 2021. Available at: www.pewresearch.org/internet/fact-sheet/internet-broadband/#whohas-home-broadband. Accessed June 30, 2021.

Robeznieks A: Why audio-only telehealth visits must continue. Chicago, IL, American Medical Association, April 5, 2021. Available at: www.ama-assn.org/practice-management/digital/why-audio-only-telehealth-visits-must-continue. Accessed July 1, 2021.

Sheeran T, Dealy J, Rabinowitz T: Geriatric telemental health, in Telemental Health: Clinical, Technical, and Administrative Foundations for Evidence-Based Practice. Edited by Myers K, Turvey CL. New York, Elsevier, 2013, pp 171–195

Speedie SM, Ferguson AS, Sanders J, et al: Telehealth: the promise of new care delivery models. Telemed J E Health 14(9):964–967, 2008 19035808

Swantek S, Bednarczyk M: COVID-19 adds a new health care gap: internet disparity. KevinMD.com, August 9, 2020. Available at: www.kevinmd.com/blog/post-author/sandra-swantek-and-magdalena-bednar. Accessed July 1, 2021.

Tomer A, Fishbane L, Siefer A, et al: How broadband can deliver health and equity to all communities. Washington, DC, Metropolitan Policy Program at Brookings, Brookings Institute, 2020. Available at: www.brookings.edu/wp-content/uploads/2020/02/20200227_BrookingsMetro_Digital-Prosperity-Report-final.pdf. Accessed June 30, 2021.

Uscher-Pines L, Sousa J, Jones M, et al: Telehealth use among safety-net organizations in California during the COVID-19 pandemic. JAMA 325(11):1106–1107, 2021 33528494

Yellowlees P, Shore J, Roberts L, et al: Practice guidelines for videoconferencing-based telemental health—October 2009. Telemed J E Health 16(10):1074–1089, 2010 21186991

Zalpuri I, Liu HY, Stubbe D, et al: Social media and networking competencies for psychiatric education: skills, teaching methods, and implications. Acad Psychiatry 42(6):808–817, 2018 30284148

CHAPTER 8

MANAGING HEALTH CARE STAFF CONCERNS DURING PANDEMICS

Acute Phase and Recovery Phase

Jonathan M. DePierro, Ph.D.
Laura Bevilacqua, M.D., Ph.D.

The authors acknowledge the contributions of the Digital Discovery Team at the Hasso Plattner Institute for Digital Health at Mount Sinai; Dr. David Putrino and his colleagues at the Mount Sinai Department of Rehabilitation and Human Performance; Dr. Jonathan Ripp and his colleagues at the Office of Well-Being and Resilience; Dr. Sabina Lim, Dr. Kimberly Klipstein, and Dr. Rachel Yehuda of the Department of Psychiatry; and Dr. Mari Umpierre and colleagues at Mount Sinai Calm. The authors also acknowledge the staff and advisers at the Mount Sinai Center for Stress, Resilience, and Personal Growth, including Dr. Craig L. Katz, Dr. Adriana Feder, Dr. Deborah B. Marin, Dr. Vansh Sharma, and Rev. Dr. Zorina Costello, and all the chaplains and support staff at the Center for Spirituality and Health.

In this chapter we provide an overview of the acute and recovery phase efforts put in place to support the mental health and resilience of health care workers during and following waves of the coronavirus SARS-CoV-2 disease (COVID-19) pandemic. Health care workers, including clinical and nonclinical staff, have encountered numerous challenges responding to the pandemic. In response, health care systems employed programming to provide for basic needs, to ensure dissemination of accurate and timely information, and to address emotional well-being. We highlight several staff support efforts in North America, including at the Mount Sinai Health System (MSHS) in New York. Lessons learned from these efforts are reviewed, with an eye toward contributing to best practices for future emergencies that lean heavily on large numbers of health care workers.

Vignette

Ms. E is a 55-year-old white woman who is married and a mother of two adult sons. She has an advanced degree in nursing and has worked as a clinical nurse for 20 years, initially in the intensive care unit but most recently in administration. Ms. E presented with no prior psychiatric history, although she experienced the sudden, traumatic loss of a loved one as a teenager. In March 2020, at the beginning of the pandemic in New York, Ms. E volunteered to work on an inpatient unit converted to care for patients with COVID-19 out of an expressed sense of duty to her junior colleagues and peers. Over the course of several months, she witnessed many patient deaths per day and felt helpless in the face of a severe illness, constantly evolving treatment guidelines, the loneliness of the patients who were dying without being able to see their loved ones, and the nearly doubled clinical workload. Many of her coworkers fell ill during this time, with one requiring intensive care. During this time, one of her sons contracted COVID-19 and was hospitalized for the first time.

In early October 2020, Ms. E's son required a second hospitalization because of post-COVID-19 respiratory complications. She then started having daily panic attacks, was sleeping no more than a few hours per night, and felt extremely fatigued, paralyzed with worry that the loss she experienced earlier in life was going to repeat itself with her son. She was plagued by intrusive images of deaths she had witnessed on her COVID-19 unit and had repeated graphic nightmares in which her son died. One of her coworkers, who had attended a grand rounds where information on the Center for Stress, Resilience, and Personal Growth (CSRPG) was presented, suggested that she contact that program to get further support. Ms. E was initially reluctant to do so because of stigma around seeking mental health care but ultimately reached out to CSRPG in late October 2020.

On initial screening with a staff social worker, Ms. E scored 15 on the nine-item Patient Health Questionnaire (PHQ-9), 14 on the seven-item

General Anxiety Disorder (GAD-7) scale, and 48 on the PTSD Checklist for DSM-5 (PCL-5), well-validated self-report symptom measures directly corresponding to established psychiatric diagnostic criteria. Her scores were indicative of clinically significant depression, generalized anxiety, and PTSD symptoms, respectively. She started weekly cognitive-behavioral therapy and medication management with CSRPG providers within a time-limited treatment frame. Ms. E worked with her therapist to identify and challenge self-blaming and catastrophic thoughts; implement an array of coping strategies, including mindfulness techniques; and engage with behavioral activation to address depressive symptoms. Ms. E had persistent thoughts of being better off dead, which were addressed in part through detailed safety planning and involvement of family members in the treatment with her permission. In addition to starting an antidepressant, Ms. E's psychiatrist ordered routine bloodwork, which identified hypothyroidism and prompted a referral to an endocrinologist.

Ms. E was highly committed to treatment, and her symptoms slowly improved. By the end of her time-limited treatment in the CSRPG service, she reported no longer having panic attacks or passive suicidal ideation. Although still reporting significant PTSD symptoms, she reported a decrease in the frequency and intensity of intrusive thoughts and nightmares and improved sleep and motivation. Her discharge symptom scores were 9 on the PHQ-9, 9 on the GAD-7, and 33 on the PCL-5. Ms. E reported improvements in her daily functioning, including being able to reach out to friends and family for support and engaging more with self-care activities. She required continued care to further process the recent and remote traumas and maintain her gains and was referred on to longer-term treatment.

The COVID-19 pandemic has presented a multifront battle for health care systems in the United States and around the globe. Rapid increases in the rates of hospitalization and need for intensive and critical care services taxed the physical and personnel resources of hospitals. Voluntary procedures were stopped, outpatient services were shuttered, and sharp attention was focused on redeploying medical and support staff from their typical duties to now supporting the care of critically ill patients. Nursing homes, where residents are in close quarters and quarantining positive cases among staff and residents was logistically challenging, became "ground zeroes" for infection (Barnett and Grabowski 2020).

In the United States, as well as in other countries, there was a rush on ventilators and personal protective equipment, with many examples of creative problem solving, including ventilators designed to be shared by multiple patients and life-supporting equipment being set up outside patient rooms to minimize staff exposures. However, as these issues were addressed, an additional front in the battle opened. Health care workers were confronted with tremendous loss of life and human suffering, including loss of friends and colleagues, and worked long hours while fearing getting sick themselves or infecting family members with the virus. Because visitation was suspended, health care workers, regardless of role and across multiple care settings, helped families of the sick connect virtually to their loved ones in the last moments of life. Support staff with little to no prior exposure to human suffering were now transporting bodies to the morgue or donning layers of protective gear to clean the hospital rooms of suspected or confirmed COVID-19-positive patients.

Studies are beginning to highlight the substantial toll the initial pandemic response took on health care workers and the potential for persistent distress. In a survey of 2,579 frontline health care workers at Mount Sinai Hospital conducted in April and May 2020, 39% met criteria for at least one mental health condition, including depression (26.6%), generalized anxiety (25.0%), and PTSD (23.3%) (Feingold et al. 2021). Risk factors for screening positive for one or more of these mental health conditions included having higher levels of prepandemic burnout, and protective factors included higher levels of perceived leadership support. Qualitative interviews conducted with nurses in geriatric nursing home settings across Europe and South America supported the high toll of emotional exhaustion and fear of personal infection, alongside a sense of duty and commitment to care for particularly vulnerable individuals (Sarabia-Cobo et al. 2021). In addition to these empirical data, the highly publicized suicide of Dr. Lorna Breen, an emergency room physician in New York City, added further urgency to the development of effective services and infrastructure to support the well-being of health care workers.

With the high level of psychosocial need in mind, in this chapter we review a range of approaches to staff support during and following peaks of the COVID-19 pandemic. With a particular focus on several hospital systems in North America that published on their efforts thus far, we highlight efforts that seem to be successful regarding uptake and others that were less used, with the hope that this review will inform institutional responses to future public health emergencies.

Prior to the pandemic, health care workers faced many occupational challenges, including burnout, depression, posttraumatic stress, and concern for elevated suicide risk. These concerns have been well-characterized for physicians, leading to the recent movement for hospital systems to have chief wellness officers and specific programming to improve the workplace experience and worker well-being for trainee and professional medical staff. Existing infrastructure, such as physician wellness programs, employee assistance programs, student and trainee mental health services, and meditation and stress reduction programs provided a vital starting place for staff support efforts that were implemented during the acute phase(s) of the pandemic and beyond. In this chapter, we describe several examples of acute and recovery phase supports provided to health care workers.

Readers should note that the COVID-19 pandemic poses challenges to traditional phase-based classification of disaster response as applied to traumatic situations such as natural disasters. For example, the fact that the pandemic has come in multiple peaks has resulted in many acute phases for individuals and institutions, stymieing efforts at personal, economic, and community recovery. Thus, conventional wisdom regarding psychosocial needs and trajectories gleaned from prior disasters may only partly apply.

ACUTE PHASE

Basic Needs

As in other disaster situations, it was quickly acknowledged that first interventions in the acute phase would address basic needs, such as housing, safety, and food (Ripp et al. 2020; Shanafelt et al. 2020). Many health care workers needed alternative housing arrangements because they worked long hours and had well-founded fears of bringing the virus home to their families; further, restaurants and food stands rapidly closed as restrictions were put in place, which, paired with high work volume, limited ready access to meals. Partnering with local businesses, many hospitals organized snack tables and food deliveries for medical units and temporary housing in hotels or dormitories for staff. Free or low-cost childcare programs also emerged; these programs became essential as schools moved to virtual instruction, but as the pandemic continued, they were often overrun by demand.

Provision of Information

On a related note, staff having access to clear information from institutional leadership has been advanced as a key driver of resilience in the face of trauma (Ripp et al. 2020). At MSHS, leadership held frequent town halls to hear staff concerns, relay information, and field questions and rounded daily on medical units. At Mount Sinai, the Office of Well-Being and Resilience organized a 24/7 resource navigation phone line, drawing on a database of continually updated internal and external resources organized by domain (e.g., housing, mental health, family supports). Further, the Office of Well-Being and Resilience assembled a single web page and a corresponding flyer for health care workers that summarized existing supports, including a brief description and contact information. Clinicians at NYU Langone Hospital have described a similar approach to increasing accessibility to information with single-page infographics (Spray et al. 2020). This consolidation of resources was essential because large health systems offer many different staff support programs, which can lead to confusion on the part of staff at times about where to get help, particularly in times of high stress.

Psychosocial Support Efforts

At MSHS, services were also put in place early on during the pandemic to address psychological needs. Staff faced exhaustion, mounting anxiety and worries, sadness and grief, and direct or indirect exposure to human suffering and life threat. Starting in March 2020, MSHS mobilized 129 mental health liaisons, internal mental health professionals who volunteered to staff a 24/7 crisis line and to provide virtual and in-person support to units and individual workers. Each provider completed a brief video-based training in psychological first aid and had the opportunity to attend weekly supervision and support meetings organized by leadership in the Department of Psychiatry. Mental health liaisons had 1,090 staff contacts between April and June 2020, including 973 individual and 117 group-based support meetings; only 77 calls were received on the highly staffed crisis phone line over the same period (Gray et al. 2021). Consistent with the initial findings of support group programming elsewhere (e.g., Spray et al. 2020 described NYU Langone Hospital's response), there was variable utilization of mental health liaison virtual support group services across the hardest-hit medical units at MSHS. One explanation for this finding is that each medical unit has its own culture around well-being and help-seeking. For that reason, close involvement of trusted peers from high-exposure units in future staff support efforts may increase utilization. At the same time, however, within MSHS many health care workers connected on their own with behavioral health services during the initial peaks of the pandemic, which may also suggest that workers were more comfortable disclosing distress on a 1:1 setting rather than in a group forum.

For many workers, faith and spirituality play a central role in their identities and how they cope with adversity. Even prior to the pandemic, the chaplains at MSHS rounded on units frequently, counseled staff, and offered Chi Time, a formalized service of tea, snacks, and calming sounds and aromas (Keogh et al. 2020). Perhaps it is not surprising then that hospital chaplains also provided a vital resource for staff during the acute phase at MSHS in March and April 2020. At MSHS, chaplains rounded on units frequently to provide in-person support and hosted virtual support groups, leading to a 120% increase in staff support activities from February ($n=391$) to the peak in April 2020 ($n=860$). Support from chaplains was particularly important as staff struggled with thoughts that they did not do enough to help their patients or grappled with their belief in a protective deity and a just world. Chaplain support may have worked to address the experience of moral injury, the pernicious belief that one acted in a way inconsistent with ethical or moral values (see DePierro et al. 2020b).

To the extent possible, programs were also established to foster self-care and a sense of momentary relaxation amid the suffering. For example, many hospitals converted spaces to provide socially distanced relaxation rooms for staff, with soothing experiences to promote a moment of pause and to manage stress. At MSHS, several multisensory *recharge rooms* were built through partnership between the Department of Rehabilitation and Human Performance and two private companies, Studio Elsewhere and Emergent Moments of Beauty and Connection (EMBC). Using readily available and relatively inexpensive supplies, one of these rooms was constructed in a converted laboratory space in approximately 4 hours (Putrino et al. 2020). Components of this room included a Google Home device to enable voice control of a high-definition projector, a scent diffuser, a Hue Bridge lighting system, and imitation plants. With respect to measurable outcomes, a 15-minute experience in this room was associated with significant declines in perceived stress, and these visits had high user experience ratings among 496 users. To date, several other rooms have been built in the MSHS, including in converted family waiting rooms on medical floors, leading to thousands of staff visits. Work is underway at Mount Sinai to maintain these spaces permanently.

POSTACUTE AND RECOVERY PHASE

Because the COVID-19 pandemic is still ongoing, *recovery* remains a challenging concept to describe for several reasons. Typically, acute-onset traumatic events, including collective traumas such as the attacks on September 11, 2001 (9/11) and individual traumas such as car accidents and unexpected losses, lead to initial distress followed by a period of re-adjustment and recovery over a period of months for most affected individuals. Yet this pattern of recovery is arguably contingent on the discrete nature of the event and may be complicated by prolonged or repeated traumas. In the United States, the first cases of COVID-19 emerged as early as January 2020, the first peak on the East Coast occurred in March and April 2020, and daily records continued to be set for new cases and deaths in the many months that followed. Recovery from this pandemic is further complicated by uncertainty, exhaustion, political discord, and the potential for dwindling staffing resources; thus, this process may unfold over a period of years rather than months.

Drawing on experiences from prior disasters, it is also clear that secondary stressors need to be identified and addressed in order to better prevent or mitigate ongoing distress among staff. The pandemic has posed many unforeseen stressors, including loss of income due to downsizing or furloughs, disruptions to usual childcare and eldercare, home-based virtual schooling, loss of access to recreational activities, and disruption of spiritual practices and rituals around mourning. A volunteer tutoring service was started by the Mount Sinai Calm program, part of the Human Resources Department at MSHS, to assist health care workers balancing their work responsibilities with home-based schooling for their children. This program matched 40 children to trained tutors by December 2020. In addition, Mount Sinai Calm partnered with Presbyterian Senior Services to help employees with eldercare responsibilities find geriatric care management services. Well-organized programming to address secondary stressors is likely to be needed well into 2022 and may contribute to improvements in staff quality of life and navigation of work-life balance concerns even beyond the pandemic.

It is also readily apparent that there is no uniform solution for all health care workers. We learned from research with workers who responded to the 9/11 terrorist attacks that those individuals with little or no prior disaster response experience (including nontraditional responders, such as construction and ironworkers, cleaners, and utilities workers) tended to have more mental health symptoms over time and fewer resources to draw on to facilitate their resilience than did traditional responders (e.g., firefighters, emergency medical technicians, police officers). Thus, we can use these observations to draw parallels between the experiences of these responders to 9/11 and health care support staff and ancillary workers, such as environmental and food service and security personnel (DePierro et al. 2020b). As a group, these workers are closely involved in the COVID-19 response but have not been a particular focus of attention in the literature, may have been underrecognized in acute and recovery phase efforts, and may have fewer economic resources and less access to care than their patient-facing clinical colleagues.

Given the need for a consolidated hub for staff support in the recovery phase and the many anticipated needs of staff over time, MSHS launched the CSRPG early on in the first wave of the pandemic in New York (DePierro et al. 2020a). This center is a resource for more than 40,000 workers in the MSHS, comprising a heterogeneous group of researchers, administrators, clinicians, students and trainees, support staff, and others. The center focuses on several avenues of staff support, many of which have been pursued by other institutions recovering from the acute impact of COVID-19. As with services implemented at other health care institutions (see, e.g., Spray et al. 2020), the center's efforts continue to evolve in response to the changing situation on the ground with the pandemic and stakeholder feedback. CSRPG services, as well as similar programming in other health systems, are described in further detail in the rest of this section.

Staff Education and Skills Building

An additional arm of service comprises efforts to engage and educate staff regarding mental health and resilience as in the following examples. One health care network in Toronto, Canada, implemented a resilience coaching program, drawing on medical units' established relationships with embedded consultation-liaison psychiatrists to educate on stress reactions, validate staff concerns, and teach coping skills (Rosen et al. 2020). Yale New Haven Health System providers deployed a series of psychoeducational and reflection-oriented town hall meetings (Krystal et al. 2021). At the CSRPG, resilience workshops draw on the work of Southwick and Charney (2018), who outlined 10 factors contributing to personal resilience from laboratory research and interviews with trauma survivors, including Vietnam-era prisoners of war. CSRPG drew on this foundation to develop a peer co-led resilience training curriculum and initially piloted an 11-session workshop series. They conducted 60-minute virtual training of more than 70 peer leaders and then began to offer virtual workshops to staff by July 2020. Although several cohorts showed consistent attendance and responded positively to this first version of the curriculum, it became clear that there were logistical barriers to regular staff attendance for others, including shifting staff responsibilities, well-needed time off, and childcare needs. Thus, they condensed the intervention to five meetings focusing on the following topics: 1) realistic optimism; 2) facing fears and active coping; 3) social support and utilizing resilient role models; 4) self-care; and 5) faith, meaning, and spirituality. Video content was developed around these topics, in part to facilitate engagement of staff who do not have the time to participate in person.

Mindfulness-based interventions provide an additional, sustainable avenue for staff education and self-care. MSHS has a long-standing meditation program that was converted to virtual format during the pandemic and has been a highly used service throughout the pandemic. The Mount Sinai Calm program held 458 meditation and yoga classes with 5,772 nonunique attendees between January and December 2020, moving to a virtual format in March; it also offered two 8-week training courses in mindfulness-based stress reduction. In addition, Krystal et al. (2021) and Klatt et al. (2020) described robust mindfulness-based support efforts at Yale New Haven Health System and The Ohio State University Wexner Medical Center, respectively, which built on existing programming and infrastructure. Overall, however, there remains a strong need for research into the efficacy of the full range of group-level interventions deployed in response to the pandemic.

Digital Health

Digital health tools also show promise in fostering resilience in health care workers. These tools have the benefit of being readily accessible, confidential, and self-guided and can include features such as text chat with peer supports or health coaches. The U.S. Department of Veterans Affairs National Center for PTSD published a free, publicly available app called COVID Coach early in the pandemic. This app provides self-screening tools and stress management resources and builds on the previously published and tested PTSD Coach app.

Inspired in part by COVID Coach, CSRPG, in partnership with the Digital Discovery Program of the Hasso Plattner Institute for Digital Health at Mount Sinai, developed an app called Wellness Hub (DePierro et al. 2020a). An initial version of the app for iOS was completed in June 2020, and an Android release was developed a few months later. The app includes several well-validated psychological symptom scales, including measures of depression, anxiety, and PTSD. Users can track their scores over time and receive automated feedback and behavioral suggestions. The app was designed to be anonymous by default to guard against privacy concerns. Brief videos on meditation and yoga, as well as content around symptom psychoeducation and resilience, are included for workers to engage with at their own pace. A journal feature allows for daily logging and tagging of user-directed activities that pertain to resilience. Wellness Hub will be used as a platform to push custom content to the MSHS workforce, with continued monitoring of engagement and efficacy. To facilitate distribution, MSHS employees can download the app via an institutionally maintained inward-facing web portal called Sinai Central. Research into the utilization and efficacy of this platform is ongoing.

Mental Health Treatment

Although the above interventions are likely to benefit most staff, the need for evidence-based psychotherapies to address persistent and more severe levels of psychological distress remains. Although there is a dearth of evidence with respect to health care worker samples specifically, existing treatment guidelines in the United States recommend cognitive-behavioral therapies to address PTSD in adults in general (for a review, see Watkins et al. 2018). These approaches focus on altering beliefs about the self, world, and others; reducing or eliminating avoidance behaviors; and placing traumatic situations into a broader life context in order to reestablish a sense of safety. Cognitive-behavioral therapies also have a compelling evidence base for depression and anxiety disorders, which are clearly prevalent among health care workers responding to the pandemic.

Utilization of mental health services is growing quickly among heath care workers. Within our MSHS ambulatory psychiatry clinics and faculty practices, more than 10,000 evaluation and treatment encounters with employees, partners, and dependents were completed between January and August 2020. Reflecting the acute impact of the first peak of the pandemic on staff, we observed a 99% increase in these behavioral health encounters from March to June 2020. To further support and extend these efforts, CSRPG started a time-limited treatment service in early October 2020. This service offers cognitive-behavioral and interpersonal psychotherapies, together with medication management if needed, to all MSHS employees. In collaboration with hospital leadership, CSRPG worked to eliminate out-of-pocket treatment costs for all MSHS health care workers in its treatment service, regardless of their insurance coverage, to the extent permissible by law.

Recommendations for Sustainable Staff Support

Many lessons have come out of the wide-ranging efforts to support health care workers that were developed or expanded during the pandemic. First, long-term support efforts will likely require transforming from a *reactive* to a *proactive* approach to the well-being of health care workers. Infusing resilience-focused instruction into graduate and medical student education, regular rounding by trusted mental health clinicians and chaplains on hospital units (including where ancillary and support staff congregate), developing and deploying digital mental health and wellness platforms, and training and supporting peer "well-being champions" within hospital departments are some methods that may communicate that staff wellness is a priority moving forward. Second, we would argue that institutions with chief wellness officers (e.g., the MSHS, Yale New Haven Health System, and The Ohio State University) may have been better positioned to leverage and scale up existing psychosocial support resources during the pandemic. These leaders can also champion robust multitiered infrastructure around staff support and positive workplace experience long after the pandemic is over. Thus, hospitals should consider enhancing leadership roles focused on well-being and resilience. There are also growing efforts to change the language on state board licensure and hospital credentialing forms regarding clinicians' mental health history, which may address fears providers may have that seeking mental health or substance use treatment will affect their job opportunities (Adibe 2021). Finally, although writers have advocated for countries worldwide to include mental health in their pandemic response plans (Brewin et al. 2020), the same recommendation should apply to local health care systems. Leadership at health care institutions is strongly encouraged to include a robust, scalable, and accessible road map for staff emotional support in their public health emergency and other disaster response plans.

It should also be noted that the financial costs of psychosocial support services are nontrivial. For example, hospital-based behavioral health services face an influx of both members of the surrounding community and health care workers themselves seeking care, requiring additional staffing, physical space, and hours of operation. The required expansion to meet this need is challenged by the financial losses incurred by the health care industry during the pandemic, including cancellations of revenue-generating elective procedures and mounting expenditures on pandemic-related supplies and personnel. With respect to psychosocial supports for health care workers, Krystal et al. (2021) have provided a useful breakdown of the provider staffing required for the comprehensive mental health support efforts at Yale University/Yale New Haven Health System. Over the long term, federal funding may prove essential in ensuring that psychosocial supports continue to be available for individuals affected by the COVID-19 pandemic, including, but not limited to, health care workers (Charney et al. 2020). This support is particularly necessary for settings that may lack resources and infrastructure around formalized staff support, including community hospitals and eldercare settings. A model for this kind of funding can be found in the James Zadroga 9/11 Health and Compensation Act of 2010, which provided for the perpetual health monitoring and treatment of responders to and survivors of the 9/11 terrorist attacks.

SUMMARY

Several psychosocial supports have been put in place during the acute and recovery phases of the COVID-19 pandemic to meet the needs of health care workers. The need for longer-term programming has become clear as all manner of health care service workers are facing a prolonged period of economic, physical, and emotional recovery related to the pandemic. Resilience-focused services, particularly those delivered in digital format, may bolster the long-term ability of health care workers to face personal and professional challenges, although further research is needed to gauge their efficacy. Over the long term, hospital systems, in close collaboration with state, local, and federal partners, should include provisions for staff psychosocial needs in public health emergency and other disaster response protocols.

KEY POINTS

- The COVID-19 pandemic added significant strain to health care workers and has brought about a multitiered psychosocial support approach incorporating basic needs, mental health services, education and outreach, and clear messaging.

- Evidence from one New York–based hospital system showed surges in staff utilization of mental health treatment and spiritual care services but lower than expected use of telephone-based crisis resources.

- Staff support efforts should include ancillary staff, who are often members of historically disadvantaged groups.

QUESTIONS FOR REVIEW

1. Which of the following was not one of the psychosocial resources described for staff support?

    A. Digital health platforms
    B. Psychological debriefing
    C. Recharge rooms and relaxation spaces
    D. Cognitive-behavioral therapy

Answer: B.

2. Which of the following are recommendations for health care systems preparing for future public health emergencies and other large-scale disasters?

    A. Designate a chief wellness officer.
    B. Proactively round on hospital units to increase knowledge of available services.
    C. Advocate for changes to reporting requirements around mental health on clinical credentialing documentation.
    D. All of the above

Answer: D.

3. A survey conducted at Mount Sinai Hospital in April and May 2020 asked frontline health care providers about symptoms of depression, anxiety, and posttraumatic stress. Overall, what percentage of the sample endorsed one or more of these concerns?

    A. 18%
    B. 59%
    C. 39%
    D. 73%

Answer: C.

ADDITIONAL RESOURCES

Abrams Z: As COVID-19 cases increase, so does trauma among health care providers. Washington, DC, American Psychological Association, June 1, 2020. Available at: www.apa.org/topics/covid-19/trauma-health-providers. Accessed November 3, 2021.

American Psychological Association: How leaders can maximize trust and minimize stress during the COVID-19 pandemic. Washington, DC, American Psychological Association, March 20, 2020. Available at: www.apa.org/news/apa/2020/03/covid-19-leadership. Accessed November 3, 2021.

Arnold KD, Skillings, JL: Treating front-line workers: a step-by-step guide. Washington, DC, American Psychological Association, May 1, 2020. Available at: www.apaservices.org/practice/news/front-line-workers-covid-19?_ga=2.162000575.2042225759.1604266504–300973343.1590361374. Accessed November 3, 2021.

Mount Sinai: Road to Resilience podcast. New York, Mount Sinai. Available at: www.mountsinai.org/about/newsroom/road-resilience.

Mount Sinai Health System: Five things to know about providing psychiatric care to COVID-19 health care workers. New York, Mount Sinai Health System, August 10, 2020. Available at: https://health.mountsinai.org/blog/five-things-to-know-about-providing-psychiatric-care-to-covid-19-heath-care-workers. Accessed November 3, 2021.

National Center for PTSD: COVID Coach app. Available at: www.ptsd.va.gov/appvid/mobile/COVID_coach_app.asp.

REFERENCES

Adibe B: Rethinking wellness in health care amid rising COVID-19–associated emotional distress. JAMA Health Forum, January 15, 2021. Available at: https://jamanetwork.com/journals/jama-health-forum/fullarticle/2775411. Accessed July 1, 2021.

Barnett ML, Grabowski DC: Nursing homes are ground zero for COVID-19 pandemic. JAMA Health Forum 1(3):e200369, 2020

Brewin CR, DePierro J, Pirard P, et al: Why we need to integrate mental health into pandemic planning. Perspect Public Health 140(6):309–310, 2020 33070716

Charney AW, Katz C, Southwick SM, et al: A call to protect the health care workers fighting COVID-19 in the United States. Am J Psychiatry 177(10):900–901, 2020 32731814

DePierro J, Katz CL, Marin D, et al: Mount Sinai's Center for Stress, Resilience and Personal Growth as a model for responding to the impact of COVID-19 on health care workers. Psychiatry Res 293:113426, 2020a 32861094

DePierro J, Lowe S, Katz C: Lessons learned from 9/11: mental health perspectives on the COVID-19 pandemic. Psychiatry Res 288:113024, 2020b 32315874

Feingold JH, Peccoralo L, Chan CC, et al: Psychological impact of the COVID-19 pandemic on frontline health care workers during the pandemic surge in New York City. Chronic Stress (Thousand Oaks) 5:2470547020977891, 2021 33598592

Gray M, Monti K, Katz C, et al: A "mental health PPE" model of proactive mental health support for frontline health care workers during the COVID-19 pandemic. Psychiatry Res 299:113878, 2021 33756208

Keogh M, Marin DB, Jandorf L, et al: Chi Time: expanding a novel approach for hospital employee engagement. Nurs Manage 51(4):32–38, 2020 32221126

Klatt MD, Bawa R, Gabram O, et al: Embracing change: a mindful medical center meets COVID-19. Glob Adv Health Med 9:2164956120975369, 2020 33354410

Krystal JH, Alvarado J, Ball SA, et al: Mobilizing an institutional supportive response for healthcare workers and other staff in the context of COVID-19: the Yale experience. Gen Hosp Psychiatry 68:12–18, 2021 33254081

Putrino D, Ripp J, Herrera JE, et al: Multisensory, nature-inspired recharge rooms yield short-term reductions in perceived stress among frontline healthcare workers. Front Psychol 11:560833, 2020 33329188

Rosen B, Preisman M, Hunter J, et al: Applying psychotherapeutic principles to bolster resilience among health care workers during the COVID-19 pandemic. Am J Psychother 73(4):144–148, 2020 32985915

Ripp J, Peccoralo L, Charney D: Attending to the emotional well-being of the health care workforce in a New York City health system during the COVID-19 pandemic. Acad Med 95(8):1136–1139, 2020 32282344

Sarabia-Cobo C, Pérez V, De Lorena P, et al: Experiences of geriatric nurses in nursing home settings across four countries in the face of the COVID-19 pandemic. J Adv Nurs 77(2):869–878, 2021 33150622

Shanafelt T, Ripp J, Trockel M: Understanding and addressing sources of anxiety among health care professionals during the COVID-19 pandemic. JAMA 323(21):2133–2134, 2020 32259193

Southwick SM, Charney DS: Resilience: The Science of Mastering Life's Greatest Challenges. New York, Cambridge University Press, 2018

Spray AM, Patel NA, Sood A, et al: Development of wellness programs during the COVID-19 pandemic response. Psychiatr Ann 50(7):289–294, 2020

Watkins LE, Sprang KR, Rothbaum BO: Treating PTSD: a review of evidence-based psychotherapy interventions. Front Behav Neurosci 12:258, 2018 30450043

GERIATRIC PSYCHIATRY AMONG OLDER ADULTS FROM DIVERSE BACKGROUNDS IN THE AGE OF COVID-19

Rita Hargrave, M.D., FAPA

Sharwat Jahan, M.D.

Kanya Nesbeth, M.D.

Yee Xiong, M.D.

Maria D. Llorente, M.D., FAPA

Ethnic/racial minority populations carry historical, genetic, and medical factors that increase their vulnerability to coronavirus SARS-CoV-2 disease (COVID-19) infection and mortality. These psychosocial, economic, and political factors are pivotal forces contributing to the disproportionate burden of COVID-19 on ethnic/racial minority older adult communities. The COVID-19 pandemic factors have resulted in worsening of mental well-being and increased anxiety, depression, xenophobia, and race-based traumatic stress for ethnic/racial minority communities of older adults affected by the COVID-19 pandemic.

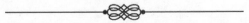

Vignette

Mr. W is a 67-year-old married African American veteran and bus driver who has presented with dyspnea, fatigue, anxiety, and body aches for the past 3 weeks, after attending a crowded memorial service for his father, who died from "breathing problems." Concerned about his potential exposure to COVID-19, Mr. W follows the Centers for Disease Control and Prevention guidelines on social distancing. However, he drives crowded buses, surrounded by passengers who do not wear masks. He wears a face mask in public spaces, despite having been stopped and questioned by police while shopping because he looked "suspicious." Mr. W uses his Veterans Affairs health care benefits, but his family is uninsured. He lives with his adult son and his 72-year-old Mexican American wife, who has obesity, diabetes mellitus, and hypertension. Mrs. W, a grocery cashier, reports symptoms similar to those of her husband. Their son, a construction foreman, denies any symptoms. Mr. W's family uses their neighborhood emergency room for health care. They are all concerned that they may lose their jobs if they test positive for COVID-19, and they are fearful that they will not receive high-quality, culturally competent care at the hospital.

DEMOGRAPHICS

The U.S. geriatric population (defined here as ages 65 and older) will continue to grow increasingly more ethnically and racially diverse. Projections estimate that from 2012 to 2060, the number of older adults will grow from 43 million to 92 million (U.S. Census Bureau 2020). By 2060, the projected demographics among Americans 65 and older will be 44% white, non-Hispanic; 27.5% Hispanic; 15.0% African American/Black; 9.1% Asian; and 0.7% American Indian/Alaska Native (AI/AN) (Administration for Community Living 2018). Between 2019 and 2040, the white (not Hispanic) population ages 65 and older is projected to increase by 29% compared with 115% for racial and ethnic minority populations: Hispanic (161%), African American (not Hispanic) (80%), American Indian and Alaska Native (not Hispanic) (67%), and Asian American (not Hispanic) (102%). Federal, state, and local agencies need to identify and address the factors that contribute to ethnic/racial disparities in social determinants of health and barriers to health care access that have been highlighted by the COVID-19 pandemic.

HISTORY OF DISPROPORTIONATE IMPACT OF PANDEMICS ON MINORITY COMMUNITIES

The *Great Dying* refers to the series of epidemics that affected the Indigenous peoples of North and South America as part of the European colonization in the late fifteenth century. Researchers have estimated that as many as 90% of these Indigenous populations were wiped out in the 100–150 years after 1492. Infectious diseases introduced by European colonizers (Berlinguer 1993; Cook 1998; Nunn and Qian 2010) resulted in an estimated 60.5 million precolonial American deaths (Koch et al. 2019). Europeans, who lived close to livestock and other mammals, became hosts for cross-species transmission of pathogens. The Europeans had developed immunity, but the Indigenous peoples had no immunity and were extremely susceptible to pathogens such as smallpox, measles, and influenza. After each epidemic, fewer Indigenous individuals survived, and mass starvation occurred. As the health of the Indigenous population declined, they became more susceptible to the next epidemic. More Indigenous peoples were killed by germs than by firearms or swords.

The 1918–1920 influenza pandemic killed 50 million people, but not everyone was equally affected (Brady and Bahr 2014; Short et al. 2018). As in the Great Dying, Indigenous peoples, especially those residing in remote areas, were at particular risk (Brady and Bahr 2014). Young people also had a higher risk of mortality, possibly because of the multiple waves of measles epidemics that preceded the influenza pandemic. Evidence suggests that measles may suppress immunity for up to 3 years afterward. Therefore, the communities whose immune systems were suppressed postmeasles during that 3-year period were more susceptible to the Spanish flu. Older adults did not have compromised immune systems because their exposure to measles (if any) occurred much earlier. African Americans had lower mortality rates than whites, thought to be due to their prior exposure to a milder strain of influenza that conferred some degree of protection (Økland and Mamelund 2019). Malnutrition also increased morbidity and mortality during this pandemic.

On October 2021 the World Health Organization reported 241,886,635 cases of COVID-19, slightly more than 3% of the world's population (World Health Organization 2021). At the time of that report there had been 4,919,755 COVID-related deaths worldwide and 6,655,399,359

Table 9–1. Risk for COVID-19 infection, hospitalization, and death by race/ethnicity

	American Indian/ Alaska Native, non- Hispanic persons	Asian, non- Hispanic persons	Black or African American, non- Hispanic persons	Hispanic or Latino persons
Cases[a]	1.7×	0.7×	1.1×	1.9×
Hospitalization[b]	3.5×	1.0×	2.8×	2.8×
Death[c]	2.4×	1.0×	2.0×	2.3×

Note. Values represent rate ratios compared with white, non-Hispanic persons.

[a]Data were reported by state and territorial jurisdictions (Centers for Disease Control and Prevention 2020b). Numbers are ratios of age-adjusted rates standardized to the 2019 U.S. intercensal population estimate. Calculations use only the 66% of case reports that have race and ethnicity; this can result in inaccurate estimates of the relative risk among groups.

[b]Data are from COVID-NET for March 1, 2020 through November 6, 2021. Numbers are ratios of age-adjusted rates standardized to the 2019 U.S. standard COVID-NET catchment population (Centers for Disease Control and Prevention 2021c).

[c]Numbers are ratios of age-adjusted rates standardized to the 2019 U.S. intercensal population estimate through November 15, 2021 (Centers for Disease Control and Prevention 2021d).

vaccine doses administered (World Health Organization 2021). However, these data likely underestimate COVID-19 infection and mortality rates among people of color because of such factors as limited testing availability in their communities, reluctance to be tested (Weinberger et al. 2020), and limited completeness and accuracy of data on race and ethnicity (World Health Organization 2021). As in other pandemics, COVID-19 is a zoonotic virus, the result of cross-species transmission. COVID-19, like other pandemic diseases, does not affect all people equally. COVID-19 infection rates are higher among older adults, especially men, those with certain comorbidities (e.g., obesity, diabetes mellitus, hypertension), and those from certain minority communities. The minority communities most affected are African Americans, Latinos, and AIs/ANs (Table 9–1) (Centers for Disease Control and Prevention 2020a). A 2020 analysis of data from 14 states reported that among AIs/ANs, COVID-19 infections rates were 3.5 times greater and mortality rates were 1.8 times higher as compared with whites (Hatcher et al. 2020). The largest reservation in the United States, the Navajo Nation, has had more per capita COVID-19-related cases and deaths than any U.S. state (Silverman et al. 2020).

SOCIAL DETERMINANTS OF HEALTH, COVID-19, AND ETHNIC/RACIAL MINORITY COMMUNITIES

"Social determinants of health (SDOH) are the conditions in the environments where people are born, live, learn, work, play, worship, and age that affect a wide range of health, functioning, and quality-of-life outcomes and risks" (Office of Disease Prevention and Health Promotion 2021). These conditions include access to daily resources, education and economic opportunities, public safety, social attitudes, and English language proficiency. Social determinants of health contribute to the increased morbidity and mortality of COVID-19 in African American, Latino, AI/AN, and Asian American/Pacific Islander (AA/PI) populations. The nature of the impact of these conditions varies depending on the unique characteristics of each community.

African Americans

In terms of daily resources, African American neighborhoods often have fewer healthy food options (Chang et al. 2020) and fewer supermarkets (Powell et al. 2007). These "food deserts" contribute to higher obesity rates in this community, a risk factor for COVID-19. In relation to education and economic opportunities, African Americans have significantly lower median yearly incomes compared with whites ($39,879 vs. $65,000) and are more likely to be essential employees who cannot telework (Funk and Tyson 2021). Regarding public safety, African Americans are less likely to have health insurance, more often live in lower-income communities, and have fewer opportunities for COVID-19 testing (Lubrano 2020) and vaccination. Regarding social attitudes, medical mistrust and vaccine hesitancy among African Americans stems from centuries of systemic racism, medical bias, and barriers to health care (Bogart et al. 2021). However, in March 2021, 61% of African Americans said they would receive or had received a COVID-19 vaccine, which was a substantial increase from the 42% acceptance rate reported in November 2020 (Funk and Tyson 2021).

Hispanics/Latinos

In terms of daily resources, many Latinos struggle with food insecurity and unhealthy food options (Velasco-Mondragon et al. 2016). Compared with non-Hispanic whites, Latinos are more likely to live in multigenerational homes, with only 15% of older Latinos living alone (Administration for Community Living 2018). In relation to educational and economic resources, Latinos are four times as likely as non-Hispanic whites to have less than a high school education and are twice as likely to live below the federal poverty threshold (Velasco-Mondragon et al. 2016). They are more often essential workers who use public transportation and are unable to telework (Velasco-Mondragon et al. 2016). Regarding public safety, Latino farm workers face occupational health hazards (e.g., exposure to pesticides and heat) and are more likely to live in communities with high levels of industrial pollution (Velasco-Mondragon et al. 2016). With respect to social attitudes, Latinos comprise more than two-thirds of the undocumented immigrants in the United States and often live with the added fear of deportation, which is a deterrent to accessing COVID-19 testing or vaccination sites (Migration Policy Institute 2021). Although 26% of Latinos reported they will get the COVID-19 vaccine, 11% stated they would get it only if it is required for work. An additional 18% stated they will decline the vaccine (Kaiser Family Foundation 2021). In terms of health care access, Latinos are more likely to lack health insurance and live in communities with limited access to COVID-19 testing and vaccinations. Finally, in relation to English language proficiency, Latinos are more likely than whites to have difficulties with English language proficiency (Velasco-Mondragon et al. 2016).

American Indians/Alaska Natives

In terms of daily resources, AI/AN communities often struggle with food insecurity (Warne and Wescott 2019). Regarding educational and economic resources, approximately 35% of AIs/ANs have not completed high school, and AIs/ANs have one of the highest unemployment rates in the United States (Education World 2021). In the Navajo Nation, 40% of people live below the poverty line (Gutman et al. 2020). Internet access is often limited or nonexistent in their neighborhoods. With respect to health care, in the AI/AN community only one-third of individuals have access to hospitals and intensive care units (Hatcher et al. 2020). Regarding public safety, AI/AN individuals often live in multigenerational households (Sequist 2020) and lack clean water, indoor plumbing, and/or electricity (Gutman et al. 2020).

Asian Americans/Pacific Islanders

AAs/PIs are a highly diverse group representing more than 40 ethnic groups, 32 languages, and wide variations in culture, sociodemographics, and migration histories (Kim et al. 2010). The relationship between social determinants of health and COVID-19 in these communities is complex (Torralba 2020). For example, in New York, AAs/PIs represent 13.9% of the population and 7.9% of COVID-related deaths (American Public Media Research Lab 2021), but in Colorado, PIs are dying at rates 16-fold higher than their population share (Arnold 2020). Inconsistent reporting of race and ethnicity among states also reduces the accuracy of comparative analysis among AA/PI communities. Many states merge data from smaller ethnic groups and classify them as *other* (American Public Media Research Lab 2021). With respect to educational and economic resources, millions of AAs/PIs are frontline essential workers employed in health care, transportation, and service industries (Asian Pacific American Labor Alliance 2021). In terms of health care, approximately 20% of AAs/PIs are uninsured (Kaholokula et al. 2020). AAs/PIs report discriminatory treatment in clinical settings and may be reluctant to seek health care services (Kaholokula et al. 2020). Regarding public safety, because AP/PI households are often multigenerational, members may have difficulty complying with social distancing and facial masking guidelines (Torralba 2020). In terms of English proficiency, one-third of AAs/PIs have limited English proficiency (Lee et al. 2018). In relation to social attitudes, thousands of COVID-related microaggressions and violence have been directed at AAs/PIs since the beginning of the pandemic (Jeung 2020), with the elderly at particular risk.

BIOLOGICAL MECHANISMS, COVID-19, AND MINORITY ELDERLY COMMUNITIES

Biological mechanisms contributing to the ethnic/racial differences in COVID-19 infection and mortality rates include genetic factors and medical comorbidities.

African Americans

Downregulation of angiotensin converting enzyme 2 (ACE2), a primary binding site for COVID-19, may increase the risk of COVID-19 infection in African Americans (Strickland et al. 2020). Genetic variations in anti-cholinesterase and interleuken-6 may also contribute to the higher rates of COVID-19 morbidity and mortality among African Americans (Vick 2020). Glucose-6-phosphate dehydrogenase (G6PD) deficiency (more common among people of African descent) may be associated with increased COVID-19 infection and mortality rates (Nkhoma et al. 2009). Obesity, hypertension, diabetes, and cardiovascular disease, which are all highly prevalent among African Americans, are significant risk factors for COVID-19 infection.

Hispanics/Latinos

Downregulated ACE2 may increase the risk of COVID-19 infection among Latinos (Strickland et al. 2020). Latinos have high rates of obesity, diabetes, cardiovascular disease, and hypertension (Velasco-Mondragon et al. 2016), known risk factors for COVID-19 infection (Centers for Disease Control and Prevention 2020b).

American Indians/Alaska Natives

A 2020 Centers for Disease Control and Prevention report revealed that data on underlying health conditions were unknown or missing for 91.6% of AI/AN patients (Hatcher et al. 2020). This absence of critical health data prevents examination of the association between premorbid medical health conditions and COVID-19 infections (Hatcher et al. 2020).

Asian Americans/Pacific Islanders

G6PD deficiency is common in persons of Asian descent (Nkhoma et al. 2009) and may make them more vulnerable to COVID-19 infection. Among Asian Americans, Filipino Americans are reported to have the highest rates of hypertension, obesity, diabetes, and cardiovascular disease (Kim et al. 2010), significant risk factors for COVID-19 infection and mortality.

COVID-19 AND MENTAL HEALTH ISSUES

COVID-19 has sparked increased psychological distress and the need for behavioral health resources, particularly among ethnic/racial communities (Centers for Disease Control and Prevention 2021a; Czeisler et al. 2020). During the pandemic, African Americans were 1.2 times more likely than whites to report anxiety or depressive disorders (Centers for Disease Control and Prevention 2021a) and 1.9 times as likely to report suicidal ideation (Czeisler et al. 2020). Latinos were 1.1 times more likely than whites to report anxiety or depressive disorder (Centers for Disease Control and Prevention 2021a) and 2.4 times as likely to report suicidal ideation (Czeisler et al. 2020).

Many ethnic/racial minority older adults experience COVID-19 as a *syndemic*. A syndemic is "a set of closely inter-twined and mutual enhancing health problems that significantly affect the overall health status of a population within the context of a perpetuating configuration of noxious social conditions (e.g. AIDS)" (Singer 1996, p. 99). Minority older adults face limited financial resources, greater medical comorbidities, and a paucity of culturally/linguistically competent mental health providers, factors that contribute to the unique mental health challenges of COVID-19 for older adults from ethnic/racial minority communities.

African Americans

African Americans, compared with whites (28% vs. 19%), more often report that COVID-19 is worsening their mental illness (Hamel et al. 2020). In addition to concerns about contracting COVID-19, African American older adults may be dealing with grief over the loss of family members and friends (Carter 2007) and anxiety related to receiving suboptimal, biased medical care (Hamel et al. 2020). Race-based traumatic stress (RBTS) is a significant contributor to overall mental health symptoms. RBTS refers to the emotional injury caused by microaggressions such as racial bias, ethnic discrimination, and hate crimes (Carter 2007). These adverse experiences may produce symptoms similar to PTSD symptoms, with associated depression, anxiety, and anger (Carter 2007). RBTS is particularly relevant to African American older adults, who often hold transgenerational histories of racially traumatic encounters that can be revived and triggered with every new episode of microaggression experienced or reported in the media (Bor et al. 2018; Laurencin and Walker 2020). The current syndemic of disproportionately high rates of COVID-19 infection and mortality, systemic racism in medical care, and racially discriminatory encounters with law enforcement may contribute to increased depression and anxiety among African American older adults (Laurencin and Walker 2020). Repeated losses of family, friends, and community members due to COVID-19 are prevalent among ethnic/racial minority older adults. African Americans are more than three times more likely than whites to know someone who has died from COVID-19 (Hamel et al. 2020). Social distancing, quarantines, and limited access to digital technology have reduced African American elders' opportunity to garner support from trusted networks (e.g., family, churches, senior centers) and may complicate and extend the bereavement process.

Hispanics/Latinos

American Latinos are a highly diverse group and exhibit variability across many dimensions, including country of origin, religious and spiritual beliefs, reasons for migrating to the United States, the migration experience, prevalence of mental illness, interpretation of treatment recommendations, and degree of acculturation (Holder-Perkins 2019). Latinos come from a collectivistic society, emphasizing the group, especially the family, over the individual. This value, known as *familismo*, is regarded as the most significant cultural value among Latinos, regardless of national origin and degree of acculturation (Hurtado 1995). A December 2020 survey by the Centers for Disease Control and Prevention (2020b) noted that nearly 40% of Latinos reported depression and anxiety. This increased psychological distress may be due to 1) Latinos (especially older adults) being concerned about their increased risk for COVID-19 infection and 2) job loss and financial and housing instability (Jacobson et al. 2020). Last, a high level of stigma is associated with mental health treatment. When Latinos do reach out for assistance, their mental health symptoms are likely to be more severe. Thus, with the increased demand for mental health services, the shortage of available culturally competent service providers is even more severe (National Alliance for the Mentally Ill 2020).

Latinos are at greater risk than are whites for developing dementia (Chen and Zissimopoulos 2018) and present to health care providers with greater degrees of cognitive and functional impairment (Alzheimer's Association 2004). Latino older adults with dementia usually live with family caregivers and are less likely to live in nursing homes. When they do live in nursing homes, the facilities are more likely to have deficiencies in performance, staffing levels, and quality of care (Fennell et al. 2010). Studies have suggested that nursing homes with high shares of African American or Latino residents were more likely to have COVID-19 infections and deaths (Paulin 2020). Latino older adults may be particularly adversely affected by the extended isolation and separation from family members during nursing home lockdowns (Paulin 2020). Last, COVID-19 is depriving Latino families of the opportunity to grieve and participate in important family and community rituals at the death of an older adult.

American Indians/Alaska Natives

Before the COVID-19 pandemic, mental health disorders were already more prevalent among AI/AN populations compared with other communities (Brave Heart et al. 2011). Intergenerational trauma has had a significant impact on the mental health of AI/AN families. Most AIs/ANs believe that historical trauma and loss of culture lie at the heart of substance abuse and mental illness in their communities (Substance Abuse and Mental Health Services Administration 2018). Researchers suggest that RBTS is the end result of decades of colonization, ethnic cleansing, genocide, forced acculturation, and loss of traditions (Ehlers et al. 2013). The mental health impact of COVID-19 on AI/AN communities is poorly understood because many studies have gaps in their data because they failed to include AI/AN individuals or because they lumped them into the *other* category (Wade 2020). AI/AN communities have taken strong measures to protect their older adults, such as restricting visitors to the reservations (Moya-Smith 2020). AI/AN older adults embody the history and resilience of the community and underscore the importance of maintaining cultural tradition and values to weather difficult periods. AIs/ANs understand the importance of maintaining connections with their heritage and communities to reduce substance use and depression. There is increasing recognition that tradition-based healing practices have a role in the mental health treatment of AI/AN individuals.

Asian Americans/Pacific Islanders

Although AP/PIs have low reported rates of mental illness compared with other older adults (Jimenez et al. 2010), COVID-19 has sparked a dramatic rise in xenophobia-related emotional distress in the community. This social phenomenon has resulted in racialized violence, discriminatory behavior, and murder directed at AAs/PIs (Budhwani and Sun 2020). By March 2021 more than 3,800 incidents of violent attacks had been reported (Stop AAPI Hate 2021). However, there has been little research on the impact of COVID-19-related xenophobia on AA/PI individuals, particularly concerning AA/PI older adults, who are often the victims of the assaults. AA/PI older adults may also be particularly vulnerable to social isolation, leading to depression and anxiety, due to their limited English language proficiency (Blacher 2017).

COVID-19 INTERVENTIONS

Effective COVID-19 health intervention requires expertise, resources, and collaboration from community and faith-based institutions, health care delivery systems, and governmental agencies (Fletcher et al. 2020). Community and faith-based organizations can 1) empower pastors and members of faith-based organizations to provide culturally sensitive health education through sermons, Bible studies, and discussion groups; 2) encourage local public health departments to provide hybrid walk-up/drive-through testing and vaccination sites near underserved communities; and 3) encourage health care providers and other community leaders to improve dissemination of COVID-19 information through social media platforms, television, and radio. State, territorial, and federal systems can support and expand telehealth services to AI/AN people through programs such as the Department of Commerce Tribal Broadband Connectivity Program (see www.grants.gov/web/grants/view-opportunity.html?oppId=333974) and the Telebehavioral Health Program (see www.ihs.gov/telehealth/telehealthprograms).

SUMMARY

COVID-19 has highlighted the long-standing disparities in medical and behavioral health care experienced by ethnic/racial minority older adults, their families, and communities. Although each group has its unique identity, history, and cultural traditions, they share similar social determinants of health, medical comorbidities, and barriers to accessing culturally competent mental health care. Future research must bring together practitioners, public health agencies, and community-based organizations for the collaborative design and implementation of effective, culturally competent interventions to address the medical, psychosocial, and behavioral health needs of ethnic/racial minority older adult communities in the face of COVID-19 and chronic health conditions.

KEY POINTS

- The COVID-19 pandemic has disproportionately affected the economic stability and physical and mental health of ethnic/racial minority communities in the United States.
- The health disparities highlighted by COVID-19 are due to the complex interplay of social determinants of health, medical comorbidities, and barriers to culturally competent physical and mental health care.

- Coordinated interventions by faith-based organizations, community agencies, and health care systems should be implemented to improve COVID-19-related public education, engagement, and access to culturally competent care for older adults from ethnic/racial minority communities.

QUESTIONS FOR REVIEW

1. Which of the following disorders has been most often associated with increased vulnerability to COVID-19 among African Americans?

    A. G6PD deficiency
    B. Sickle cell anemia
    C. Insulin resistance
    D. Hypocalcemia
    E. Vitamin B_{12} deficiency

Answer: A.

2. *Familismo* among Latinos describes which of the following?

    A. The importance of family relationships
    B. Extreme anxiety experienced at family gatherings
    C. Values and expectations concerning female gender roles
    D. The importance of male gender roles
    E. The experience of the spirit leaving the body after a frightening event

Answer: A.

3. Which of the following ethnic/racial minority populations of older adults is projected to have the greatest increase by 2030?

    A. Hispanics/Latinos
    B. Whites
    C. African Americans
    D. Asian Americans/Pacific Islanders
    E. Native Americans/Alaskan Natives

Answer: A.

ADDITIONAL RESOURCES

American Psychological Association: African American older adults and COVID-19 webinar. Washington, DC, APA Office on Aging, July 8, 2020. Available at: www.youtube.com/watch?v=1-qVFttDf_wandfeature=youtu.be. Accessed July 2, 2021.

American Public Media Research Lab: The color of coronavirus: COVID-19 deaths by race and ethnicity in the U.S. St. Paul, MN, American Public Media Research Lab, March 5, 2021. Available at: www.apmresearchlab.org/covid/deaths-by-race. Accessed February 15, 2021.

Center for American Indian Health: COVID-19 resources for Native American communities. Baltimore, MD, Center for American Indian Health, 2021. Available at: https://caih.jhu.edu/resource-library/. Accessed January 18, 2021.

Centers for Disease Control and Prevention: Community engagement of African Americans in the era of COVID-19: considerations, challenges, implications, and recommendations for public health. Atlanta, GA, Centers for Disease Control and Prevention, August 13, 2020. Available at: www.cdc.gov/pcd/issues/2020/20_0255.htm. Accessed December 5, 2020.

League of United Latin American Citizens: Coronavirus resources. Washington, DC, League of United Latin American Citizens, 2021. Available at: https://lulac.org/covid19/. Accessed December 5, 2020.

Mental Health America: Native and Indigenous communities and mental health. Alexandria, VA, Mental Health America, 2021. Available at: www.mhanational.org/issues/native-and-indigenous-communities-and-mental-health. Accessed January 10, 2021.

National Asian Pacific Center on Aging: COVID-19—what you need to know. Seattle, WA, National Asian Pacific Center on Aging, 2021. Available at: www.napca.org/resource/covid19-whatyouneedto know. Accessed December 6, 2020.

National Council on Aging: Recursos para adultos mayores y sus cuidadores. Arlington, VA, National Council on Aging, March 5, 2021. Available at: www.ncoa.org/article/covid-19-recursos-para-adultos-mayores-y-sus-cuidadores. Accessed December 5, 2020.

Roessel MH, Nahulu L, Zein M: Culturally competent care for geriatric Indigenous peoples, in Culture, Heritage, and Diversity in Older Adult Mental Care. Edited by Llorente MD. Washington DC, American Psychiatric Association Publishing, 2019, pp 115–127

University of Michigan, Michigan Medicine, Department of Psychiatry: Psychiatric resources for COVID-19: impact on special populations, Asian American communities. Ann Arbor, University of Michigan, 2021. Available at: https://medicine.umich.edu/dept/psychiatry/ michigan-psychiatry-resources-covid-19/healthcare-providers/ covid-19-mental-health-toolkit/impact-special-populations/asian-american-communities. Accessed December 9, 2020.

REFERENCES

Administration for Community Living: 2017 profile of older Americans. Washington, DC, Administration for Community Living, April 2018. Available at: https://acl.gov/sites/default/files/Aging%20and%20Disability%20in%20America/2017OlderAmericansProfile.pdf. Accessed February 15, 2021.

Alzheimer's Association: Hispanics/Latinos and Alzheimer's disease. Chicago, IL, Alzheimer's Association, May 18, 2004. Available at: www.alz.org/media/Documents/alzheimers-hispanics-latinos-r.pdf. Accessed January 10, 2021.

American Public Media Research Lab: The color of coronavirus: COVID-19 deaths by race and ethnicity in the U.S. St. Paul, MN, American Public Media Research Lab, March 5, 2021. Available at: www.apmresearchlab.org/covid/deaths-by-race. Accessed February 15, 2021.

Arnold E: COVID-19 rates disproportionately higher among Blacks, Hispanics, Pacific Islanders. Highland Ranch Herald, April 14, 2020

Asian Pacific American Labor Alliance: Protecting Asian American and Pacific Islander working people. Washington, DC, Asian Pacific American Labor Alliance, 2021. Available at: www.apalanet.org/uploads/8/3/2/0/83203568/aapi_covid-19_guidance.pdf. Accessed February 16, 2021.

Berlinguer G: The interchange of disease and health between the Old and New Worlds. Int J Health Serv 23(4):703–715, 1993 8276530

Blacher K: Asian Americans and Pacific Islanders in the United States aged 65 years and older: population, nativity and language. Data brief. Seattle, WA, National Asian Pacific Center for Aging, 2017. Available at: https://napca.org/wp-content/uploads/2017/10/65-population-report-FINAL.pdf. Accessed December 28, 2020.

Bogart LM, Ojikutu BO, Tyagi K, et al: COVID-19 related medical mistrust, health impacts, and potential vaccine hesitancy among black Americans living with HIV. J Acquir Immune Defic Syndr 86(2):200–207, 2021 33196555

Bor J, Venkataramani AS, Williams DR, et al: Police killings and their spillover effects on the mental health of Black Americans: a population-based, quasi-experimental study. Lancet 392(10144):302–310, 2018 29937193

Brady BR, Bahr HM: The influenza epidemic of 1918–1920 among the Navajos: marginality, mortality and the implications of some neglected eyewitness accounts. Am Indian Q 38(4):459–491, 2014

Brave Heart MYH, Chase J, Elkins J, et. al: Historical trauma among Indigenous peoples of the Americas: concepts, research, and clinical considerations. J Psychoactive Drugs 43(4):282–290, 2011 22400458

Budhwani H, Sun R: Creating COVID-19 stigma by referencing the novel coronavirus as the "Chinese virus" on Twitter: quantitative analysis of social media data. J Med Internet Res 22(5):e19301, 2020 32343669

Carter RT: Racism and psychological and emotional injury: recognizing and assessing race-based traumatic stress. Counseling Psychologist 35(1):13–105, 2007

Centers for Disease Control and Prevention: Your health. Atlanta, GA, Centers for Disease Control and Prevention, 2020a. Available at: www.cdc.gov/coronavirus/2019-ncov/your-health/index.html. Accessed: October 24, 2021.

Centers for Disease Control and Prevention: COVID-19 hospitalization and death by race/ethnicity. Atlanta, GA, Centers for Disease Control and Prevention, 2020b. Available at: www.cdc.gov/coronavirus/2019-ncov/covid-data/investigations-discovery/hospitalization-death-by-race-ethnicity.html Accessed January 10, 2021.

Centers for Disease Control and Prevention: Anxiety and depression: household pulse survey. Atlanta, GA, Centers for Disease Control and Prevention, June 30, 2021a. Available at: www.cdc.gov/nchs/covid19/pulse/mental-health.htm. Accessed January 10, 2021.

Centers for Disease Control and Prevention: Hospitalization and death by race/ethnicity. Atlanta, GA, Centers for Disease Control and Prevention, 2021b. Available at: www.cdc.gov/coronavirus/2019-ncov/covid-data/investigations-discovery/hospitalization-death-by-race-ethnicity.html. Accessed November 16, 2021.

Centers for Disease Control and Prevention: Hospitalization surveillance network COVID-NET. Atlanta, GA, Centers for Disease Control and Prevention, 2021c. Available at: www.cdc.gov/coronavirus/2019-ncov/covid-data/covid-net/purpose-methods.html. Accessed November 16, 2021.

Centers for Disease Control and Prevention: Provisional COVID-19 deaths: distribution of deaths by race and Hispanic origin. Centers for Disease Control and Prevention. Atlanta, GA, Centers for Disease Control and Prevention. 2021d. Available at: https://data.cdc.gov/NCHS/Provisional-COVID-19-Deaths-Distribution-of-Deaths/pj7m-y5uh. Accessed November 16, 2021.

Chang RC, Penaia C, Thomas K: Count Native Hawaiian and Pacific Islanders in COVID-19 data—it's an OMB mandate. Health Affairs Blog, August 27, 2020. Available at: www.healthaffairs.org/do/10.1377/hblog20200825.671245/full/. Accessed July 1, 2021.

Chen C, Zissimopoulos JM: Racial and ethnic differences in trends in dementia prevalence and risk factors in the United States. Alzheimers Dement (NY) 4:510–520, 2018 30364652

Cook ND: Born to Die: Disease and New World Conquest. New York, Cambridge University Press, 1998

Czeisler ME, Lane RI, Petrosky E, et al: Mental health, substance use, and suicidal ideation during the COVID-19 pandemic—United States, June 24–30, 2020. MMWR Morb Mortal Wkly Rep 69(32):1049–1057, 2020 32790653

Education World: Reporters' notebook: Native Americans struggle, build pride. Education World, 2021. Available at: www.educationworld.com/a_issues/schools/schools012.shtml. Accessed February 2, 2020.

Ehlers CL, Gizer IR, Gilder DA, et al: Measuring historical trauma in an American Indian community sample: contributions of substance dependence, affective disorder, conduct disorder and PTSD. Drug Alcohol Depend 133(1):180–187, 2013 23791028

Fennell ML, Feng Z, Clark MA, et al: Elderly Hispanics more likely to reside in poor-quality nursing homes. Health Aff (Millwood) 29(1):65–73, 2010 20048362

Fletcher FE, Allen S, Vickers SM, et al: COVID-19's impact on the African American community: a stakeholder engagement approach to increase public awareness through virtual town halls. Health Equity 4(1):320–325, 2020 32775941

Funk C, Tyson A: Growing share of Americans say they plan to get a COVID-19 vaccine—or already have. Washington, DC, Pew Research Center, March 5, 2021. Available at: www.pewresearch.org/science/2021/03/05/growing-share-of-americans-say-they-plan-to-get-a-covid-19-vaccine-or-already-have/. Accessed July 1, 2021.

Gutman M, Rodriguez L, Shakya T: Navajo Nation: where COVID-19 claims whole families. ABC News, May 21, 2020. Available at: https://abcnews.go.com/US/navajo-nation-covid-19-claims-families/story?id=70787562. Accessed March 18, 2021.

Hamel L, Lopes L, Munana C, et al: KKF/The Undefeated survey on race and health. KKF, 2020. Available at: www.kff.org/racial-equity-and-health-policy/report/kff-the-undefeated-survey-on-race-and-health/. Accessed January 26, 2021.

Hatcher SM, Agnew-Brune C, Anderson M: COVID among American Indian and Alaska Native persons—23 states, January 31–July 13, 2020. MMWR Morb Mortal Wkly Rep 69(34): 1166–1169, 2020 32853193

Holder-Perkins V: Cultural competency and Latino elders, in Culture, Heritage, and Diversity in Older Adult Mental Health Care. Edited by Llorente MD. Washington, DC, American Psychiatric Association Publishing, 2019, pp 161–180

Hurtado A: Variations, combinations, and evolutions: Latino families in the United States, in Understanding Latino Families: Scholarship, Policy, and Practice. Edited by Zambrana RE. Thousand Oaks, CA, Sage, 1995, pp 40–61

Jacobson G, Feder J, Radley DC: COVID-19's impact on older workers: employment, income, and Medicare spending. New York, Commonwealth Fund, Issue Briefs, October 6, 2020. Available at: www.commonwealthfund.org/publications/issue-briefs/2020/oct/covid-19-impact-older-workers-employment-income-medicare. Accessed February 5, 2021.

Jeung R: Incidents of coronavirus discrimination. Los Angeles, CA, Asian Pacific Policy and Planning Council, 2020. Available at: www.asianpacificpolicyand planningcouncil.org/wp-content/uploads/A3PCON_Public_Weekly_Report_3.pdf. Accessed July 2, 2021.

Jimenez DE, Alegría M, Chen CN, et al: Prevalence of psychiatric illnesses in older ethnic minority adults. J Am Geriatr Soc 58(2):256–264, 2010 20374401

Kaholokula JK, Samoa RA, Miyamoto RES, et al: COVID-19 special column: COVID-19 hits native Hawaiian and Pacific Islander communities the hardest. Hawaii J Health Soc Welf 79(5):144–146, 2020 32432218

Kaiser Family Foundation: Vaccine hesitancy among Hispanic adults. Baltimore, MD, Kaiser Family Foundation, January 14, 2021. Available at: www.kff.org/coronavirus-covid-19/poll-finding/vaccine-hesitancy-among-hispanic-adults/. Accessed March 16, 2021.

Kim G, Chiriboga DA, Jang Y, et al: Health status of older Asian Americans in California. J Am Geriatr Soc 58(10):2003–2008, 2010 20929469

Koch A, Brierly C, Maslin MM, et al: Earth system impacts of the European arrival and Great Dying in the Americas after 1492. Quat Sci Rev 207:13–36, 2019

Laurencin CT, Walker JM: A pandemic on a pandemic: racism and COVID-19 in Blacks. Cell Syst 11(1):9–10, 2020 32702320

Lee J, Ramakrishnan K, Wong J: Accurately counting Asian Americans is a civil rights issue. Ann Am Acad Pol Soc Sci 677(1):191–202, 2018

Lubrano A: High-income Philadelphians getting tested for coronavirus at far higher rates than low-income residents. Knight-Ridder/Tribune Business News, April 6, 2020. Available at: https://search.proquest.com/docview/2386189605. Accessed on February 2, 2021.

Migration Policy Institute: Profile of the unauthorized population: United States. Washington, DC, Migration Policy Institute, 2021. Available at: www.migrationpolicy.org/data/unauthorized-immigrant-population/state/US. Accessed February 12, 2021.

Moya-Smith S: Coronavirus takes more than Native Americans' lives. Killing our elderly erases our culture. NBC News, April 22, 2020. Available at: www.nbcnews.com/think/opinion/coronavirus-takes-more-native-americans-lives-killing-our-elderly erases-ncna1189761. Accessed January 10, 2021.

National Alliance for the Mentally Ill: Mental health services for Latinos are in low supply, higher demand due to COVID-19. Arlington, VA, National Alliance for the Mentally Ill, October 23, 2020. Available at: www.nami.org/Press-Media/In-The-News/2020/Mental-health-services-for-Latinos-are-in-low-supply-higher-demand-due-to-COVID-19?feed=In-the-news. Accessed January 10, 2021.

Nkhoma ET, Poole C, Vannappagari V, et al: The global prevalence of glucose-6-phosphate dehydrogenase deficiency: a systematic review and meta-analysis. Blood Cells Mol Dis 42(3):267–278, 2009 19233695

Nunn N, Qian N: The Columbian exchange: a history of disease, food, and ideas. J Econ Perspect 24:163–188, 2010

Office of Disease Prevention and Health Promotion: Healthy People 2030: social determinants of health. Rockville, MD, Office of Disease Prevention and Health Promotion, 2021. Available at: https://health.gov/healthypeople/objectives-and-data/social-determinants-health. Accessed July 1, 2021.

Økland H, Mamelund SE: Race and 1918 influenza pandemic in the United States: a review of the literature. Int J Environ Res Public Health 16(14):2487, 2019 31336864

Paulin E: Is extended isolation killing older adults in long-term care? Washington, DC, AARP, September 3, 2020. Available at: www.aarp.org/caregiving/health/info-2020/covid-isolation-killing-nursing-home-residents. Accessed October 24, 2021.

Powell LM, Auld MC, Chaloupka FJ, et al: Associations between access to food stores and adolescent body mass index. Am J Prev Med 33(4)(suppl):S301–S307, 2007 17884578

Sequist T: The disproportionate impact of Covid-19 on communities of color. NEJM Catalyst, July 6, 2020. Available at: https://catalyst.nejm.org/doi/full/10.1056/CAT.20.0370. Accessed January 10, 2021.

Short KR, Kedzierska K, van de Sandt CE: Back to the future: lessons learned from the 1918 influenza pandemic. Front Cell Infect Microbiol 8:343, 2018 30349811

Silverman H, Toropin K, Sidner S, Perrot L: Navajo Nation surpasses New York State for the highest COVID-19 infection rate in the US. Atlanta, GA, CNN, May 18, 2020. Available at: www.cnn.com/2020/05/18/us/navajo-nation-infection-rate-trnd/index.html. Accessed: October 24, 2021.

Singer M: A dose of drugs, a touch of violence, a case of AIDS: conceptualizing the SAVA syndemic. Free Inq Creat Sociol 24(2):99–110, 1996

Stop AAPI Hate: Stop AAPI Hate national report. San Francisco, CA, Stop AAPI Hate, 2021. Available at: https://secureservercdn.net/104.238.69.231/a1w.90d.myftpupload.com/wp-content/uploads/2021/03/210312-Stop-AAPI-Hate-National-Report-.pdf. Accessed March 20, 2021.

Strickland OL, Powell-Young Y, Reyes-Miranda C, et al: African-Americans have a higher propensity for death from COVID-19: rationale and causation. J Natl Black Nurses Assoc 31(1):1–12, 2020 32853490

Substance Abuse and Mental Health Services Administration: Behavioral Health Services for American Indians and Alaska Natives. TIP 61. Rockville, MD, Substance Abuse and Mental Health Services Administration, 2018. Available at: https://store.samhsa.gov/sites/default/files/d7/priv/tip_61_aian_full_document_020419_0.pdf. Accessed January 10, 2021.

Torralba E: COVID-19 exposes how Native Hawaiians and Pacific Islanders face stark health care disparities. UCLA Newsroom, August 26, 2020. Available at: https://newsroom.ucla.edu/stories/covid-19-stark-differences-NHPI. Accessed October 24, 2021.

U.S. Census Bureau: Demographic turning points for the United States: population projections for 2020 to 2060. Washington, DC, U.S. Census Bureau, February 2020. Available at: www.census.gov/library/publications/2020/demo/p25-1144.html#:~:text=Beyond%202030%2C%20the%20U.S.%20population,400%20million%20threshold%20in%202058. Accessed February 28, 2021.

Velasco-Mondragon E, Jimenez A, Palladino-Davis AG, et al: Hispanic health in the USA: a scoping review of the literature. Public Health Rev 37:31, 2016 29450072

Vick DJ: Glucose-6-phosphate dehydrogenase deficiency and COVID-19 infection. Mayo Clin Proc 95(8):1803–1804, 2020 32680625

VOA News: 10% of world's population may have been infected with coronavirus, WHO says. VOA News, October 5, 2020. Available at: www.voanews.com/covid-19-pandemic/10-worlds-population-may-have-been-infected-coronavirus-who-says. Accessed January 10, 2021.

Wade L: COVID-19 data on Native Americans is a "national disgrace." This scientist is fighting to be counted. Science Magazine, 2020. Available at: www.sciencemag.org/news/2020/09/covid-19-data-native-americans-national-disgrace-scientist-fighting-be-counted. Accessed January 10, 2021.

Warne D, Wescott S: Social determinants of American Indian nutritional health. Curr Dev Nutr 3 (suppl 2):12–18, 2019 31453425

Weinberger DM, Chen J, Cohen T, et al: Estimation of excess deaths associated
    with the COVID-19 pandemic in the United States, March to May 2020.
    JAMA Intern Med 180(10):1336–1344, 2020 32609310
World Health Organization: WHO coronavirus (COVID-19) dashboard. Geneva,
    World Health Organization, 2021. Available at: https://covid19.who.int.
    Accessed October 24, 2021.

CHAPTER 10

SOCIAL DETERMINANTS OF COVID-19 MORBIDITY AND MORTALITY

Linda Nix, M.D, M.P.H.
Emily Tan, B.A.
Nhi-Ha Trinh, M.D., M.P.H.
Iqbal "Ike" Ahmed, M.D., FRCPsych (UK)

The coronavirus SARS-CoV-2 disease (COVID-19) pandemic has exposed and exacerbated the long-standing impact of social determinants of health (SDOH) for individuals with medical and psychiatric disorders. SDOH have had a major impact on worsening of morbidity and mortality during the COVID-19 pandemic. Three groups have disproportionately suffered from the effects of SDOH: 1) ethnic/racial minorities, 2) the socioeconomically disadvantaged, and 3) older adults, especially those living in residential care homes and nursing homes. SDOH and COVID-19 together have led to a perfect storm of widespread devastation from the COVID-19 pandemic. Future directions for improving access to interventions and addressing SDOH are discussed.

Vignette

Mrs. K, a 78-year-old Micronesian woman, is hospitalized after being brought to a Honolulu hospital with fever and respiratory symptoms. Testing for COVID-19 infection by nasal swab confirms suspicion of COVID-19 infection. Mrs. K quickly develops high fever and respiratory distress and is intubated in the intensive care unit. Her condition worsens in a matter of days, and she is pronounced dead secondary to complications of COVID-19 infection. Her medical history includes obesity, diabetes, hypertension, and osteoarthritis. She lived with three children and four grown grandchildren in a three-bedroom apartment in a poor neighborhood where a number of other Micronesian families live after moving from Micronesia. Her children and grandchildren work in the service industries, mainly as cooks, janitors, and hotel workers. She had not seen a physician for more than a year and was not consistently taking her medications because of financial reasons. Contact tracing reveals that at least two other family members had symptoms of COVID-19 infection but did not need hospitalization.

Data reported by the state Department of Health show that the recent COVID-19 surge in Hawaii has disproportionately affected non-Hawaiian Pacific Islanders, who account for just 4% of the state population but 30% of all cases in the state (Thomas 2020). Under the category of Pacific Islanders, Micronesians are one of the most vulnerable minority groups residing in Hawaii. Although Pacific Islanders come to Hawaii to work, raise families, and contribute to the social fabric, data show that Micronesians in particular experience poorer health and greater poverty than any other Pacific Islander group. The reason is a range of external factors, including the severe impacts of U.S. militarism, systemic racism, cultural erasure or disconnect, and language barriers. Other SDOH also influence access to health care for the Micronesian community. For example, many Micronesians are poor, working-class people who are frontline workers at the airport, hotels, fast food restaurants, and car rental agencies. This exposes them to people who may have transmissible infections such as COVID-19 (Thomas 2020).

The pandemic of COVID-19 infection has shone an even more glaring spotlight on the impact of SDOH on the medical and psychiatric morbidity and mortality outcomes from infection in older adults both in the United States and globally. SDOH affect health outcomes for both medical and psychiatric disorders (Compton and Shim 2015). Social determinants that have been implicated include being part of a disadvantaged minority or immigrant group or other marginalized population, systemic and structural racism, poverty, adversities in the living environment (including crowding, pollution, and climate change), and limited access to health care. In addition to older age itself, SDOH can increase the likelihood of several health conditions, including obesity, diabetes, chronic respiratory disorders, cardiovascular and cerebrovascular disorders, and dementia, which themselves have been identified as risk factors in contracting COVID-19 infection and resulting in poorer outcomes. Three groups have disproportionately suffered the health burden: 1) ethnic/racial minorities, 2) the socioeconomically disadvantaged, and 3) older adults, especially those living in residential care homes and nursing homes (Ali et al. 2020).

The intersectionality of older age, SDOH, and COVID-19 has led to a perfect storm of widespread devastation from the COVID-19 pandemic.

We discuss SDOH and health disparities affecting health care outcomes of both psychiatric and medical disorders and then move to discussing the impact of SDOH on COVID-19 in older adults, particularly greater exposure to the virus, the presence of risk factors from other SDOH-associated medical illnesses, and poorer outcomes in older adults. In addition, disparities in access to care and prevention through vaccination are discussed. We conclude with possible strategies to address SDOH and reduce the disparities in outcomes and health care.

SCOPE OF THE PANDEMIC FOR MARGINALIZED POPULATIONS

Both U.S. data and international data suggest that the COVID-19 pandemic has had a greater impact on minority populations (Ali et al. 2020). In early 2020, COVID-19 hot spots in predominantly Black counties in the United States experienced mortality risk that was sixfold higher than in predominantly white counties (Yancy 2020). Meanwhile, in the United Kingdom, Black and Asian cases were reported to represent almost twice their population share (Intensive Care National Audit and Research Centre 2020).

The most recent Centers for Disease Control and Prevention (CDC) data showed that between 2019 and the first half of 2020, life expectancy decreased 2.7 years for the non-Hispanic Black population (from 74.7 to 72.0) (Arias et al. 2021). It decreased by 1.9 years for the Hispanic population (from 81.8 to 79.9) and by 0.8 year for the non-Hispanic white population (from 78.8 to 78.0). This disparity is presumed to be due to the impact of the COVID-19 pandemic disproportionately affecting minority populations. Race and ethnicity are risk markers for other underlying conditions that affect health, including socioeconomic status, access to health care, and exposure to the virus via occupation, for example, frontline, essential, and critical infrastructure workers (Centers for Disease Control and Prevention 2020).

SOCIAL DETERMINANTS OF HEALTH

The World Health Organization (2008) defines SDOH as the conditions in which people "are born, grow, live, work, and age." Social determinants are shaped by the multilevel distribution of money, power, and resources; they can include the distribution of wealth and other forms of opportunity within society, access to and quality of education for children and employment for adults, health care access and quality, economic stability, and the neighborhood built environment, as well as the characteristics of housing and other societal infrastructure (Centers for Disease Control and Prevention 2020). Understanding the ways in which health is influenced by these societal variables and conditions helps frame the importance of striving for health equity within the realms of governance and encourages us all to consider the health impacts of societal policies (Compton and Shim 2015).

Prior to the COVID-19 pandemic, there was increasing recognition of the importance of SDOH on both physical and mental health. Healthy People 2020 created a *place-based* organizing framework, reflecting five key areas of SDOH: economic stability, education, social and community context, health and health care, and neighborhood and built environment (Office of Disease Prevention and Health Promotion 2021a). Investing in resources in these areas can enhance quality of life and exert significant influence on population health outcomes. Examples of these resources include safe and affordable housing, access to education, public safety, availability of healthy foods, local emergency and health services, and environments free of life-threatening toxins. More recently, Healthy People 2030 highlighted the importance of addressing SDOH by including "social and physical environments that promote good health for all" as one of the four overarching goals for the decade (Office of Disease Prevention and Health Promotion 2021b).

SDOH have been shown to have tremendous impacts on physical health and mental health (Figure 10–1). An example that starkly illustrates this impact is the matter of income inequality (Compton and Shim 2015). Income inequality is associated with premature mortality (Kondo et al. 2009), and there is a correlation between income distribution of countries and average life expectancies (Wilkinson 1992). Income inequality is also a social determinant of mental health, leading to poorer mental health, increasing risk for and incidence of mental illnesses and substance use disorders (SUDs), and worsening course and outcome among people affected by mental illnesses or substance use disorders (Compton and Shim 2015). It is important to understand the impact of SDOH not only to improve individual, community, and population health but also to advance health equity across the board. In the context of the COVID-19 pandemic, certain vulnerable communities have been disproportionately affected. As articulated by historian Frank M. Snowden, "Epidemic diseases are not random events that af-

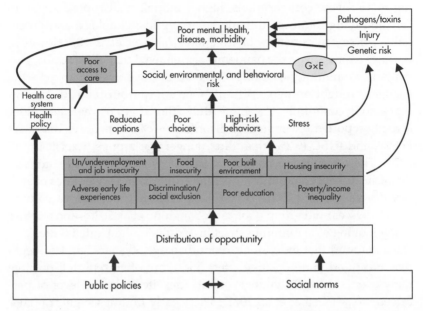

FIGURE 10–1. Conceptualizing the social determinants of mental health.

G×E=gene-by-environment interaction.
Source. Compton MT, Shim RS: The social determinants of mental health. Focus 13(4):419–425, 2015. Copyright American Psychiatric Association © 2015. Used with permission.

flict societies capriciously and without warning. On the contrary, every society produces its own specific vulnerabilities," and times of crisis, such as the COVID-19 pandemic, act like "a mirror for humanity" (Chotiner 2020).

SOCIAL DETERMINANTS OF HEALTH AND COVID-19

Age

Among the clearest SDOH associated with increased morbidity and mortality during the COVID-19 pandemic is age. U.S. adults ages 65 and older accounted for approximately 80% of COVID-19 deaths as of December 2020 (Centers for Disease Control and Prevention 2019). As seen during the early spread of COVID-19, older adults experienced disproportionately greater adverse effects from the pandemic, including more severe complications, higher mortality, disrupted access to care and daily routines, difficulty adapting to technology, and potentially worse consequences of isolation (Vahia et al. 2020). However, findings from early in the pandemic also showed that older adults, particularly community-dwelling older adults, were adaptable to the changes brought on by COVID-19. One study from June 2020 found that among community-dwelling adults, those ages 65 years and older actually reported fewer anxiety disorders (6.2%), depressive disorders (5.8%), and PTSD (9.2%) than did younger age groups (Czeisler et al. 2020). These results are similar to those of two international studies: a Spanish study of community-dwelling adults found lower rates of anxiety, depression, and PTSD in a 60- to 80-year-old group compared with a 40- to 59-year-old group (González-Sanguino et al. 2020), and another study looking at community-dwelling adults in the United States and Canada found that individuals older than age 60 years had less negative affect and more positive affect and more often reported positive daily events than did younger adults, despite a similar level of perceived stress (Klaiber et al. 2021). These early findings suggest higher resilience to the mental health effects of COVID-19 among community-dwelling older individuals, which may be explained partially by older adults' lower stress reactivity and better emotional regulation and well-being, along with the role that wisdom may play (Vahia et al. 2020).

Access to Health Care

There are many examples of how disparities in ability to access health care during the pandemic not only affect accurate data collection in assessing the extent of health care delivery inequity but may also be a factor in worse morbidity and mortality among vulnerable populations. Compared with non-Hispanic white people, African Americans are less likely to have health insurance (U.S. Census Bureau 2019). A study of commercially insured and Medicare Advantage enrollees from January to June 2020 found that telemedicine use was lower in communities with higher rates of poverty and in more rural areas, which is an example of what is termed the *digital divide* (Patel et al. 2021). Foreign-born noncitizens have historically avoided accessing health care for fear of being deported or risking their future legal resident status on the basis of the federal public charge regulations (Bernstein et al. 2019; Sommers et al. 2020), which could explain some of the poorer health outcomes among populations with higher percentages of noncitizens. Black patients are vulnerable to the impact of implicit and explicit health care biases, which are more likely to affect decision-making in times of emotional stress, such as during the COVID-19 surges, when providers and health care systems were stretched to capacity (Kirksey et al. 2021). One study from April and May 2020 data found that Latino adults reported a higher prevalence of psychosocial stress related to not having enough food or stable housing compared with adults in other ethnic groups (McKnight-Eily et al. 2021). All of these disparities contribute significantly to morbidity and mortality.

Social Distancing

Homeless and Prison Populations

The ability to physically distance can be thought of as an issue of privilege that is simply inaccessible to some communities (Yancy 2020). A particularly vulnerable population is individuals experiencing homelessness, who are at higher risk of COVID-19 transmission due to crowded living spaces and scarce access to COVID-19 screening and testing (Tsai and Wilson 2020). A staggering study from early on in the pandemic tested more than 400 individuals residing in a Boston shelter and found that 36% had a positive COVID-19 polymerase chain reaction test (Baggett et al. 2020). Similarly, incarcerated populations are more vulnerable to COVID-19 exposure because of overcrowding and limited access to resources. An investigation by The Marshall Project and the Associated Press projected that an average of one in every five state and federal prisoners in the United States would have tested positive for COVID-19, with more than 1,700 deaths in that population as of mid-December 2020 (Schwartzapfel et al. 2020). Because African Americans are incarcerated at more than five times the rate of whites and receive longer sentences (Sentencing Project 2018), they are at even greater risk of COVID-19 exposure. For example, in Michigan, Black prisoners represented 49% of positive COVID-19 tests, whereas Black community residents accounted for 31% of the positive tests (Schwartzapfel et al. 2020).

Long-Term Facilities

Although Chapter 5, "Geriatric Mental Health Care: Lessons From a Pandemic," addresses long-term care during the pandemic, it is important to additionally address the role that SDOH play for individuals living in long-term care facilities during the COVID-19 pandemic. Long-term care facilities have been identified as one of the most racially segregated sectors of health care (Rahman and Foster 2015), and this segregation has been known to result in worse outcomes for older adults who are a part of Black, Indigenous, and people of color (BIPOC) communities

(Mack et al. 2020). Individuals living in these facilities rely on care from essential workers, many of whom are people of color who rely on public transportation to get to work and live in underserved neighborhoods disproportionately affected by COVID-19, which places both the care workers and residents at higher risk of infection and mortality (Shippee et al. 2020).

Employment

Another important source of inequity during the COVID-19 pandemic is employment and how it affects people's abilities to physically distance and avoid COVID-19 exposure. Although African Americans account for just 13.4% of the U.S. population, they account for 17.1% of the service sector, including cashiers, bus drivers, taxi drivers, housekeepers, janitorial staff, and sanitation workers, all occupations that are less likely than office-based jobs to be able to translate to work-from-home positions (U.S. Bureau of Labor Statistics 2021). Essential frontline workers are more likely to have lower educational attainment, self-identify as members of racial and ethnic minority groups, be socioeconomically disadvantaged, and identify as immigrants (Blau et al. 2020). These workers tend to have jobs with low decision latitude and high job demands but often have fewer labor protections and may be more likely to have associated psychiatric disorders (Stansfeld et al. 1999). In addition to having to be present at work, many of these individuals require public transit to get to work. All of these factors contribute to increased risk for these already vulnerable workers (Clark 2017).

Differences in COVID-19 outcomes across races may be related to the complex interaction of SDOH, including socioeconomic disparities, barriers to accessing care, and higher prevalence of medical comorbidities (Tai et al. 2021). These populations may be at increased risk of exposure through their workplaces and crowded living conditions, including refugee camps (Greenaway et al. 2020).

MEDICAL COMORBIDITIES, COVID-19, AND SOCIAL DETERMINANTS OF HEALTH

Asthma

Most of the medical comorbidities that are associated with higher morbidity and mortality from COVID-19 are highly linked to underlying socioeconomic differences and other types of inequalities. This is particularly true for underlying chronic respiratory conditions such as asthma or chronic obstructive pulmonary disease (Abrams and Szefler 2020), for which there may be additive or even multiplicative effects on COVID-19 morbidity (Abrams and Szefler 2020). Although the CDC recognizes asthma as a risk factor for COVID-19 morbidity (Centers for Disease Control and Prevention 2019), the poorer outcomes in people with asthma may be related to the association of worse asthma morbidity (including poorer asthma control and increased emergency department [ED] visits for asthma) seen in those affected by SDOH such as poverty, smoke exposure, and non-Hispanic Black race (Federico et al. 2020).

Smoking

Smoking, as a comorbidity, is twice as common in individuals with psychiatric illness compared with adults without psychiatric illness (Gfroerer et al. 2013; Lasser et al. 2000) and is notably higher in individuals diagnosed with schizophrenia (Vanable et al. 2003). An early systematic review found that current or former smokers were more likely to have severe COVID-19 symptoms (relative risk 1.4) and an increased risk of intensive care unit admission, mechanical ventilation, and death related to COVID-19 (relative risk 2.4) compared with nonsmokers (Vardavas and Nikitara 2020).

Mental Health

COVID-19 itself has been associated with worse mental health, including depression, suicide, anxiety disorders, and SUDs (Czeisler et al. 2020). People with serious mental illnesses and SUDs have been shown to be at greater risk of contracting COVID-19 (Ettman et al. 2020). Ettman and colleagues found that not only were prevalence rates of depression higher across all severity levels during COVID-19 compared with rates of depression prior to the pandemic in the United States (including prevalence rates of severe depression increasing from 0.7% to 5.1%) but also certain populations, such as those with lower incomes and greater stress levels associated with the pandemic, had even more pronounced depressive symptoms (Ettman et al. 2020).

One study from June 2020 found that 40.9% of U.S. adult respondents to a survey reported mental or behavioral health concerns during the pandemic, with 13.3% saying they had increased or initiated substance use (Czeisler et al. 2020). Another study used surveys from April and May 2020 and found self-reported prevalence of current depression in 28.6% of respondents, initiation or increasing substance use in 18.2%, and suicidal thoughts or ideation in 8.4% (McKnight-Eily et al. 2021). A South Korean study found that among people who were hospitalized during the 3 years prior to the study, individuals with psychotic features were nearly four times more likely to have COVID-19 (Lee et al. 2020).

Another U.S. study reviewed records for 61 million adults and found that individuals who had received a recent diagnosis of a mental illness had an increased risk for COVID-19 infection, an effect strongest in depression (adjusted odds ratio [AOR] 7.64) and schizophrenia (AOR 7.34) (Wang et al. 2021c). Further, African Americans had higher odds of COVID-19 infection than did whites, with the highest disparity for depression (AOR 3.78). This study also found worse outcomes among individuals with both a recent diagnosis of a mental illness and COVID-19 infection: this group was hospitalized at a rate of 27.4% compared with a hospitalization rate of 18.6% for COVID-19 patients without any mental illness. Among patients with COVID-19 who had a recent diagnosis of mental illness, the hospitalization rate for African Americans was even higher at 33.6% compared with a rate of 24.8% for whites. Mortality rates were also found to be higher for patients with mental illness; those with mental illness died at a rate of 8.5% compared with 4.7% among COVID-19 patients without any mental illness (Wang et al. 2021c).

In a large U.K. study using U.S. data that also used propensity score matching, there was an observed higher incidence of COVID-19 in individuals diagnosed with a psychiatric illness during the past year (relative risk 1.65). The main focus of the study was comparing hazard ratios of having a psychiatric diagnosis in the 14–90 days following six health events ranging from influenza or other respiratory illness to other infections or long bone fractures (Taquet et al. 2021). From a subset of 44,779 patients with a COVID-19 diagnosis and no previous psychiatric illness, the incidence of new psychiatric illness after 90 days was 5.8%, higher than all studied similarly acute health events with hazard ratio between 1.58 and 2.24. Incidence of anxiety was 4.7%, followed by depression at 2%. When further expanding the patient population to target the rate of all psychiatric illnesses (including relapses) by day 90 after a COVID-19 diagnosis, the probability increased to 18.1%, with anxiety at 12.8% and mood disorders at 9.9% (Taquet et al. 2021).

Schizophrenia

Researchers in New York City studied 7,348 patients for 45 days after their COVID-19 diagnosis and found that among those who had a prior diagnosis of a schizophrenia spectrum disorder there was an increased risk of mortality (OR 2.67) even after adjusting for demographics and medical comorbidities (Nemani et al. 2021). This was not the case with those who had a diagnosis of mood or anxiety spectrum disorders.

Substance Use Disorders

A retrospective case-control study from June 15, 2020, in patients with a new diagnosis of SUD within the previous year found that this population had an AOR of being diagnosed with COVID-19 of 8.7, with an even stronger association among those with opioid use disorder, with an AOR of 10.244 (Wang et al. 2021b). The study found that patients with a SUD had significantly higher prevalence of several known COVID-19 risk factors (chronic kidney, liver, and lung diseases; cardiovascular diseases; type 2 diabetes; obesity; and cancer), and among people with recent SUD diagnoses, African Americans had an AOR of 2.2 of contracting COVID-19 compared with whites, with an even greater effect in those with opioid use disorder (AOR 4.162). The study also found worse morbidity and mortality among patients with SUD (hospitalization rate of 41% and mortality rate of 9.6%) compared with those without SUD (hospitalization rate of 30% and mortality rate of 6.6%). African Americans with SUD and COVID-19 had worse outcomes compared with whites with SUD and COVID-19 (hospitalization rate of 50.7% vs. 35.2% and death rate of 13% vs. 8.6%, respectively). The study also found that among patients with recent SUD diagnoses, senior citizens were more likely to develop COVID-19 (AOR 1.3) and African Americans were more likely to develop COVID-19 compared with whites (2.1).

Overdoses

In a study that evaluated nearly 20 million U.S. ED visits from December 30, 2018, to October 10, 2020, although total ED visits decreased after COVID-19 mitigation measures were implemented, the median visit counts for suicide attempts and all overdose types (prescription or illicit substances, including opioids) were significantly higher (Holland et al. 2021). During this same period, visit counts for physical intimate partner violence were also significantly higher (Gosangi et al. 2021). Opioid overdoses, in particular, exhibited the most consistent increases in visit counts. Reasons for this increase could include changes in the illicit drug supply during the pandemic, more free time, use of opioids in a more isolated or higher-risk fashion increasing the likelihood of an overdose, or the reduction of access to naloxone or other risk reduction services. These results demonstrate that although ED visits decreased, visits for these outcomes did not decrease to the same extent as overall ED visits, raising concern that suicide attempts, overdoses, and violence remain an issue during the pandemic (Holland et al. 2021).

Dementia

Dementia has been strongly associated with other known COVID-19 risk factors such as cardiovascular diseases, diabetes, obesity, and hypertension (Baumgart et al. 2015; Nelis et al. 2019; Schubert et al. 2006). A retrospective case-control study representing 20% of the U.S. population found that patients with dementia had a twofold increased association with COVID-19 infection, with a hospitalization risk of 59% and a 6-month mortality risk of 21% (Wang et al. 2021a). The study further found that Black individuals with dementia had close to nearly a three times higher risk of death compared with whites with dementia (AOR 2.86) even after controlling for COVID-19 risk factors, suggesting that other factors such as access to health care, socioeconomic status, and social adversity may have contributed to this significant racial disparity. Of note, the study also found that the impact of dementia on the risk for COVID-19 infection persisted even after controlling for nursing home care (Wang et al. 2021a).

MORTALITY

In August 2020, a *New York Times* analysis used CDC estimates comparing death rates in the United States during the previous 5 years and found that at least 200,000 more people had died than would have been expected between March and late July 2020; however, accounting for the deaths directly attributable to COVID-19 leaves approximately 60,000 more deaths that occurred during that time period (Lu 2020). These excess deaths were also discovered by an analysis of a similar time period using data from the National Center for Health Statistics that found 225,000 additional deaths, 65% of which were estimated to be attributable to COVID-19 (Woolf et al. 2020). The remaining 35% were thought to be not directly related to COVID-19, but rather were related to other conditions such as diabetes, heart disease, Alzheimer's disease, and cerebrovascular disease. Although the excess deaths from the former analysis may include nonrespiratory complications of COVID-19, the remaining additional deaths may have been from societal disruptions that reduced or delayed access to health care and worsening medical conditions associated with SDOH (Cooper and Williams 2020).

A British study found that mortality risk from COVID-19 among ethnic minority groups was twice that of white patients after controlling for age, sex, income, education, housing tenure, and neighborhood level of deprivation (Public Health England 2020). Another U.K. study found that racial/ethnic disparities persisted after accounting for occupational exposure, population density, household composition, and preexisting health conditions (Government Equalities Office et al. 2020). Razai et al. (2021) argued that racism on societal and individual levels has both direct and indirect negative effects on health, contributing to many of the sustained disparities among ethnic groups even after controlling for known risk factors from SDOH.

An American research duo used pandemic data through December 2020 to estimate life expectancy among different groups using four scenarios (one with no COVID deaths and the others with low to high mortality projections) and found drastic disparities across race and ethnicities. Although overall they found a 1.13-year reduction in life expectancy at birth, causing the lowest life expectancy of any year since 2003, they found Black populations to have an estimated 2.10-year reduction and Latinx populations to have an estimated 3.05-year reduction, along with a nearly 40% increase in Black-white life expectancy gap, from 3.6 to 5 years (Andrasfay and Goldman 2021).

FUTURE DIRECTIONS

Interventions

Strategies and tools are available to reduce the incidence and impact of COVID-19 in communities with increased burden from SDOH. First, addressing the intersectionality of SDOH, older age, risk factors for COVID-19 infection, and access to care issues can reduce the impact of the disease on vulnerable populations. Other strategies may involve community engagement, education, advocacy, political action, and using the social determinants framework as a guide to address structural and systemic racism and poverty and to provide timely and targeted preventive interventions in a way that ensures equal access (Compton and Shim 2020).

Community-Based Participatory Research

Community-based participatory research (CBPR) is a partnership approach to conducting research that seeks to equitably involve all members of a community: community members themselves, organizational representatives, and academic researchers. Within the domain of public health, CBPR holds promise in supporting collaborative interventions that involve both scientific researchers and community members to address the spread of disease and conditions that disproportionately affect communities affected by SDOH (National Institute on Minority Health and Health Disparities 2018). When communities are involved in CBPR, their input into the project helps ensure that interventions created are responsive to and appropriate for the community's needs. The COVID-19 pandemic presents an opportunity to participate in CBPR projects and protocols that develop COVID-19-related interventions for communities, especially given that COVID-19 disproportionately affects historically marginalized communities and those affected by SDOH. Despite the challenges of in-person CBPR protocols in the time of the pandemic, movement toward a virtual or online CBPR framework is feasible and efficacious (Valdez and Gubrium 2020).

Lessons Learned

Vaccine Distribution

Jean-Jacques and Bauchner (2021) outlined four guidelines for making COVID-19 vaccine distribution more equitable: 1) prioritize distribution to zip codes most severely affected by COVID-19 and with high indexes of economic hardship, 2) partner with local institutions and organizations that have already built trust in the community, 3) prioritize distribution via mobile outreach solutions to people with mobility or other transportation barriers, and 4) simplify registration procedures to accommodate noncitizens and individuals who have limited technology comfort or limited English proficiency or literacy.

Four Domains of Intervention

Metzl et al. (2020) urged us to use the coming months and years to rehaul the U.S. health care system to address inequities by redesigning the health care delivery and educational systems through a lens of health equity and racial justice. Metzl and Hansen (2014) urged for structural competency, which uses principles from sociology, economics, urban planning, and other disciplines, to be taught to health care professionals and other key players in health care systems to "recognize ways that institutions, neighborhood conditions, market forces, public policies, and health care delivery systems shape symptoms and diseases" (p. 231). Metzl et al. (2020) suggested four domains of intervention: promoting truth and reconciliation, reimagining infrastructure, democratizing information, and educating.

SUMMARY

SDOH have significantly affected health outcomes for both medical and psychiatric disorders in the COVID-19 pandemic. SDOH such as older age and belonging to a historically marginalized group increase the likelihood of health conditions such as obesity, diabetes, chronic respiratory disorders, cardiovascular and cerebrovascular disorders, and dementia, which themselves have been identified as risk factors in contracting COVID-19 infection and resulting in poorer outcomes. The COVID-19 pandemic has brought to light the impact of SDOH on the medical and psychiatric morbidity and mortality outcomes for older adults, among others, both in the United States and globally. Most of the medical comorbidities that are associated with higher morbidity and mortality from COVID-19 are highly linked to underlying socioeconomic differences and other types of inequities. COVID-19 has also been associated with worsening mental health outcomes in depression, suicide, anxiety disorders, and SUDs. Using the SDOH framework as a guide, clinicians and researchers can work to address structural and systemic racism and poverty and create interventions targeted to COVID-19 and to prevent future pandemics.

KEY POINTS

- Social determinants of health (SDOH) affect health outcomes for both medical and psychiatric disorders. In addition to older age itself, SDOH can increase the likelihood of several health conditions, including obesity, diabetes, chronic respiratory disorders, cardiovascular and cerebrovascular disorders, and dementia, which themselves have been identified as risk factors in contracting COVID-19 and resulting in poorer outcomes.

- Although SDOH and health care disparities affected communities long before the COVID-19 pandemic, the pandemic has both highlighted and exacerbated the impact of SDOH on medical and psychiatric morbidity and mortality, especially among marginalized and vulnerable communities. In general, pandemics and other times of crisis tend to act like a mirror, reflecting already existing vulnerabilities and inequities in society.

- In moving toward a postpandemic world, it is important to implement strategies and tools to reduce the incidence and impact of COVID-19 in communities that are most affected by SDOH. At the forefront of this effort is vaccine distribution; health care systems and providers should consistently strive for equitable COVID-19 vaccine distribution by prioritizing communities with limited access to health care and/or technology, partnering with communities to better address their needs, and communicating health information in a clear and accessible way.

QUESTIONS FOR REVIEW

1. According to Healthy People 2020, which of the following is a key area of social determinants of health (SDOH)?

    A. Recreational setting
    B. Community design
    C. Economic stability
    D. Exposure to toxic substances
    E. Physical barriers, especially for people with disabilities

Answer: C.

2. Which of the following statements about dementia has *not* been supported by early COVID-19 data on morbidity and mortality?

    A. Black individuals with dementia have a significantly higher risk of death from COVID-19 compared with white individuals with dementia.
    B. Dementia is associated with increased COVID-19 infection only in individuals living in skilled care facilities and not in community-dwelling individuals.
    C. Dementia has been strongly associated with multiple known COVID-19 risk factors.
    D. A diagnosis of dementia was found to be an independent risk factor in increasing risk of COVID-19 infection, hospitalization, and mortality at 6 months after COVID-19 infection.

Answer: B.

3. Which of the following is a SDOH risk factor increasing morbidity and mortality for COVID-19?

    A. Younger age
    B. Living in multigenerational households
    C. Living in rural areas
    D. Female sex

Answer: B.

ADDITIONAL RESOURCES

American Psychiatric Association: Social determinants of health. Washington, DC, American Psychiatric Association, 2020. Available at: www.psychiatry.org/File%20Library/Psychiatrists/Directories/Library-and-Archive/resource_documents/Resource-Document-2020-Social-Determinants-of-Health.pdf. Accessed July 3, 2021.

American Psychiatric Association: COVID-19 pandemic guidance document: the role of the psychiatrist in the equitable distribution of the Covid-19 vaccine. Washington, DC, American Psychiatric Association, 2021. Available at: www.psychiatry.org/File%20Library/Psychiatrists/APA-Guidance-Psychiatrists-Role-in-Equitable-Distribution-COVID-19-Vaccine.pdf. Accessed July 3, 2021.

Compton MT, Shim RS: Mental illness prevention and mental health promotion: when, who, and how. Psychiatr Serv 71(9):981–983, 2020 32867610

Shim RS, Vinson SY: Social (In)Justice and Mental Health. Washington, DC, American Psychiatric Association Publishing, 2021

REFERENCES

Abrams EM, Szefler SJ: COVID-19 and the impact of social determinants of health. Lancet Respir Med 8(7):659–661, 2020 32437646

Ali S, Asaria M, Stranges S: COVID-19 and inequality: are we all in this together? Can J Public Health 111(3):415–416, 2020 32578185

Andrasfay T, Goldman N: Reductions in 2020 US life expectancy due to COVID-19 and the disproportionate impact on the Black and Latino populations. Proc Natl Acad Sci USA 118(5):e2014746118, 2021 33446511

Arias E, Tejada-Vera B, Ahmad F, Kochanek KD: Provisional life expectancy estimates for 2020. Vital Statistics Rapid Release Rep No 15. Hyattsville, MD, National Center for Health Statistics, July 2021

Baggett TP, Keyes H, Sporn N, et al: Prevalence of SARS-CoV-2 infection in residents of a large homeless shelter in Boston. JAMA 323(21):2191–2192, 2020 32338732

Baumgart M, Snyder HM, Carrillo MC, et al: Summary of the evidence on modifiable risk factors for cognitive decline and dementia: a population-based perspective. Alzheimers Dement 11(6):718–726, 2015 26045020

Bernstein H, Gonzalez D, Karpman M, et al: One in seven adults in immigrant families reported avoiding public benefit programs in 2018. Washington, DC, Urban Institute, May 22, 2019. Available at: www.urban.org/research/publication/one-seven-adults-immigrant-families-reported-avoiding-public-benefit-programs-2018. Accessed April 25, 2021.

Blau FD, Koebe J, Meyerhofer PA: Who are the essential and frontline workers? Cambridge, MA, National Bureau of Economic Research, 2020. Available at: www.nber.org/papers/w27791. Accessed July 3, 2021.

Centers for Disease Control and Prevention: NCHHSTP social determinants of health. Atlanta, GA, Centers for Disease Control and Prevention, December 19, 2019. Available at: www.cdc.gov/nchhstp/socialdeterminants/index.html. Accessed April 25, 2021.

Centers for Disease Control and Prevention: Health equity considerations and racial and ethnic minority groups. Atlanta, GA, Centers for Disease Control and Prevention, April 12, 2020. Available at: www.cdc.gov/coronavirus/2019-ncov/community/health-equity/race-ethnicity.html. Accessed April 25, 2021.

Chotiner I: How pandemics change history. The New Yorker, March 3, 2020. Available at: www.newyorker.com/news/q-and-a/how-pandemics-change-history. Accessed April 26, 2021.

Clark HM: Who rides public transportation. Washington, DC, American Public Transportation Association, January 2017. Available at: /www.apta.com/wp-content/uploads/Resources/resources/reportsandpublications/Documents/APTA-Who-Rides-Public-Transportation-2017.pdf. Accessed April 26, 2021.

Compton MT, Shim RS: The social determinants of mental health. Focus 13(4):419–425, 2015

Compton MT, Shim RS: Mental illness prevention and mental health promotion: when, who, and how. Psychiatr Serv 71(9):981–983, 2020 32867610

Cooper LA, Williams DR: Excess deaths from COVID-19, community bereavement, and restorative justice for communities of color. JAMA 324(15):1491–1492, 2020 33044518

Czeisler MÉ, Lane RI, Petrosky E, et al: Mental health, substance use, and suicidal ideation during the COVID-19 pandemic—United States, June 24–30, 2020. MMWR Morb Mortal Wkly Rep 69(32):1049–1057, 2020 32790653

Ettman CK, Abdalla SM, Cohen GH, et al: Prevalence of depression symptoms in US adults before and during the COVID-19 pandemic. JAMA Netw Open 3(9):e2019686, 2020 32876685

Federico MJ, McFarlane AE II, Szefler SJ, et al: The impact of social determinants of health on children with asthma. J Allergy Clin Immunol Pract 8(6):1808–1814, 2020 32294541

Gfroerer J, Dube S, King B, et al: Vital signs: current cigarette smoking among adults aged ≥ 18 years with mental illness—United States, 2009–2011. MMWR Morb Mortal Wkly Rep 62(5):81–87, 2013 23388551

González-Sanguino C, Ausín B, Castellanos MÁ, et al: Mental health consequences during the initial stage of the 2020 Coronavirus pandemic (COVID-19) in Spain. Brain Behav Immun 87:172–176, 2020 32405150

Gosangi B, Park H, Thomas R, et al: Exacerbation of physical intimate partner violence during COVID-19 pandemic. Radiology 298(1):E38–E45, 2021 32787700

Government Equalities Office, Race Disparity Unit, and Badenoch K: Quarterly report on progress to address COVID-19 health inequalities. HM Government, October 22, 2020. Available at: www.gov.uk/government/publications/quarterly-report-on-progress-to-address-covid-19-health-inequalities. Accessed April 3, 2021.

Greenaway C, Hargreaves S, Barkati S, et al: COVID-19: Exposing and address-ing health disparities among ethnic minorities and migrants. J Travel Med 27(7):taaa113, 2020 32706375

Holland S, Jones C, Vivolo-Kantor AM, et al: Trends in ED visits for mental health, overdose, and violence outcomes before and during the COVID-19 pandemic. JAMA Psychiatry 78(4):327–379, 2021

Intensive Care National Audit and Research Centre: COVID-19 report. London, Intensive Care National Audit and Research Cetnre, 2020. Available at: www.icnarc.org/our-audit/audits/cmp/reports. Accessed February 24, 2021.

Jean-Jacques M, Bauchner H: Vaccine distribution—equity left behind? JAMA 325(9):829–830, 2021 33512381

Kirksey L, Tucker DL, Taylor E Jr, et al: Pandemic superimposed on epidemic: Covid-19 disparities in Back Americans. J Natl Med Assoc 113(1):39–42, 2021 32747313

Klaiber P, Wen JH, DeLongis A, et al: The ups and downs of daily life during COVID-19: age differences in affect, stress, and positive events. J Gerontol B Psychol Sci Soc Sci 76(2):e30–e37, 2021 32674138

Kondo N, Sembajwe G, Kawachi I, et al: Income inequality, mortality, and self rated health: meta-analysis of multilevel studies. BMJ 339(7731):b4471, 2009 19903981

Lasser K, Boyd JW, Woolhandler S, et al: Smoking and mental illness: a population-based prevalence study. JAMA 284(20):2606–2610, 2000 11086367

Lee SW, Yang JM, Moon SY, et al: Association between mental illness and COVID-19 susceptibility and clinical outcomes in South Korea: a nationwide cohort study. Lancet Psychiatry 7(12):1025–1031, 2020 32950066

Lu D: The true coronavirus toll in the U.S. has already surpassed 200,000. New York Times, August 12, 2020. Available at: www.nytimes.com/interactive/2020/08/12/us/covid-deaths-us.html. Accessed April 25, 2021.

Mack DS, Jesdale BM, Ulbricht CM, et al: Racial segregation across U.S. nursing homes: a systematic review of measurement and outcomes. Gerontologist 60(3):e218–e231, 2020 31141135

McKnight-Eily LR, Okoro CA, Strine TW, et al: Racial and ethnic disparities in the prevalence of stress and worry, mental health conditions, and increased substance use among adults during the COVID-19 pandemic—United States, April and May 2020. MMWR Morb Mortal Wkly Rep 70(5):162–166, 2021 33539336

Metzl JM, Hansen H: Structural competency: theorizing a new medical engage-ment with stigma and inequality. Soc Sci Med 103:126–133, 2014 24507917

Metzl JM, Maybank A, De Maio F: Responding to the COVID-19 pandemic: the need for a structurally competent health care system. JAMA 324(3):231–232, 2020 32496531

National Institute on Minority Health and Health Disparities: Community-based participatory research program (CBPR). Bethesda, MD, National In-stitute on Minority Health and Health Disparities, October 2, 2018. Avail-able at: www.nimhd.nih.gov/programs/extramural/community-based-participatory.html. Accessed July 3, 2021.

Nelis SM, Wu Y-T, Matthews FE, et al: The impact of co-morbidity on the quality of life of people with dementia: findings from the IDEAL study. Age Age-ing 48(3):361–367, 2019 30403771

Nemani K, Li C, Olfson M, et al: Association of psychiatric disorders with mortality among patients with COVID-19. JAMA Psychiatry 78(4):380–386, 2021 33502436

Office of Disease Prevention and Health Promotion: Healthy People 2020: social determinants of health. Rockville, MD, Office of Disease Prevention and Health Promotion, 2021a. Available at: www.healthypeople.gov/2020/topics-objectives/topic/social-determinants-of-health/objectives. Accessed April 25, 2021.

Office of Disease Prevention and Health Promotion: Healthy People 2030: social determinants of health. Rockville, MD, Office of Disease Prevention and Health Promotion, 2021b. Available at: https://health.gov/healthypeople/objectives-and-data/social-determinants-health. Accessed July 1, 2021.

Patel SY, Mehrotra A, Huskamp HA, et al: Variation in telemedicine use and outpatient care during the COVID-19 pandemic in The United States. Health Aff (Millwood) 40(2):349–358, 2021 33523745

Public Health England: Disparities in the risk and outcomes of COVID-19. Public Health England, August 2020. Available at: https://assets.publishing.service.gov.uk/government/uploads/system/uploads/attachment_data/file/908434/Disparities_in_the_risk_and_outcomes_of_COVID_August_2020_update.pdf. Accessed July 2, 2021.

Rahman M, Foster AD: Racial segregation and quality of care disparity in US nursing homes. J Health Econ 39:1–16, 2015 25461895

Razai MS, Kankam HKN, Majeed A, et al: Mitigating ethnic disparities in Covid-19 and beyond. BMJ 372:m4921, 2021 33446485

Schubert CC, Boustani M, Callahan CM, et al: Comorbidity profile of dementia patients in primary care: are they sicker? J Am Geriatr Soc 54(1):104–109, 2006 16420205

Schwartzapfel B, Park K, Demillo A: 1 in 5 prisoners in the U.S. has had COVID-19. New York, The Marshall Project, December 18, 2020. Available at: www.themarshallproject.org/2020/12/18/1-in-5-prisoners-in-the-u-s-has-had-covid-19. Accessed April 25, 2021.

Sentencing Project: Report to the United Nations on racial disparities in the U.S. criminal justice system. Washington, DC, The Sentencing Project, April 19, 2018. Available at: www.sentencingproject.org/publications/un-report-on-racial-disparities/. Accessed April 25, 2021.

Shippee TP, Akosionu O, Ng W, et al: COVID-19 pandemic: exacerbating racial/ethnic disparities in long-term services and supports. J Aging Soc Policy 32(4–5):323–333, 2020 32476614

Sommers BD, Allen H, Bhanja A, et al: Assessment of perceptions of the public charge rule among low-income adults in Texas. JAMA Netw Open 3(7):e2010391, 2020 32667651

Stansfeld SA, Fuhrer R, Shipley MJ, et al: Work characteristics predict psychiatric disorder: prospective results from the Whitehall II study. Occup Environ Med 56(5):302–307, 1999 10472303

Tai DBG, Shah A, Doubeni CA, et al: The disproportionate impact of COVID-19 on racial and ethnic minorities in the United States. Clin Infect Dis 72(4):703–706, 2021 32562416

Taquet M, Luciano S, Geddes JR, et al: Bidirectional associations between COVID-19 and psychiatric disorder: retrospective cohort studies of 62 354 COVID-19 cases in the USA. Lancet Psychiatry 8(2):130–140, 2021 33181098

Thomas D: Why Micronesians are being disproportionately affected by COVID-19. Honolulu, Hawai'i Budget and Policy Center, August 19, 2020. Available at: www.hibudget.org/blog/micronesians-disproportionately-affected-covid-19. Accessed April 25, 2021.

Tsai J, Wilson M: COVID-19: a potential public health problem for homeless populations. Lancet Public Health 5(4):e186–e187, 2020 32171054

U.S. Bureau of Labor Statistics: Employed persons by detailed occupation, sex, race, and Hispanic or Latino ethnicity. Washington, DC, U.S. Bureau of Labor Statistics, January 22, 2021. Available at: www.bls.gov/cps/cpsaat11.htm. Accessed April 25, 2021.

U.S. Census Bureau: Health insurance coverage in the United States 2018. Washington, DC, U.S. Census Bureau, November 8, 2019. Available at: www.census.gov/library/publications/2019/demo/p60-267.html. Accessed July 2, 2021.

Vahia IV, Jeste DV, Reynolds CF III: Older adults and the mental health effects of COVID-19. JAMA 324(22):2253–2254, 2020 33216114

Valdez ES, Gubrium A: Shifting to virtual CBPR protocols in the time of corona virus/COVID-19. Int J Qual Methods 19:1609406920977315, 2020

Vanable PA, Carey MP, Carey KB, et al: Smoking among psychiatric outpatients: relationship to substance use, diagnosis, and illness severity. Psychol Addict Behav 17(4):259–265, 2003 14640821

Vardavas CI, Nikitara K: COVID-19 and smoking: a systematic review of the evidence. Tob Induc Dis 18:20, 2020 32206052

Wang Q, Davis PB, Gurney ME, et al: COVID-19 and dementia: analyses of risk, disparity, and outcomes from electronic health records in the US. Alzheimers Dement Feb 9, 2021a 33559975 Epub ahead of print

Wang QQ, Kaelber DC, Xu R, et al: COVID-19 risk and outcomes in patients with substance use disorders: analyses from electronic health records in the United States. Mol Psychiatry 26(1):30–39, 2021b 32929211

Wang Q, Xu R, Volkow ND: Increased risk of COVID-19 infection and mortality in people with mental disorders: analysis from electronic health records in the United States. World Psychiatry 20(1):124–130, 2021c 33026219

Wilkinson RG: Income distribution and life expectancy. BMJ 304(6820):165–168, 1992 1637372

Woolf SH, Chapman DA, Sabo RT, et al: Excess deaths from COVID-19 and other causes, March–July 2020. JAMA 324(15):1562–1564, 2020 33044483

World Health Organization: Closing the gap in a generation: health equity through action on the Social determinants of health: final report of the Commission on Social Determinants of Health. Geneva, World Health Organization, 2008. Available at: www.who.int/publications/i/item/WHO-IER-CSDH-08.1. Accessed April 26, 2021.

Yancy CW: COVID-19 and African Americans. JAMA 323(19):1891–1892, 2020 32293639

CHAPTER 11

THE EFFECT OF COVID-19 ON RESEARCH

Tales From a Pandemic

Maria Loizos, Ph.D.
Judith Neugroschl, M.D.

The coronavirus SARS-CoV-2 disease (COVID-19) pandemic has disproportionately affected older adults and therefore has had an enormous impact on every aspect of aging clinical research from recruitment to study procedures to retention to outcomes. We review some of the challenges in continuing research in Alzheimer's disease and the steps taken to minimize disruptions.

Vignette

Mrs. J, a cognitively intact 76-year-old widowed Latina from East Harlem, New York City, was scheduled for her annual visit for cognitive testing and a physician evaluation on March 20, 2020. Because of the COVID-19 pandemic, all in-person research was halted, and Mrs. J worried that she would miss her yearly visit. Medical staff were able to rapidly restructure the cognitive testing battery and change the entire visit and evaluation forms to be done over the phone. Because Mrs. J did not have internet access, research staff reached her via her landline on March 30 and were able to perform the full adapted battery, take a careful history, and ask about targeted neurological symptoms. Her visit underwent a clinical consensus conference over the telephone with a neuropsychologist and geriatric psychiatrist and was submitted to the national Alzheimer's subject database. Mrs. J continued to be cognitively intact, although her depression score was mildly elevated (Geriatric Depression Scale=6/15, mildly depressed) and she was feeling isolated because her children were living in New Jersey. She was making a plan to move to her daughter's home the following week, where she would continue to quarantine.

In the early days of the COVID-19 pandemic in New York, shelter-in-place guidelines were enacted, and clinical research was halted by the Icahn School of Medicine at Mount Sinai's institutional review board on March 15, 2020. Clinical research is a collaborative process with researchers and staff working with volunteers who have put enormous efforts into participating in ongoing research funded through the government, private institutions, and companies. However, in the face of the pandemic, we were in a bind. We could not put our participants at risk, but abandoning the research would be to devalue the enormous efforts and contributions that they had given. We therefore needed to quickly change our research efforts to remote platforms to be able to meet the needs of our participants as well as maintain the aims of the research as much as was feasible.

To review the effect of COVID-19 on clinical research, we are using New York City and, specifically, the Mount Sinai's Alzheimer's Disease Research Center (ISMMS ADRC) as an exemplar of how clinical research was performed during the pandemic. In this chapter we explore the varied effects of the pandemic on clinical research: development of new compounds, enrollment, retention, actual conducting of research, patient safety, and outcomes. It will likely take years to fully appreciate the impact of COVID-19, particularly as it relates to underrepresented groups. COVID-19 affects older adults and people of color more (in terms of both frequency of infection and severity of disease; Rhodus et al. 2020; Yancy 2020). Both of these groups are underrepresented in clinical research generally, and COVID-19 will likely compound these disparities.

IMPACT OF THE PANDEMIC ON RESEARCH OPERATIONS

When the COVID-19 pandemic was declared and cases were rising in New York City, all in-person research was halted to protect the safety of ISMMS ADRC staff and participants and to respect the public health imperative to minimize disease spread (Parry 2020). Staff transitioned to working remotely, with institutional resources such as information technology support, remote access guides, and videoconferencing accounts. It was necessary to track study participants, access data, and manage workflow while ensuring appropriate data security. A significant investment of information technology and personnel time was required to create new mechanisms to permit anonymized sharing of documents. This allowed clinical research coordinators to determine which participants were due for assessment, had completed assessments, had undergone a consensus diagnostic conference, and were ready to be submitted to the national database.

Because in-person testing was no longer feasible, the ISMMS ADRC determined that remote testing was in the best interest of older participants and staff (Nicol et al. 2020). In order to ensure that all participants had equal access to testing, we decided to administer the testing battery via telephone rather than using video. This format meant using a modality that was already familiar to our participants instead of spending time teaching a new assessment method (e.g., videoconferencing) that may not be accessible to all. Additionally, videoconferencing was subject to speech delays due to internet connectivity, which could compromise the participant's ability to accurately hear certain tasks and interfere with timed tasks. Avoiding closed captioning was also important because it could compromise the validity of verbal memory tasks. Thus, electronic versions of our cognitive battery were adapted for the telephone and went through multiple rounds of formatting and testing to ensure their usability and functionality.

IMPACT ON PARTICIPANT SAFETY, OPERATIONS, AND ENGAGEMENT

Because of the varying infection rates across the country, there was no unified approach from leadership on how to conduct clinical research during the pandemic. The ISMMS ADRC advocated for patient safety to sponsors (i.e., pharmaceutical companies and national Alzheimer's consortia) who were based in other parts of the country and outside COVID-19 hot spots. This included requesting modifications to research plans (e.g., changing to a hybrid model or going completely remote) and support for technology to facilitate remote data collection (e.g., tablets).

Once it was determined that a primarily remote model was to be adopted for our longitudinal research, another challenge encountered was contacting participants to participate. Some of our older participants moved out of New York City to stay with family during the pandemic, making it difficult to reach them. Participants who were used to receiving calls from our hospital system were wary of answering calls from staff working remotely and calling from unfamiliar or blocked numbers. This added to the difficulty of scheduling appointments. One solution for these challenges was to leave messages with a callback number or find additional ways to contact participants either by email or via their study partner. Once participants were contacted to schedule their visit, some wished to delay their participation until we were back in the office—it became clear that participating in research is a social event for many older adults, and the loss of face-to-face contact was noted as a reason some were hesitant to participate remotely. As the pandemic dragged on, most were willing to have a virtual visit.

Although we enacted a plan at the ISMMS ADRC to conduct research remotely to keep participants safe, one concern was that older adults would be less familiar with and have less access to technology. Interestingly, of the English-speaking subjects who agreed to participate in the telephone testing and clinician visit for our longitudinal study, the vast majority were using technology: 86% used a smartphone, 76% used a laptop, and 51% used a tablet, with <1% using no technology. Use of devices for text, instant messaging, and email (92%) and news and information (86%) was surprisingly common. Only 37% of participants had participated in a telehealth visit, but this number is likely to increase as the pandemic continues.

With regard to demographics and diversity, the subjects who participated in our telephone assessments and completed our technology use questionnaire were more educated than our overall cohort (mean 17 years vs. 15 years) and represented a higher percentage of non-Hispanic whites (65% vs. 51%). Because it took time to translate, edit, and review Spanish versions of the questionnaire, the data on non-English-speaking participants are being collected only now. It will be crucial to explore technology access and use in the full range of diverse subjects in our cohort because the differences in our sample demographics seen here underscore the challenges that we face during the pandemic to embrace equity and equal access to research for diverse participants.

As the pandemic continued, there was ongoing discussion about remaining completely remote or embracing a hybrid model. For each study and each subject visit, the individual components were examined closely to identify aspects that could be done remotely (e.g., interviews, certain cognitive tests). Evaluations that required in-person contact included specific cognitive measures requiring writing, drawing, or interactive coordinator feedback; components of the physical and neurological exams; and procedures such as blood draws, checking vital signs, infusions, and imaging. Small, windowless testing rooms needed to be abandoned for other spaces such as negative pressure rooms and larger rooms that allowed for social distancing. New cleaning protocols were embraced, and therefore, greater time between patient visits was needed in, for example, the imaging suite. Adequate personal protective equipment (PPE), including eye coverings and additional masks, needed to be procured.

Although testing was conducted primarily via telephone, for some of our interventional trials, videoconferencing was necessary for collecting certain trial data such as results of neurological examinations and specific cognitive testing measures. Some older adults were already using various videoconferencing platforms to communicate with friends and family and were therefore familiar with the technology. For others, it was necessary for research coordinators to walk participants through the process of downloading the platform and assisting with any connectivity issues. At times a family member or close contact was needed to assist with the process. Other issues, particularly for underrepresented or diverse groups, included phone plans with limited minutes as well as limited availability of Wi-Fi. In those instances, an hour-long telehealth visit by phone was not feasible. Coordinators tried to help the subjects find safe and free Wi-Fi and direct them to free e-phone service through an app.

ARE THE DATA BEING COLLECTED COMPARABLE?

Moving our research to remote platforms leaves many unanswered questions. The comparability of remote assessments with in-person testing is a concept that is still being evaluated. With regard to remote cognitive assessments, issues concerning cheating (e.g., writing down word lists), lack of nonverbal cues, and different testing conditions (e.g., noise or distractions at home vs. in a clinical setting) were noted. Managing anxiety as well as encouragement also needed to be considered as potential confounders. Although research on the reliability of remote cognitive assessment visits is available (Cullum et al. 2006, 2014), much of this research was conducted while the patient was in a clinic setting and not while the participant was at home alone. Further research will need to be conducted to assess comparability between at-home and in-person testing. Additionally, assessing neurological symptoms (e.g., signs of rigidity, gait) is more difficult remotely than in person, although research indicates adequate reliability of remote neurological visits (Awadallah et al. 2018).

It is also important to underscore the disproportionate effect of COVID-19 on minorities. Inequities in the social determinants of health, such as poverty and health care access, negatively affect these communities (Kim and Bostwick 2020; Sood and Sood 2021; Yancy 2020). Beyond the obvious impact on communities and the differential impacts on health and health outcomes, this pandemic may have further implications on research by diverse participants. Will willingness to participate be affected by chronic illnesses, greater risk of infection, and confidence in the ability of medical and research communities to ensure safety? Will underrepresented communities, particularly those with lower levels of education or less access to technology, be excluded from research because they are unable to participate for technology or logistical reasons? Will these communities be further disenfranchised because reaching them for recruitment requires more creativity and effort on the part of researchers?

IMPACT ON RETENTION

Throughout the pandemic, Alzheimer's disease centers across the country prioritized reaching out to their communities and providing support to participants who were struggling with the local effects of COVID-19. Our ADRC developed a COVID-19 questionnaire in order to explore changes in mood, anxiety, and caregiving challenges. The impact on our participants was substantial. Of the 195 subjects who completed the questionnaire, 30% reported the loss of a family member or close friend to COVID-19, 23% were worried about financial stability, 46% reported anxiety, and 27% self-characterized as depressed. In response, our ADRC social worker contacted participants who were having difficulties and provided support and connections to services as necessary.

Another challenge in research that was heightened by the pandemic was retention of participants. A yearly event held by our ADRC to increase engagement as well as to give thanks for participation in our center is Participant Appreciation Day (PAD). PAD is usually a full-day event filled with guest lecturers, lunch, and activities for participants and their friends and families. To maintain engagement, a shortened PAD was held virtually over a videoconferencing platform. Participants were invited via email or phone and were provided links to the event or a phone number to call. Coordinators were on hand to assist with any connectivity issues prior to and on the day of the event. Reaching out to subjects without email or other technology has represented a challenge requiring significant staff time. However, with the success of the initial program, further educational sessions are planned over the year.

IMPACT ON RECRUITMENT INTO RESEARCH

Bringing new participants into research essentially stalled during the pandemic. Until vaccines have been widely distributed and the virus is truly contained, outreach and enrollment will remain a safety challenge. Even with greater knowledge and availability of PPE, issues of safety with evaluation and study procedures continue to limit recruitment efforts. This in turn will hamper the collection and interpretation of data and therefore slow down the availability of study outcomes, handicapping the acquisition of new knowledge in the field. Studies that required extensive in-person assessments (either physical evaluations, blood draws, or other biomarker acquisition and/or in-person cognitive testing protocols) still remain difficult to recruit for, and negotiations continue with centralized sponsoring organizations to advocate for more hybrid measures to ensure safety. In our center, new evaluations were completely halted except for one study for which the procedures (a behavioral-experiential intervention) could be implemented remotely.

Outreach activities to share research opportunities have been essentially halted, or if they take place, they are in the context of virtual talks. This, again, likely disadvantages underrepresented minority participants, whose participation is so crucial in ensuring that the results of studies are generalizable. In our active longitudinal cohort, which tracks the memory health and/or cognitive decline of diverse elders over time, historically, 26% of non-Hispanic Blacks and 38% of Hispanics were recruited through in-person community memory talks.

GENERAL IMPLICATIONS

Effect on Functioning of Clinical Research Operations

The financial impact of the pandemic on research centers will become clearer over time. Particularly for industry-sponsored trials, sites are reimbursed by per subject fees to support the research infrastructure. Patients were not being seen in person, recruitment was halted, and reimbursement for remote assessments was budgeted at lower levels;

therefore, sites will likely face financial difficulties, especially those whose primary funding depends on industry-sponsored trials. However, federal funding was not halted and was disbursed. If staff had to be laid off, that action will slow down reopening efforts, when it is safe to do so.

Effect on Research Results

There are many unanswerable questions concerning the effect of this pandemic on research outcomes and interpretability. Will attrition in ongoing clinical trials lead to a decrease in sample size and therefore make it harder to interpret trial results? Will symptoms from intercurrent COVID-19 infections have an impact on outcome measures? Because there have been reports of some people feeling "foggy" for an extended period after a COVID-19 infection, could that fogginess have an effect on cognitive outcome measures (Columbia University Irving Medical Center 2020)? Because some individuals who have had COVID-19 infections have lingering physical symptoms, will inclusion of these participants affect our understanding of the potential safety of medications under study?

Long-Term Effect on Research Pipeline

There are many unknowns related to the downstream effects on research from nonfederal funding. For example, the Leukemia and Lymphoma Society had to cancel a large portion of its promised funding because of financial losses due to COVID-19, which affected many laboratories, research fellows, and cancer researchers (Cahan 2020; Harris 2020). It is unclear how many other nonprofits, which may rely on donations and may fund small, more speculative pilot projects that in turn may seed future research, were affected (Radecki and Schonfeld 2020). Bench research, which fuels the ideas that later are translated to clinical research, was significantly affected when the pandemic caused labs to close. For example, mice that are used in studying certain diseases have complex genetic breeding programs to make them appropriate to study how genes affect disease. Because many scientists were unable to go to their labs in March and April, mouse strains had to be euthanized, which may set back basic research for months or even years (Grimm 2020).

SUMMARY

In this chapter we described the effect of COVID-19 on clinical research through the lens of the Icahn School of Medicine Alzheimer's Disease

Research Center. Conducting research during a pandemic has presented serious challenges on multiple levels of clinical research, including enrollment, retention, patient safety, conducting the research itself, outcome measures, and, probably, future research. Conducting research via telehealth, although a feasible option that prioritizes patient and staff safety, will require future work to determine whether data are comparable between in-person and remote visits. The full magnitude of the effect that COVID-19 has had on research is presently unclear, and it likely will take years to fully understand its impact. What is clear is the negative effect of COVID-19 on older adults as well as people of color because these effects are not limited to the frequency of infection and severity but also will likely magnify the underrepresentation of these groups in clinical research. Additionally, there are long-term effects on research from the rescinding of promised funding, which could stall or set back research discoveries for many years. Despite these challenges, the determination and creativity of researchers and subjects have led to the creation of new protocols and therefore the continued collection of data. This determination and creativity will ultimately help shape research for years to come. The expansion of telehealth and, hopefully, the confirmation of the reliability of remote data collection will allow for greater participation in research by older adults in general and leave us in a position to manage future pandemics in a more seamless manner. Familiarity with protocols to prevent viral spread, having adequate stockpiles of PPE, and a greater cultural acceptance of mask wearing will help minimize viral spread and allow research to continue.

KEY POINTS

- The COVID-19 pandemic significantly affected research operations and will have lasting effects on basic and clinical research.

- Centers were able to adapt to remote or hybrid research to try to mitigate the effects of the pandemic.

- In addition to having safety concerns and dealing with the effects of COVID-19 infection, study participants were and are under enormous stress, with associated anxiety and depression, which could also have an effect on cognitive research outcomes.

- It is unlikely that we have begun to fully appreciate the long-term effects of the pandemic on research operations and outcomes, especially with regard to marginalized groups,

QUESTIONS FOR REVIEW

1. What patient concerns regarding the COVID-19 pandemic should be considered when discussing cognitive research outcomes?

    A. Cognitive sequelae associated with COVID-19
    B. Lack of access to personal protective equipment (PPE)
    C. Continued stress and associated depression and anxiety, which can have long-term impacts on cognition
    D. A and C

Answer: D.

2. How can research prepare to prevent interruptions in future pandemics?

    A. Revert back to prepandemic practices; future pandemics are unlikely.
    B. Use a hybrid model of data collection, ensure that data collected remotely are reliable, and ensure access to adequate protocols and PPE.
    C. Hospitals and supply chains will prepare; research can rely on other system preparedness.
    D. Transition all research to an outside setting to avoid possibility of impacts from a future pandemic.

Answer: B.

3. How did the COVID-19 pandemic affect the research pipeline?

    A. Pilot and speculative research may have been compromised because some foundations suffered financial reversals.
    B. Basic science research was halted for months in major centers, leading to setbacks (e.g., experiments that were halted midway, mouse strains that had to be euthanized).
    C. Clinical research outcomes may be compromised by loss of data or participants and negative effects on cognition caused by the virus. These concerns may make it difficult to interpret outcomes of clinical trials and therefore may slow the pipeline to approved treatments.
    D. All of the above

Answer: D.

REFERENCES

Awadallah M, Janssen F, Körber B, et al: Telemedicine in general neurology: interrater reliability of clinical neurological examination via audio-visual telemedicine. Eur Neurol 80(5–6):289–294, 2018 30783053

Cahan E: COVID-19 cancels charity galas and walks. Science is paying the price. Science, June 24, 2020. Available at: www.sciencemag.org/news/2020/06/covid-19-cancels-charity-galas-and-walks-science-paying-price. Accessed July 6, 2021.

Columbia University Irving Medical Center: Even mild cases can cause "COVID-19 fog." New York, Columbia University Irving Medical Center, September 21, 2020. Available at: www.cuimc.columbia.edu/news/even-mild-cases-can-cause-covid-19-fog. Accessed July 6, 2021.

Cullum CM, Weiner MF, Gehrmann HR, et al: Feasibility of telecognitive assessment in dementia. Assessment 13(4):385–390, 2006 17050908

Cullum CM, Hynan LS, Grosch M, et al: Teleneuropsychology: evidence for video teleconference-based neuropsychological assessment. J Int Neuropsychol Soc 20(10):1028–1033, 2014 25343269

Grimm D: "It's heartbreaking." Labs are euthanizing thousands of mice in response to coronavirus pandemic. Science, March 23, 2020. Available at: www.sciencemag.org/news/2020/03/it-s-heartbreaking-labs-are-euthanizing-thousands-mice-response-coronavirus-pandemic. Accessed July 6, 2021.

Harris AL: COVID-19 and cancer research. Br J Cancer 123(5):689–690, 2020 32591747

Kim SJ, Bostwick W: Social vulnerability and racial inequality in COVID-19 deaths in Chicago. Health Educ Behav 47(4):509–513, 2020 32436405

Nicol GE, Piccirillo JF, Mulsant BH, et al: Action at a distance: geriatric research during a pandemic. J Am Geriatr Soc 68(5):922–925, 2020 32207542

Parry M: As coronavirus spreads, universities stall their research to keep human subjects safe. The Chronicle of Higher Education, 2020. Available at: www.chronicle.com/article/as-coronavirus-spreads-universities-stall-their-research-to-keep-human-subjects-safe. Accessed July 6, 2021.

Radecki J, Schonfeld R: The impacts of COVID-19 on the research enterprise: a landscape review. Ithaka S+R, 2020. Available at: https://sr.ithaka.org/publications/the-impacts-of-covid-19-on-the-research-enterprise. Accessed July 6, 2021.

Rhodus EK, Bardach SH, Abner EL, et al: COVID-19 and geriatric clinical trials research. Aging Clin Exp Res 32(10):2169–2172, 2020 32939681

Sood L, Sood V: Being African American and rural: a double jeopardy from COVID-19. J Rural Health 37(1):217–221, 2021 32362036

Yancy CW: COVID-19 and African Americans. JAMA 323(19):1891–1892, 2020 32293639

CHAPTER 12

SOCIAL ISOLATION AND LONELINESS IN OLDER ADULTS DURING THE COVID-19 PANDEMIC

Susan W. Lehmann, M.D.
Mari Umpierre, Ph.D., LCSW
Shehan Chin, LMSW
Janet Baek, M.D.

Social isolation, loneliness, and depression in older adults are associated with negative health and mental health outcomes. These outcomes are as detrimental to overall health as the effects of smoking and obesity. During the pandemic, social and physical distancing rules exacerbated social isolation and loneliness for many older adults. In this chapter we review interventions and strategies that could help to mitigate the health risks associated with the disruption of social connectedness among older adults, including establishing service delivery models and partnerships between community organizations and clinicians and incorporating technology to help maintain social connections, social routines, and social activities among this vulnerable group.

Vignette

Ms. A is a 70-year-old widowed African American woman with a history of schizoaffective disorder, PTSD, alcohol use disorder, and moderate hearing loss. Her psychiatrist of 20 years at the community mental health clinic retired abruptly during the pandemic. Ms. A is limited to phone appointments with her new psychiatrist because she does not have a camera or reliable internet for telehealth. She lives alone in a subsidized apartment. Her two adult children live far away and are frequently unavailable. She previously relied on her church community and Alcoholics Anonymous meetings for social support, but she is unable to attend either during the pandemic. She finds it challenging to engage in phone conversations or socially distanced meetings with masks because of her hearing loss. She feels isolated and anxious at home. She stays in bed into the early afternoon on most days.

BACKGROUND

Loneliness and Social Isolation Among Older People

Even prior to the coronavirus SARS-CoV-2 disease (COVID-19) pandemic, older people were increasingly at risk of being socially isolated. The National Health and Aging Trends Study released a 2020 report prior to the pandemic showing that 24% of community-dwelling adults ages 65 and older in the United States were socially isolated (Cudjoe et al. 2020). Other contributors to social isolation and loneliness among older people are decreasing economic and social resources, functional limitations, death of loved ones, and changes to family structures. Older people are more at risk for detrimental effects of social isolation and loneliness because of generally poorer health compared with younger people.

Association With Health Outcomes

Among older people, social isolation is a risk factor for negative health outcomes, mortality, depression, and cognitive decline (Courtin and Knapp 2017). Health risks associated with social isolation and loneliness have been shown to be as detrimental as the effects of smoking and obesity (Holt-Lunstad et al. 2010). Depression, cardiovascular health, and quality of life have been most studied. Social isolation and loneliness are independent risk factors for coronary artery disease, stroke, depression, anxiety, and suicide (Donovan and Blazer 2020).

At-Risk Groups

In the report "Social Isolation and Loneliness in Older Adults: Opportunities for the Health Care System," many additional risk factors for social isolation and loneliness among the elderly were identified (National Academies of Sciences, Engineering, and Medicine 2020). They included depression, anxiety, and cognitive deficits. These factors are often bidirectional in the sense that significant depressive and anxiety symptoms can lead to social withdrawal and vice versa. Studies have shown mixed results in terms of gender differences in the impact of loneliness and isolation. Some studies have shown that men are more negatively affected, and others have shown that women are more sensitive to the biological impact of loneliness (Hackett et al. 2012; Zebhauser et al. 2014). It is possible that men and women experience different types of loneliness, which may affect their mental and physical health differently.

A study by Ayalon and Shiovitz-Ezra (2011) found that among people ages 50 and older, loneliness is a major risk factor for passive suicidality. This effect was not found in people older than age 75. In a review article, Courtin and Knapp (2017) found a number of studies showing that certain groups are at higher risk of isolation and loneliness and subsequent adverse health outcomes. These groups included older people with a history of cancer, substance use, HIV, institutionalization, and work as unpaid caregivers. Individuals who identify as LGBTQ+ or other marginalized groups are more likely to report loneliness (Anderson and Thayer 2018). Racial and ethnic differences in social isolation and loneliness are an area needing further investigation.

SOCIAL ISOLATION, LONELINESS, AND THE COVID-19 PANDEMIC: RECENT LITERATURE

The COVID-19 pandemic has had a disproportionately deleterious impact on older adults from multiple perspectives, but its impact on loneliness and social isolation has been particularly harsh. These two concepts are linked but not identical. *Social isolation* identifies a physical state of aloneness and lack of social contacts, whereas *loneliness* describes the distraught subjective feeling of deprivation due to perceived lack of social closeness. The impact of COVID-19 on social isolation and loneliness has been a focus of concern for geriatric clinicians and re-searchers since the onset of the pandemic (Wu 2020). Prior to the onset of the pandemic, older adults living in the community and in long-term care facilities enjoyed a wide variety of social activities with family, friends, and faith communities. Many older adults also benefited from se-nior centers, medical day care programs, Meals on Wheels food delivery service, and respite care. Access to all these opportunities for social contact was drastically curtailed by measures to contain the spread of the virus.

During the pandemic, the public health mandate for social and physical distancing as a critical approach to deter spread of the COVID-19 contagion has led to local and national policies that have caused or ex-acerbated social isolation and loneliness for older adults. Nursing homes and assisted living facilities throughout the world have insti-tuted restrictions in their visitor policies during the pandemic. At times, as weather and local coronavirus community positivity rates allowed, families who had been prohibited from visiting their family members in nursing homes and assisted living facilities indoors have been invited to visit with their loved ones in outdoor on-site spaces. When commu-nity coronavirus positivity rates have been high, residents have been re-stricted to their rooms or apartments, and communal dining and group activities have been suspended. During these most restricted periods, family and other visitors have been prohibited from entering the facilities, and residents have been limited to using phones and electronic devices to keep in communication with family.

Visitor policies for acute hospital patients have fluctuated over the past year as well, depending on local coronavirus positivity rates. During periods of COVID-19 virus surge, acute hospital policies have instituted bans on visitors for patients in all hospital units, including medical units, intensive care units, emergency departments, and psy-chiatry units. Although all of these restrictions are understandable and appropriate from a medical point of view, there has been considerable concern about the possible negative impact on the mental health of older adults. During the pandemic, numerous news reports have fea-tured stories of older adults and their families experiencing emotional distress at the inability to be with each other during hospitalizations and worrying that social isolation and loneliness could be contributing to worsening of cognitive and emotional functioning, as well as general well-being, of older adults. Indeed, in most cases, family visits have been allowed only for hospitalized patients who are determined to be dying. A report from Norway described how at the start of the COVID-19 pandemic, all nursing homes were closed for visits, and staff at the University of Bergen used alternative means of communication to facilitate connection between residents and families, such as video calling and tablets (Husebø and Berge 2020). Similar approaches have been used in other countries, including the United States.

A number of recent studies have looked at the impact of social isolation and loneliness due to COVID-19 on older adults, and the emerging data are painting a picture of significant concern. Early during the pandemic, a study of 93 cognitively intact older adults in the United States compared their responses on measures asking about their social networks, subjective loneliness, and depression during the pandemic with responses they had given on the measures 6–9 months prior to the pandemic. The researchers found that after onset of the pandemic, older adults reported higher levels of both depression and loneliness. Individuals who felt less close to their social network were especially likely to experience increases in both loneliness and depression (Krendl and Perry 2021). A similar study of community-dwelling elders older than age 60 in Austria compared responses on measures of loneliness obtained via a telephone survey prior to the pandemic with responses on the same measures assessed early in the COVID-19 pandemic (Heidinger and Richter 2020). The authors found a significant increase in reported loneliness in the peripandemic period. A study of 277 older adult Israelis who completed a web-based questionnaire asking questions about loneliness, anxiety, and depressive and peritraumatic distress symptoms found a relationship between loneliness and psychiatric symptoms and subjective age (Shrira et al. 2020). Interestingly, individuals in that study who experienced an older subjective age (i.e., felt older than their chronological age) were more likely to affirm adverse effects related to loneliness, suggesting to the authors that these individuals may be at higher risk for negative health consequences related to loneliness.

In a longitudinal study of 151 community-dwelling older adults in the San Francisco Bay area, investigators contacted participants for a phone survey every 2 weeks during a shelter-at-home order due to the pandemic. More than half of the respondents reported worsened loneliness and worsened feelings of depression. Although overall rates of loneliness improved over the 4- to 6-week period, feelings of loneliness persisted for some individuals, especially those with poor emotional coping and those who had difficulty using new technologies (Kotwal et al. 2021). The authors reported that nearly 80% of participants had minimal video interactions and 40% used internet socializing infrequently, which contributed to feelings of isolation. They further noted that social isolation was also associated with difficulty in accessing personal care assistance for meal preparation, bathing, and transportation.

A recent study using an online survey examined anxiety about developing COVID-19, proactive coping, and stress related to COVID-19 among 515 adults, ages 20–79. The authors reported that although there were no age differences in stress levels, anxiety related to developing COVID-19 was greater for older adults compared with younger adults, but proactive coping strategies were associated with less COVID-19 stress for older adults than for younger people (Pearman et al. 2021). These results suggest that opportunities to strengthen proactive coping skills may be especially beneficial for older adults in dealing with the mental health challenges of the pandemic.

A report from Spain noted that older adults who engaged in higher levels of physical activity during the nationwide lockdown due to COVID-19 reported lower levels of depressive symptoms and higher levels of psychological well-being on scales measuring resilience and optimism (Carriedo et al. 2020). The authors suggested that regular physical activity could help promote resilience to stress in healthy older adults and could help them cope with challenges such as those posed by the pandemic lockdown.

Before the current pandemic, there were few randomized controlled trials of interventions for loneliness and social isolation in older adults. One of these prepandemic studies showed that teledelivered interventions focused on behavioral activation could be effective (N.G. Choi et al. 2020). Not surprisingly, promoting the use of social media and video visits to help older adults combat loneliness and isolation has been a focus of recommendations during the pandemic (Hajek and König 2020), although a Cochrane review did not find conclusive evidence that video calls reduce loneliness in older adults (Noone et al. 2020). A major limitation is that many older adults lack access to these technologies or skill in using them. Older adults who live in economically disadvantaged neighborhoods may lack access to the internet as well (Donovan and Blazer 2020).

Emerging from these reports is the clear need to screen older adults not only for feelings of isolation and loneliness but also for access to, and comfort with, available technology. During the pandemic, a plethora of online resources have become available, but they are useful only if the older adult is able to successfully use them. Assessment needs to include a review of the older adult's ability to use a smartphone, laptop, or tablet and the ability to use the internet. It is also important to screen for additional possible consequences of social isolation, including diminished access to groceries and pharmacy medications and to determine whether assistance is needed with meal preparation.

SOCIAL ISOLATION AND LONELINESS: ASSESSMENTS AND SCREENINGS

Smith et al. (2020) identified measures designed to evaluate and assess concepts associated with isolation and loneliness. They recommend using assessment tools when services and solutions are available and to postpone screenings and assessments until services are in place (Table 12–1).

STRATEGIES AND INTERVENTIONS: EXAMPLES FROM THE FIELD

Digital Literacy and Technology Use Support

Research suggests that technology can create opportunities for social connectedness, helping alleviate social isolation and loneliness (Barbosa Neves et al. 2019). Unfortunately, many older adults, before and during the pandemic, did not have the digital literacy skills, the hardware, and/or the infrastructure to use technology as a resource. A growing number of local and national organizations, including community-based agencies such as Search and Care (www.searchandcare.org), have focused on teaching older adults to become comfortable with technology use by providing digital literacy services in addition to traditional care and case management services before and during the pandemic. The fact that these services have been added by care management agencies to their menu of services is an indication of how critical it is for older adults to be able to use technology.

Digital literacy and technology use, including video visits with family members (Hajek and König 2020), can help decrease loneliness and isolation. However, to get older adults started with the use of technology, in-person training and support are often required. Support from a digital navigator along with education and training has been investigated by LaMonica et al. (2021), who indicated that training services should be tailored to the individual needs of the users.

Candoo Tech (www.candootech.com) is a for-profit organization that provides tech support and digital literacy and education for older adults in two formats: do-it-yourself and structured group classes. For

Table 12–1. Tools for evaluating concepts associated with isolation and loneliness

Measure	Description
Berkman-Syme Social Network Index	The Berkman-Syme Social Network Index measures social integration versus isolation by looking at marital status, frequency of contact with other people, participation in religious activities, and participation in other club or organization activities (Berkman and Syme 1979).
Duke Social Support Index (DSSI)	The 35-item DSSI measures multiple dimensions of social support among older adults. The 23-item and 11-item versions have been used for chronically ill and frail older adults (Koenig et al. 1993).
UCLA Loneliness Scale	The UCLA Loneliness Scale consists of 20 items and was designed to measure subjective feelings of loneliness as well as feelings of social isolation. Participants rate each item on a scale from 1 (Never) to 4 (Often) (Russel 1996; Russell 1980).
Lubben Social Network Scale–6 (LSNS-6)	The LSNS-6 was designed to gauge social isolation in older adults by measuring the number and frequency of social contacts with friends and family members and the perceived social support received from these sources (Lubben et al. 2006).
De Jong Gierveld Loneliness Scale	The 6-item De Jong Gierveld Loneliness Scale measures both emotional loneliness and social loneliness (De Jong-Gierveld and Kamphuls 1985; Gierveld and Tilburg 2006). Social loneliness occurs when someone is missing a wider social network, and emotional loneliness is caused when someone is missing an "intimate relationship."
Cornwell Perceived Isolation Scale	The Cornwell Perceived Isolation Scale measures social isolation by evaluating social disconnectedness (Cornwell and Waite 2009).
Campaign to End Loneliness Measurement Tool	The main purpose of this tool is to measure the impact of the intervention associated with the Campaign to End Loneliness. The tool was developed "in partnership with over 50 older people, service providers, commissioners and housing associations" (Goodman et al. 2015, p. 34).

those who want to learn independently, free resources, guides, and downloadable instruction packets are offered. For those who prefer didactic instruction, group classes and personalized instruction services are available and include annual memberships and ongoing access to tech support.

During the pandemic, Papa (www.joinpapa.com), a for-profit organization, addressed the gap in in-person tech support services for older adults by matching older adults with students of nursing, medicine, and other health professions. The cost of services is covered by some employers and by health insurance plans, including Medicare and Medicaid. Papa employees, also known as Papa Pals, offer a variety of services (e.g., tech support, socialization, transportation to medical appointments, grocery shopping) for a fee. Carefully following public health recommendations, Papa Pals successfully delivered their services during the pandemic in 12 states.

Virtual Senior Centers: Resources for Social Connection

In New York City, senior centers closed in-person operations in March 2020 and partially reopened in September 2021. During this time the centers swiftly adapted to the new normal by providing programs and services virtually and over the phone. Staff members incorporated technical support and education into their offerings to keep older adults engaged and socially connected. Senior Planet (https://seniorplanet.org), in collaboration with AARP (www.aarp.org), provided a free technology hotline that was available 9–5 Eastern Daylight Time, delivered programs virtually to nationwide audiences, and operated four senior centers. The in-person centers, located in New York City; Plattsburgh, New York; Montgomery County, Maryland; and San Antonio, Texas, operated in a modified manner to comply with social distancing rules. Senior Planet also partnered with a large number of organizations nationally and locally, including the Department for the Aging (DFTA) in New York City (www1.nyc.gov/site/dfta/index.page), to address and mitigate the impact of the pandemic nationwide.

In New York City, PSS (https://pssusa.org), a not-for-profit organization that operates 10 senior centers, modified their services to keep members engaged by delivering craft supplies and activities (e.g., puzzles, word searches), along with pantry boxes (with personal protective equipment and other supplies), to participants' homes. All of PSS's centers provided opportunities for member interaction through telephone calls (using apps such as WhatsApp) and/or new technologies (such as Zoom) for virtual learning. Through PSS Life! University, the organization provided virtual programs, including classes, support groups, wellness events, and joint enrichment opportunities for older adults and their care partners and/or family members. Like these senior centers, many others across the country modified their services, breaking down geographic boundaries. A list of selected senior centers is given in Table 12–2.

Table 12–2. Selected senior centers

Center	Description
Self-help virtual senior centers (https://vscm.selfhelp.net)	Founded 10 years ago to combat isolation and loneliness through online learning for homebound older adults in New York City, their services now are available nationwide.
LiveOn NY (www.liveon-ny.org/virtual-activities)	Their mission is to help New Yorkers age with confidence, grace, and vitality through advocacy, policy work, and individual support and services.
JASA Senior Centers (https://jasa.org/events)	Founded in 1968, the centers provide support services to promote aging with purpose and help older adults maintain autonomy, ensuring they can live in their homes and communities.
SAGE Centers virtual programs (https://sagenyc.org/nyc/centers/calendar.cfm?center=midtown)	The centers' mission is to make aging better for LGBTQ+ older adults nationwide through service, advocacy, and education.
New York City senior centers, Department for the Aging (www1.nyc.gov/site/dfta/services/find-help.page)	NYC Department for the Aging is committed to helping older adults in New York City age in their homes and communities. In partnership with local community agencies, they operate services in a large group of senior centers and provide advocacy and resources.

Volunteering and Volunteers for Mutual Aid, Support, and Intergenerational Connections

In New York City, Friendly Visiting and Friendly VOICES, two volunteer programs designed to build friendships and decrease social isolation among older adults, are operated by the city's DFTA (www1.nyc.gov/site/dfta/index.page). These programs train and match volunteers, who are often older adults themselves, to connect with other older adults on a weekly basis. The Friendly Visiting program trains volunteers to conduct in-person visits to older adults in their homes, and Friendly VOICES trains them to keep in touch over the phone. During the COVID-19 pandemic, all volunteers kept in touch via phone or video calls exclusively. A public service announcement recorded by Lin-Manuel Miranda encourages program participation and volunteering (https://soundcloud.com/user-531949329/dfta-social-isolation-psa).

In Chicago, volunteer students (medicine, neuroscience, and genetic counseling) developed and implemented Seniors Overcoming Social Isolation (SOS), a telephone outreach program, to address social isolation among older adults in the community during the pandemic (Office et al. 2020). Primary care providers identified older adults at risk and referred them to a volunteer coordinator who, in turn, assigned them to volunteer student callers. Callers engaged older adults in conversations to explore unmet needs, provide information about how to access concrete resources, and offer opportunities for social connection and companionship. The volunteers reported bidirectional benefits (Office et al. 2020): older adults were receptive to engaging in social conversations with a focus on reminiscing about their pasts, and students found the experience inspiring and gratifying.

Advice to Families, Friends, Neighbors, and Communities

The Centers for Disease Control and Prevention (CDC) and the World Health Organization suggest that families stay in touch with older members and check in with them regularly over the phone. In addition, the CDC recommends the design and implementation of a care plan with health promotion and disease prevention information along with information on how to access medications, personal protective equipment, and food and toiletries (Centers for Disease Control and Prevention 2021; World Health Organization 2020).

In New York City, the DFTA encourages family members, neighbors, and friends to check in on older New Yorkers over the telephone. DFTA's website encourages all New Yorkers to promote connection and interaction with older family members, friends, and/or neighbors and to regularly stay in touch via weekly10-minute calls. The New York City Department for the Aging provides simple steps and guidance to maximize this effort (see www1.nyc.gov/site/dfta/index.page)

Life story building studies have shown that elders who are given the opportunity to tell their life story in a rich and meaningful way report high mental well-being (Lai et al. 2018). Engaging in reminiscence may be another way to support connection and tap into an older adult's resilience and resourcefulness during touch base and wellness calls.

E. Y. Choi et al. (2020) and N. G. Choi et al. (2020) conducted studies looking at loneliness and isolation during the COVID-19 pandemic and concluded that to address loneliness and isolation, the quality of social interactions is more important than their quantity. Thus, families and friends are encouraged to intentionally plan phone calls or video chats, to participate together in virtual activities, and to use these activities as opportunities for meaningful interactions. The Metropolitan Opera Nightly Opera Stream (https://metoperafree.brightcove-services.com/?videoId= 6222600039001) and the Metropolitan Museum of Art offer free performances as well as 360-degree virtual tours of specific exhibitions (www.metmuseum.org/events/whats-on) and are examples of online cultural programs to be shared with older adults for recreation and leisure.

During the pandemic, governments around the world, social media, and news outlets, as well as some political figures, identified COVID-19 as a disease of older adults (Ayalon et al. 2021). As the virus continued to spread and researchers learned more about the disease, it became clear that COVID-19 affects people of all ages (Fraser et al. 2020). Nevertheless, COVID-19 continues to be perceived by many as a disease of elderly people. Although older adults need to be protected and helped to remain safe, it is important to recognize as well that many are resilient and resourceful (MacLeod et al. 2016).

Older adults reported feeling protected and valued when family members took the initiative of buying food for them and when they received information about, and access to, senior hours at grocery stores and senior food delivery services (Monahan et al. 2020). A practical way to support older adults during the pandemic and beyond may involve the provision of concrete help and safety in combination with social support. Concrete help may include assessing the older adult's ability to live independently in the community. Families should engage in exploratory conversations to maximize the older adult's participation in establishing plans for safety, balancing the need for protection with the need to preserve autonomy and independence.

In partnership with Candoo Tech, PSS Circle of Care provides orientation and information to families on the use of technology as a resource to increase social connections and to promote health and safety with and for older adults. The information is posted on their website along with a webinar and video available free of charge to the public (https://pssusa.org). This webinar may be used as a resource to guide families and older adults on the selection of products and services to help older adults to live safely and independently in their own homes.

Advice to Clinicians, Collaborations, and Partnerships With Community Agencies

The COVID-19 pandemic helped to uncover and identify the need for collaborations and partnerships between clinical providers and community-based organizations to deliver care to older adults living in the community (Smith et al. 2020). In Mannheim, Germany, psychologists and psychiatrists specializing in geriatric mental health designed and operated a geriatric helpline that went live on April 13, 2020. It was implemented to address the possible consequences of social isolation (e.g., the need to access groceries and medicines, the need for assistance with activities of daily living), to provide information about COVID-19, to deliver counseling and support, and to better understand the impact of lockdown measures on mental health–related issues in older adults within the local population. Not surprisingly, loneliness was identified as a psychosocial stressor by most helpline callers who were referred to and accepted counseling services (Ayalon et al. 2021).

The vignette presented at the start of the chapter highlights how the pandemic disrupted the patient's access to treatment and support services, which in turn increased her risks for poor health and mental health outcomes. Table 12–3 illustrates potential psychosocial interventions that could have been delivered to this patient in partnership with a psychosocial care provider from a local community-based organization. The proposed interventions incorporate resources that promote, strengthen, and maximize adaptation and coping.

Providing a combination of personalized and comprehensive clinical and psychosocial care to this vulnerable group of patients may positively affect their health and mental health outcomes. Thus, we recommend that clinical providers become familiar with local senior service organizations in the communities in which they practice. These organizations are prepared to provide a variety of services to their clients, including education and support with technology use. Because older adults without access to technology were at an increased risk for poor mental health outcomes during the pandemic, providing older adults with a pathway to access digital literacy resources would be of great benefit.

The loneliness epidemic in combination with the COVID-19 pandemic has brought enormous challenges that will need to be managed one patient at a time, using a variety of approaches and flexible methods delivered by care teams of clinicians, family members, community workers, and intergenerational volunteers, including older adults themselves.

Table 12-3. Psychosocial interventions that promote adaptation and coping for Ms. A

Presenting problems	Interventions
Schizoaffective disorder, PTSD, alcohol use disorder, moderate hearing loss Transition to a new provider Adjustment to telehealth Lack of access to support services Adult children frequently unavailable	Psychosocial care will be provided by a community-based agency such as Search and Care (www.searchandcare.org) rooted in the patient's community. Care provider is familiar with resources available at the local level.
Lack of access to meals and/or groceries, pharmacy medications, COVID-19-appropriate PPE, hearing aids, a sound amplification system for the telephone, and a tablet or smartphone with a video camera and internet broadband to optimize participation in telehealth services, AA meetings, religious services, and a virtual senior center Lack of family support and involvement	Psychosocial care provider will assess Ms. A's ability to adapt to the COVID-19 pandemic, focusing on access to groceries and the ability to prepare meals, to obtain and take medications regularly, and to access and use appropriate PPE. Provider will help Ms. A access services and resources needed to maximize well-being and social connectedness, including access to hardware (smartphone, computer, or tablet) that will allow participation in a virtual senior center, in religious activities, and in AA meetings. Psychosocial care provider could explore and assess Ms. A's relationships with her children with the goal of expanding her support network.

Note. AA=Alcoholics Anonymous; COVID-19= coronavirus SARS-CoV-2 disease; PPE=personal protective equipment.

SUMMARY

In this chapter we provided an overview of the recent literature addressing the impact of the loneliness epidemic and the COVID-19 pandemic on the health and mental health outcomes of older adults. We provided an overview of local and national programs as well as of services and resources that helped older adults remain socially connected while physically distanced and sheltering at home. We also illustrated the importance of digital literacy for older adults' overall well-being. Finally, we highlighted the importance of using multiple strategies at the individual, family, and community levels to address psychosocial needs and improve health and mental health outcomes, as well as quality of life for older adults, during the pandemic and beyond.

KEY POINTS

- Before the onset of the COVID-19 pandemic, older adults were at increasingly high risk of being socially isolated. In 2020 they endured the social isolation and loneliness epidemic exacerbated by the public health mandate for social and physical distancing to prevent the spread of the COVID-19 virus and faced higher risks to their health and mental health outcomes than any other group.

- As the COVID-19 pandemic continues in combination with the social isolation and loneliness epidemic, incorporating new technologies and establishing service delivery models and partnerships between community organizations and clinicians could help improve health and mental health outcomes as well as overall well-being among older adults.

- Older adults who lack skills and access to technology for social media and videoconferencing are at increased risk for worse mental health due to social isolation and loneliness during a pandemic.

QUESTIONS FOR REVIEW

1. Social isolation in older adults during a pandemic has been associated with further difficulty in which of the following areas?

  A. Personal care
  B. Transportation
  C. Meal preparation
  D. Grocery shopping
  E. All of the above

Answer: E.

2. Which of the following has been found to be an outcome associated with social isolation and loneliness among older adults?

  A. Depression
  B. Coronary artery disease

C. Stroke
D. All of the above

Answer: D.

3. As the world continues to endure the COVID-19 pandemic, what can be done to help improve the health and mental health outcomes for this vulnerable group?

   A. Encourage older adults to increase their digital literacy.
   B. Establish service delivery models and partnerships between community organizations and clinicians.
   C. A and B
   D. Encourage older adults to rely on their family members for support.

Answer: C.

REFERENCES

Anderson GO, Thayer C: Loneliness and social connections: a national survey of adults 45 and older. AARP Research, September 2018. Available at: https://doi.org/10.26419/res.00246.001. Accessed October 29, 2021.

Ayalon L, Shiovitz-Ezra S: The relationship between loneliness and passive death wishes in the second half of life. Int Psychogeriatr 23(10):1677–1685, 2011 21777504

Ayalon L, Chasteen A, Diehl M, et al: Aging in times of the COVID-19 pandemic: avoiding ageism and fostering intergenerational solidarity. J Gerontol B Psychol Sci Soc Sci 76(2):e49–e52, 2021 32296840

Barbosa Neves B, Franz R, Judges R, et al: Can digital technology enhance social connectedness among older adults? A feasibility study. J Appl Gerontol 38(1):49–72, 2019 29166818

Berkman LF, Syme SL: Social networks, host resistance, and mortality: a nine-year follow-up study of Alameda County residents. Am J Epidemiol 109(2):186–204, 1979 425958

Carriedo A, Cecchini JA, Fernandez-Rio J, et al: COVID-19, psychological well-being and physical activity levels in older adults during the nationwide lockdown in Spain. Am J Geriatr Psychiatry 28(11):1146–1155, 2020 32919872

Centers for Disease Control and Prevention: Older adults: older unvaccinated adults are more likely to be hospitalized or die from COVID-19. Atlanta, GA, Centers for Disease Control and Prevention, March 17, 2021. Available at: www.cdc.gov/coronavirus/2019-ncov/need-extra-precautions/older-adults.html. Accessed July 6, 2021.

Choi EY, Farina M, Wu Q, et al: COVID-19 social distancing measures and loneliness among older adults. Innov Aging 4(suppl 1):939, 2020

Choi NG, Pepin R, Marti CN, et al: Improving social connectedness for homebound older adults: randomized controlled trial of tele-delivered behavioral activation versus tele-delivered friendly visits. Am J Geriatr Psychiatry 28(7):698–708, 2020 32238297

Cornwell EY, Waite LJ: Social disconnectedness, perceived isolation, and health among older adults. J Health Soc Behav 50(1):31–48, 2009 19413133

Courtin E, Knapp M: Social isolation, loneliness and health in old age: a scoping review. Health Soc Care Community 25(3):799–812, 2017 26712585

Cudjoe TKM, Roth DL, Szanton SL, et al: The epidemiology of social isolation: National Health and Aging Trends Study. J Gerontol B Psychol Sci Soc Sci 75:107–113, 2020 29590462

De Jong-Gierveld J, Kamphuls F: The development of a Rasch-type loneliness scale. Appl Psychol Meas 9(3):289–299, 1985

Donovan NJ, Blazer D: Social isolation and loneliness in older adults: review and commentary of a National Academies report. Am J Geriatr Psychiatry 28(12):1233–1244, 2020 32919873

Fraser S, Lagacé M, Bongué B, et al: Ageism and COVID-19: what does our society's response say about us? Age Ageing 49(5):692–695, 2020 32377666

Gierveld JDJ, Tilburg TV: A 6-item scale for overall, emotional, and social loneliness: confirmatory tests on survey data. Res Aging 28(5):582–598, 2006

Goodman A, Wrigley J, Silversides K, et al: Measuring Your Impact on Loneliness in Later Life. London, Campaign to End Loneliness, 2015

Hackett RA, Hamer M, Endrighi R, et al: Loneliness and stress-related inflammatory and neuroendocrine responses in older men and women. Psychoneuroendocrinology 37:1801–1809, 2012 22503139

Hajek A, König HH: Social isolation and loneliness of older adults in times of the COVID-19 pandemic: can use of online social media sites and video chats assist in mitigating social isolation and loneliness? Gerontology 67(1):121–124, 2020 33264778

Heidinger T, Richter L: The effect of COVID-19 on loneliness in the elderly: an empirical comparison of pre-and peri-pandemic loneliness in community-dwelling elderly. Front Psychol 11:585308, 2020 33101154

Husebø BS, Berge LI: Intensive medicine and nursing home care in times of SARS CoV-2: a Norwegian perspective. Am J Geriatr Psychiatry 28(7):792–793, 2020 32381282

Holt-Lunstad J, Smith TB, Layton JB: Social relationships and mortality risk: a meta-analytic review. PLoS Med 7(7):e1000316, 2010 20668659

Koenig HG, Westlund RE, George LK, et al: Abbreviating the Duke Social Support Index for use in chronically ill elderly individuals. Psychosomatics 34(1):61–69, 1993 8426892

Kotwal AA, Holt-Lunstad J, Newmark RL, et al: Social isolation and loneliness among San Francisco Bay area older adults during the COVID-19 shelter-in-place orders. J Am Geriatr Soc 69(1):20–29, 2021 32965024

Krendl AC, Perry BL: The impact of sheltering in place during the COVID-19 pandemic on older adults' social and mental well-being. J Gerontol B Psychol Sci Soc Sci 76(2):e53–e58, 2021 32778899

Lai CKY, Igarashi A, Yu CTK, et al: Does life story work improve psychosocial well-being for older adults in the community? A quasi-experimental study. BMC Geriatr 18(1):119, 2018 29769035

LaMonica HM, Davenport TA, Roberts AE, et al: Understanding technology preferences and requirements for health information technologies designed to improve and maintain the mental health and well-being of older adults: participatory design study. JMIR Aging 4(1):e21461, 2021 33404509

Lubben J, Blozik E, Gillmann G, et al: Performance of an abbreviated version of the Lubben Social Network Scale among three European community-dwelling older adult populations. Gerontologist 46(4):503–513, 2006 16921004

MacLeod S, Musich S, Hawkins K, et al: The impact of resilience among older adults. Geriatr Nurs 37(4):266–272, 2016 27055911

Monahan C, Macdonald J, Lytle A, et al: COVID-19 and ageism: how positive and negative responses impact older adults and society. Am Psychol 75(7):887–896, 2020 32672988

National Academies of Sciences, Engineering, and Medicine: Social Isolation and Loneliness in Older Adults: Opportunities for the Health Care System. Washington, DC, National Academies Press, 2020

Noone C, McSharry J, Smalle M, et al: Video calls for reducing social isolation and loneliness in older people: a rapid review. Cochrane Database Syst Rev 5(5):CD013632, 2020 32441330

Office EE, Rodenstein MS, Merchant TS, et al: Reducing social isolation of seniors during COVID-19 through medical student telephone contact. J Am Med Dir Assoc 21(7):948–950, 2020 32674825

Pearman A, Hughes ML, Smith EL, et al: Age differences in risk and resilience factors in COVID-19-related stress. J Gerontol B Psychol Sci Soc Sci 76(2):e38–e44, 2021 32745198

Russel D: UCLA Loneliness Scale Version 3 (description of measure). J Pers Soc Psychol 39:3–4, 1996

Russell JA: A circumplex model of affect. J Pers Soc Psychol 39(6):1161–1178, 1980

Shrira A, Hoffman Y, Bodner E, et al: COVID-19-related loneliness and psychiatric symptoms among older adults: the buffering role of subjective age. Am J Geriatr Psychiatry 28(11):1200–1204, 2020 32561276

Smith ML, Steinman LE, Casey EA: Combatting social isolation among older adults in a time of physical distancing: the COVID-19 social connectivity paradox. Front Public Health 8:403, 2020 32850605

World Health Organization: Coronavirus disease (COVID-19) advice for the public. Geneva, World Health Organization, 2020. Available at: www.who.int/emergencies/diseases/novel-coronavirus-2019/advice-for-public. Accessed July 6, 2021.

Wu B: Social isolation and loneliness among older adults in the context of COVID-19: a global challenge. Glob Health Res Policy 5:27, 2020 32514427

Zebhauser A, Hofmann-Xu L, Baumert J, et al: How much does it hurt to be lonely? Mental and physical differences between older men and women in the KORA-Age Study Int J Geriatr Psychiatry 29(3):245–252, 2014 23804458

CHAPTER 13

THE COVID-19 ECONOMY

Mental Health Impact on Older Adults

Sarah E. LaFave, Ph.D., M.P.H., R.N.
Robert P. Roca, M.D., M.P.H., M.B.A.

Pandemics adversely affect the economy, and economic downturns adversely affect general and mental health across the age spectrum. Older adults in the United States are somewhat insulated from the full force of recessions by federal programs such as Social Security and Medicare, but many older adults, particularly those with the least wealth, are at risk for financial strain and its adverse impact on health during pandemics. There are several pathways by which financial strain may affect mental health. Knowledge of these pathways may enable us to address and mitigate the impact of financial strain in clinical work and policy making.

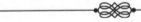

Vignette 1

In March 2020, the household of Mrs. L, a 70-year-old empty nester, and her husband suddenly grew to a household of six as her 96-year-old mother, who had resided in assisted living, and a pregnant daughter and newly unemployed son-in-law, who had been living in New York City, came to live with them until the pandemic subsided. Her retired brother came as well to help care for their mother. Household expenses skyrocketed overnight for Mr. and Mrs. L, and many household expenses (e.g., rent, assisted living fees) continued unabated for the others. Mr. and Mrs. L had the advantage of income from ongoing postretirement employment. Mrs. L's mother received ongoing Social Security payments to support her and provide some assistance to Mr. and Mrs. L. In addition, the daughter had her maternity leave income, and the son-in-law was receiving federally enhanced unemployment income. Without Mrs. L's ongoing employment income as well as the contributions from the visiting parties—much of which came from government programs, including federal stimulus checks—the increase in household expenses would have put Mr. and Mrs. L at risk for financial strain. As it was, the new situation created stress for the family because federal relief programs were constantly under debate during the period, and some income sources, such as the unemployment benefits, were temporary.

The coronavirus SARS-CoV-2 disease (COVID-19) pandemic is first and foremost a public health event with devastating impact on the millions who become ill and those who care for them. But it also is a potent disrupter of the world economy and, as a result, has profoundly affected even those spared the medical consequences of contagion. Increased unemployment and expenses, reduced availability of essential goods, and uncertainty about the adequacy of savings and the fate of investments increased the risk for financial strain among people of all ages, including older adults. In this chapter we review the economic impact of past pandemics, the impact of past economic downturns on older adults, the adverse health effects of financial strain, and both clinical and social policy interventions that may reduce those effects now and during future pandemics.

ECONOMIC FALLOUT OF PAST PANDEMICS

In the second quarter of the fourteenth century the world was ravaged by the Black Death, a devastating disease caused by the bacterium *Yersinia pestis* and transmitted to humans by fleas borne by infected rats. Millions of people died worldwide. The economic effects were complex and phasic. At the height of the pandemic, economic activity ground to a halt as a large fraction of the productive labor force perished. Then, as the pandemic subsided and productivity struggled to recover, laborers in the dramatically diminished postpandemic workforce found themselves in demand, and wages rose significantly. The increase in wages was sufficient to prompt the promulgation of ordinances designed to limit further increases in payment for labor in England. Earlier pandemics, such as the Antonine Plague (second century, Roman Empire) and the Justinianic Plague (sixth through eighth centuries) appear to have exerted similar upward pressure on wages and resulted in short-term reductions in wealth inequality and gains for the common man (Scheidel 2018).

The 1918–1920 influenza pandemic provides a more recent and better-documented example of the complex economic effects of these public health calamities. Much of what is known is culled from the print media of the era, and much of that is anecdotal. The *Arkansas Gazette* reported declines in retail sales for many establishments (33% for grocery stores, 50% for department stores), whereas sales of pharmaceuticals and mattresses increased. The *Memphis Commercial Appeal* reported reductions in industrial productivity, mining activity, and the capacity to handle telephone calls because of influenza outbreaks among factory workers, miners, and telephone operators (Garrett 2008).

The limited academic research on the economics of the 1918 pandemic yields two findings. First, on the basis of the experience with past pandemics, it was expected that the pandemic-related reduction in the size of the workforce would lead in the short term to an increase in wages for labor. In fact, Garrett (2008) found that states and cities with higher rates of influenza mortality had greater wage growth in the period between 1914 and 1918 (two to three percentage points, for a 10% increase in per capita mortality) than did states and cities with lower mortality rates. Second, there were also apparent long-term economic consequences of the influenza pandemic. Evidence derived from census data showed that cohorts in utero during the pandemic had poorer educational attainment, more physical disability, and lower incomes than expected (Almond 2006).

IMPACT OF PAST ECONOMIC DEPRESSIONS AND RECESSIONS ON OLDER ADULTS

Pandemics of the past have had profound adverse economic effects. A review of recent economic downturns unrelated to pandemics provides insight into the impact of such downturns, whatever their cause, on the health and well-being of the affected populations, including older adults.

The Great Depression of the 1930s

The stock market crash of 1929 led to financial panic and a cascade of events that caused banks to fail and businesses to close. Fortunes were lost, millions of people became unemployed, and suicide rates rose (Tapia Granados and Diez Roux 2009). Although everyone suffered, the impact on older adults was particularly significant:

> As the economic crisis worsened, many employers were reluctant to re-hire or keep on older workers. Widespread bank failures often wiped out savings accumulated over a lifetime of labor. At a time when home ownership was a long and arduous process for working-class families, poor employment prospects and the loss of savings brought the threat of foreclosure. Given the inability of private and public aid organizations to provide adequate relief, those in need were forced to rely on the assistance of friends and relatives. Even those older Americans who managed to avoid the immediate impact of the Depression often had less fortunate kin, resulting in the day-to-day stress of providing economic assistance or sharing living space. (Encyclopedia.com 2019)

The policy response to this crisis involved the creation of a host of federal programs collectively called the New Deal, including Social Security, and, decades later, an additional suite of federal programs dubbed the Great Society, including Medicare and Medicaid. These policy innovations would help mitigate the impact of future downturns on older adults.

The Great Recession of 2008

The Great Recession of 2008 was ushered in by the collapse of an inflated housing market propped up by risky loans that had been bundled into complex and poorly understood investment instruments. As borrowers unable to keep up with mortgages beyond their means defaulted on their loans and as the institutions that had been buying these bundled loans stopped doing so, the institutions holding this bad debt began to fail. The effects included bankruptcies, spikes in unemployment, and a stock market crash that greatly reduced the value of pension funds and retirement accounts. The crisis called for dramatic action on the part of the Federal Reserve (e.g., interest rates were reduced to historic lows) and the federal government (e.g., the Troubled Asset Relief Program [TARP]).

The impact on older adults included decreased total net wealth and increased levels of poverty. The decrease in total net wealth varied by age and employment status. The decrease was most pronounced (13%)

among retired older adults between ages 60 and 74 and least pronounced (4%) among retired adults older than age 75, perhaps because members of the older cohort were more likely to own their homes and had more conservative investments. The percentage of older adults falling below the federal poverty line grew from about 5% to just over 7%. Not surprisingly, those most at risk for poverty were those with the lowest total wealth prior to the recession, regardless of age and retirement status (Cohen et al. 2020).

The economic disruption associated with the Great Recession adversely affected mental health at the population level. One sign of this impact was the international rise in suicide rates among men. In North, South, and Central America, the suicide rate among men during the recession was 6.4% higher than expected. The steepest increase in rate (5.2% more than the expected rate) was among men ages 45–64 years, but the rate among men ages 65 years and older also significantly increased (3.2% more than the expected rate). The suicide rate among women did not rise significantly during this period (Chang et al. 2013). It has been speculated that the increase in suicide rates among men, particularly middle-age men, may have been linked to unemployment, but recent analyses suggest that the apparent link between unemployment and suicide may, in fact, be mediated by poverty. Rates of poverty, rather than unemployment, have been shown to be linked to suicide rates at the county level for all population groups (Kerr et al. 2017).

THE COVID-19 ECONOMY

COVID-19 has been called the "$16 trillion virus" (Cutler and Summers 2020). Fear of contagion on the part of individuals, along with governmental measures taken to control the spread of infection (e.g., quarantines, business closures), dramatically reduced activity in many sectors of the economy, resulting in lost revenue, business closures, and unemployment. The travel, leisure, and hospitality sectors were especially hard-hit. In anticipation of these effects, the equity markets plunged, dramatically reducing the holdings of pension funds and the value of retirement accounts invested in stocks.

Governmental interventions in the form of stimulus packages (e.g., Coronavirus Aid, Relief, and Economic Security [CARES] Act) and action by the Federal Reserve (e.g., holding interest rates at historic lows) eased the economic impact of the pandemic to some degree, leading to reductions in unemployment and a dramatic turnaround in the stock market. But the recovery was K shaped, favoring those who were better educated, could work from home, and/or had financial resources invested in the resurgent equity markets. In contrast, those who were less well educated, did not enjoy pandemic-proof employment or income, and did not have investments in equity markets continued to struggle. Older adults were present in both groups.

Effects on Employment Income

Many older adults need employment income to make ends meet. This group, of course, includes individuals who have not yet reached retirement age, as well as many adults ages 66 years and older for whom income from Social Security, even when supplemented by retirement savings, is not sufficient to meet their financial needs. Working older adults who become ill with COVID-19 are unable to work while ill and may lack sufficient sick leave or disability coverage to provide income throughout the often protracted recovery period. Individuals who care for them may also need to stay home from work during the convalescent period, further compounding the reduction in household income. The financial impact of this sudden income loss is especially severe for the 40%–50% of older adults without emergency savings (Li and Mutchler 2020).

Individuals who do not become ill face the threat of loss of employment. Unemployment reached the unprecedented level of 14.7% in April 2020 and was still elevated at 6.7% in November 2020. The unemployment rate was particularly high among those in the leisure and hospitality industries (39.3% in April and 15% in November), although other industries requiring close in-person contact (e.g., mining) also saw persistently elevated rates (19%). Other relatively disadvantaged groups included workers without a high school degree (21%), teenagers (37% among girls and 29% among boys), Black Americans (17% vs. 14% for white Americans), and Hispanics (19% vs. 14% for non-Hispanics) (Congressional Research Service 2020).

In general, unemployment rates were higher among young workers and women early in the pandemic. Table 13–1 shows monthly unemployment rates by sex and age. Peak unemployment rates were highest for teenagers (28.6% among boys and 36.6% among girls) and lowest among adults between the ages of 25 and 54 (12.1% among men and 13.7% among women). They were similar or somewhat higher among men and women older than age 55 (12.1% and 15.5%, respectively) (Congressional Research Service 2020).

These data show that older workers, although clearly adversely affected by the pandemic, fared better than their younger counterparts in the job market. But there are important caveats to this generalization.

Table 13–1. Unemployment rates during the COVID pandemic by age (%)

| | Ages 16–19 | | Ages 20–24 | | Ages 25–54 | | Ages 55 and older | |
	Women	Men	Women	Men	Women	Men	Women	Men
Pre-COVID-19	11.0	13.5	6.5	6.8	3.0	3.0	2.4	2.6
April 2020	36.6	28.6	28.0	23.5	13.7	12.1	15.5	12.1
November 2020	12.8	15.2	9.3	11.7	5.8	6.3	5.8	5.8

Source. Congressional Research Service 2020.

First, the unemployment rates were higher for nonwhite people and Hispanics than for non-Hispanic white people at the unemployment peak in the spring of 2020 and at all points thereafter (Congressional Research Service 2020). There is every reason to believe that this racial disparity occurred across the age spectrum. Second, the reduction in unemployment did not indicate that workers reentering the workforce were necessarily returning to employment at their pre-COVID-19 level. Older reemployed workers often do not find full-time work, may not be able to match their former earnings, and may not find jobs with employer-sponsored health benefits (Farber 2017; Johnson and Kawachi 2007).

Effects on Investments and Retirement Income

There was a dramatic drop in all stock market indexes in March 2020, resulting in sudden and significant losses for pension funds and retirement accounts. Investors who did not respond by moving out of equities saw a very substantial recovery in their retirement accounts by the end of 2020. On the other hand, those who moved out of equities precipitously lost out on the steep gains that occurred later in the spring and thereafter.

Early in the COVID-19 pandemic, some employers, especially in the travel and retail sectors, stopped contributing to employees' retirement plans. It is likely that individuals fortunate enough to remain employed reduced their own contributions to their retirement accounts. The impact of these reductions will endure indefinitely for all workers but will be particularly harmful to older workers, who will have fewer years of future employment during which to make up the shortfall, possibly delaying retirement.

Effects on Expenses

Medicare provides substantial protection against catastrophic medical expenses for eligible older adults. This benefit is not generally available to older adults younger than 65 unless they have a qualifying disability. The "young old" adults who became unemployed as a result of the pandemic found themselves, like their younger counterparts, without employer-based health benefits. The alternatives included paying expensive Consolidated Omnibus Budget Reconciliation Act (COBRA) premiums to retain their employer-sponsored coverage temporarily or going to the health insurance exchanges to obtain individual policies for themselves and their dependents. In either case, the out-of-pocket costs were substantially higher than the employee portion of the employer-based plans that covered them while they were employed.

Even older adults with health care coverage were at risk of unexpected health care expenses. Health care providers, faced with new operating expenses driven by the need for enhanced sanitizing procedures and personal protective equipment, sometimes tacked "COVID fees" onto their bills (Kliff and Silver-Greenberg 2020). These fees were generally not covered by health insurance, particularly when associated with services for which Medicare offers no benefit, such as dental care and services at assisted living facilities. These fees might be assessed on a one-time-only basis (e.g., a $900 charge for masks, cleaning supplies, and meal delivery at an assisted living facility) or on a per service basis (e.g., a $60 charge added to an ambulance bill, a $45 charge added to a dental care bill).

The broad economic and social impact of the pandemic sometimes forced households to consolidate, and as occurred during the Great Depression, some older adults found themselves opening their homes to their suddenly unemployed adult children, their families, and other relatives. With the sudden growth of these households came unexpected increases in household expenses that potentially strained the budgets of the hosts, particularly if, like half of older adults, they had no emergency savings and/or, like many minority older adults, little in the way of liquid assets (Li and Mutchler 2020).

PANDEMIC ECONOMICS AND HEALTH

It is clear that past pandemics caused widespread and painful economic disruption as the pandemic diseases spread throughout the population and that their adverse economic impact extended into subsequent generations. Short-lived increases in wages for labor did not compensate for these devastating effects. Historically, older adults were particularly vulnerable to the repercussions of economic calamities, but social policy innovations introduced in the wake of the Great Depression reduced the vulnerability of older adults to more recent economic downturns such as the Great Recession of 2008. Nonetheless, many older adults, particularly ethnic and racial minorities, those with the least savings and net wealth, and those dependent on employment income, may find themselves struggling to make ends meet in the face of falling income and rising expenses. This predicament creates financial strain and may cause adverse general and mental health effects that compound the health risks associated with the pandemic disease itself.

FINANCIAL STRAIN AND OLDER ADULT HEALTH

Financial strain is the "subjective perception of economic pressure" associated with a mismatch between income and expenses (Asebedo and Wilmarth 2017). It is generally operationalized through a series of questions ascertaining the level of difficulty paying bills for essential goods and services. Financial strain may occur because income is objectively low, expenses are objectively high, or both. However, although financial strain generally occurs when income is quantitatively inadequate to meet expenses, it is not defined in objective economic terms. It is, rather, a psychological variable influenced by values, expectations, and perceptions as well as objective financial conditions.

Financial strain has been linked to a number of health consequences among older adults, including disability (Matthews et al. 2005), psychological distress (Ferraro and Su1999), and even mortality (Szanton et al. 2008). Importantly, because financial strain reflects a person's subjective *perception* of his or her financial situation, it may be a particularly important predictor of psychological stress and mental health. During past crises, including the Great Recession, older adults experienced poor mental health outcomes, including increased anxiety and depression, that were more strongly associated with increased financial strain than with objective measures of financial well-being such as income and net worth (Wilkinson 2016). Given the established relationship between mental health and financial strain and the impact of the COVID-19 pandemic on the financial condition of all demographic groups, including older adults, it is important to consider the pathways by which financial strain may influence mental health outcomes and to develop strategies to mitigate the impact.

POTENTIAL MECHANISMS BY WHICH FINANCIAL STRAIN MAY IMPACT HEALTH

Financial strain may influence health through several pathways. First, and perhaps most obvious, financial strain may result in reduced access to health-promoting resources, including fresh foods, preventive health care treatment, stable housing, and leisure activities that promote social and physical health. People experiencing financial strain may be less able to afford these healthy resources; for example, a person may rely on food banks if experiencing food insecurity, making it more difficult to regularly obtain fresh foods (Prayogo et al. 2018).

Similarly, a person may choose to forgo health care treatment because of the expense of co-pays and transportation to appointments. As telehealth becomes increasingly prevalent and particularly relied on during crises such as the COVID-19 pandemic, people experiencing financial strain may also experience a lack of access to health care due to a lack of access to the internet. More than 40% of community-dwelling Medicare beneficiaries lack access to high-speed internet at home (Roberts and Mehrotra 2020). That number may increase during crises, when older adults are making difficult choices about how to use limited funds.

In addition, people experiencing financial strain are more likely to live in low-income neighborhoods that have disproportionately poor access to health-promoting resources. For example, grocery stores are less likely to open in low-income neighborhoods, resulting in residents living in food deserts and relying on packaged and unhealthy foods. There is also significantly less public spending on green space in low-income neighborhoods, limiting access to parks and sidewalks for safe and enjoyable walking and exercise.

People experiencing financial strain may also have less expendable time to spend engaging in physical activity or socializing because of time spent working extra jobs, navigating public transportation, and other "time taxes" associated with the stress of making ends meet. This lost time for self-care and social health may, in turn, affect a person's overall health and well-being. These factors may contribute to the association between financial strain and negative health behaviors such as poor diet (Nelson et al. 2008), missed doses of prescribed medications (Osborn et al. 2017), and inadequate physical activity (Komazawa et al. 2021).

People experiencing financial strain not only have reduced access to healthy goods but also have increased exposure to unhealthy goods and toxins. For example, studies demonstrate that there is more marketing of tobacco, fast food, alcohol, and other unhealthy goods in low-income neighborhoods. People living in low-income neighborhoods are also more likely to be exposed to environmental toxins such as lead in water and ground soil, industrial plants, and toxic waste sites. These factors may contribute to the association between financial strain and substance use as well as other adverse health outcomes (Kendzor et al. 2010; Shaw et al. 2011).

Another mechanism by which financial strain may affect health is through the inflammatory stress process. All of the experiences described above, as well as the general stress of worrying about making ends meet, may contribute to a chronically heightened stress response in people experiencing financial strain. Research demonstrates that financial strain is linked to an increase in oxidative stress, inflammatory cytokines, and hemoglobin A1c (Cutrona et al. 2015; Gémes et al. 2008; Palta et al. 2015; Samuel et al. 2020; Walker et al. 2021). Abnormal changes in all these biomarkers predict poor health outcomes, including disability, obesity, functional limitations, increased health care utilization, nursing home admissions, and mortality. This body of research suggests that in addition to financial strain indirectly affecting physiology through its impact on access to resources and exposure to toxins, it may also directly affect physiology through the stress response. This is particularly concerning in the context of a crisis like the COVID-19 pandemic when acute global stressors collide with long-term household-level stressors.

Although we are too close to the COVID-19 pandemic to fully understand its effects on financial strain and health, initial research suggests that this crisis has disproportionately affected and widened disparities among older people. At the same time that older adults are concerned about their increased risk for severe disease due to the virus, they are experiencing the stress of social isolation, and they are experiencing economic stress due to job loss, lack of savings, and concerns about pension funding shortfalls (Li and Mutchler 2020; Whitehead and Torossian 2021). Many of the usual support systems that older adults rely on, such as senior centers, sandwich generation family caregivers, and senior housing providers, may be less accessible because of quarantine and social distancing requirements. They may also themselves be facing additional stressors during the pandemic and be less able to provide support. For example, senior housing providers are experiencing unprecedented financial hardship during the pandemic, straining their ability to support residents, which could, in turn, add to the burden of the pandemic for older people (LeadingAge 2020). These pandemic stressors are of particular concern given their potential to exacerbate existing inequalities among low-income and racial and ethnic minority older adults.

ADDRESSING OLDER ADULT FINANCIAL STRAIN DURING THE PANDEMIC AND BEYOND

Implications for Clinical Care

Clinicians have opportunities to investigate, address, and mitigate the effects of financial strain on the older adults they treat. Providers should consider screening for financial strain at each visit. A well-validated quick nine-question survey developed by Pearlin and colleagues (1981) can elucidate a patient's stress related to finances and open the door to conversations about social resources and supportive services. The screener asks about the person's ability to afford a home, furniture, car, food, medical care, clothing, and leisure activities and to pay bills (Pearlin et al. 1981). Some researchers and providers even find value in using a single question from Pearlin and colleagues' survey (Szanton et al. 2008). It asks, "At the end of the month do you end up with some money left over, just enough to make ends meet, or not enough money to make ends meet?" (Pearlin et al. 1981). This question, of course, requires providers to be prepared to support patients with resource navigation. Practices should maintain current databases of local resources such as food banks and their eligibility criteria and hours of operation. Practices should also ensure that providers are familiar with and able to connect patients to organizations that can assist with resource navigation, such as the local Area Agency on Aging. Practice-level changes such as partnerships with local social service providers, inclusion of social workers and nurse navigators on the team, and staff training in social determinants of health are positive first steps that can help providers respond to patient reports of financial strain.

It is also important for clinicians to recognize that financial strain may occur even when financial conditions are not objectively dire. For example, it may occur as a result of a psychiatric disorder such as major depression with delusions.

Vignette 2

Mr. C, an 80-year-old retired business executive, was admitted to a psychiatric unit after attempting suicide. He had been in good health and had no history of psychiatric illness or treatment. He lived with his wife of many years and had close relationships with his children. During the weeks before admission, Mr. C became severely depressed and began ruminating about the security of his retirement savings. Despite the efforts of his family and financial advisers to reassure him that his money was secure, he was convinced that he was on the verge of poverty and would have nothing to pass on to his children if he did not die soon. Spurred on by this delusion, Mr. C went to the city harbor with the intention of drowning himself. His delusions of impending poverty and his suicidality subsided in response to treatment for depression.

This case illustrates that subjective financial insecurity may be a *result* of a psychiatric disorder as well as a *cause* of psychological distress. In such cases, treatment of the primary disorder is of paramount importance.

Implications for Policy

COVID-19 exposed structural weaknesses in the financial safety net supporting older adults. Adopting policies that address these weaknesses will reduce financial strain in the waning days of the COVID-19 pandemic and prepare us for the next public health emergency.

First, policy innovations should be directed at preserving income. Many "retired" older adults depend on incomes from jobs in retail, a sector that has been severely affected by the pandemic. Policy solutions could take the form of government aid and loans to retail businesses and immediate and sufficient unemployment benefits for retail workers, such as those enacted in an ad hoc fashion early in the pandemic. In addition, the current Social Security system should be reformed to ensure that benefits keep pace more adequately with inflation.

Second, policies easing expenses for older adults should be implemented. Preserving and enhancing programs that older adults depend on, such as the Supplemental Nutrition Assistance Program (SNAP), Meals on Wheels, senior centers, volunteer caregiver programs, and affordable housing and transportation, should be policy priorities. The national Community Care Corps program funds programs that provide nonmedical volunteer support to older adults aging in place such as companionship, transportation, and help with groceries and household chores. Supporting national service programs such as these, which typically have wide bipartisan support, would help ensure that communities have infrastructure in place to support older residents in times of need.

In addition, policies allowing for the reduction or deferral of out-of-pocket medical expenses should be adopted. During the COVID-19 crisis, Medicare beneficiaries have reported increased difficulty affording copays, prescription drugs, and other medical cost sharing (Davis and Willink 2020). Implementing policies that would allow for flexibility during a crisis would not only help reduce financial strain but could have a direct impact on avoidable emergency care and nursing home use associated with the crisis.

SUMMARY

Pandemics throughout history have had severe and enduring adverse economic effects that have compounded the devastation wrought by the pandemic diseases themselves. Economic disruptions on the scale produced by pandemics have well-documented effects on the general and mental health of all segments of the population, including older adults. Older adults in the United States are somewhat insulated from the full force of recessions by federal programs such as Social Security and Medicare, but many older adults, particularly those with the least wealth, are at risk for financial strain and its adverse impact on health during pandemics. Older adults who are ethnic or racial minorities are often at particular risk because structural racism contributes to significant racial disparities in wealth accumulation. Financial strain—the perception of financial pressure—may affect health through several mechanisms, including limiting access to health-promoting resources, increasing exposure to unhealthy conditions, and inducing physiological stress reactions that promote disease. Knowledge of these mechanisms may enable us to address and mitigate the impact of financial strain due to pandemics in clinical work and policy making.

KEY POINTS

- Past pandemics have had complex, phasic, and enduring adverse economic effects.

- In the United States, older adults, particularly those with the least wealth, have been especially vulnerable to past economic downturns. The impact has been softened in recent decades by federal programs such as Social Security and Medicare for those fortunate to have access to them, although the programs have not kept pace with the cost of living for those for whom they are a primary income source.

- The well-documented health effects of financial strain compound the health risks directly associated with the pandemic disease itself for older adults and must be taken into account by clinicians and policy makers.

QUESTIONS FOR REVIEW

1. Financial strain is operationalized for research and clinical use as which of the following?

    A. The ratio of a person's monthly income to monthly expenses
    B. A person's total debt subtracting total assets
    C. The extent to which a person's income falls below the federal poverty level
    D. The subjective perception a person has about his or her ability to make ends meet

Answer: D.

2. Older adults may be less vulnerable to contemporary financial crises compared with historical crises as a result of which of the following?

    A. They are more likely to live in long-term care settings than at home.
    B. They have access to government programs, including Social Security and Medicare.
    C. They are less likely to be supporting younger generations of family.
    D. They rarely depend on wages from jobs for income during retirement years.

Answer: B.

3. Older adults may be at particular risk for financial strain during financial crises because of which of the following?

    A. Unexpected expenses, such as medical costs, may increase.
    B. Access to usual sources of low- or no-cost support may be limited.
    C. They may experience a decrease in income due to lost wages or investment losses.
    D. All of the above

Answer: D.

REFERENCES

Almond D: Is the 1918 influenza pandemic over? Long-term effects of in utero influenza exposures in the post-1940 US population. Journal of Political Economy 114:672–712, 2006

Asebedo SD, Wilmarth MJ: Does how we feel about financial strain matter for mental health? Journal of Financial Therapy 8(1):5, 2017

Chang SS, Stuckler D, Yip P, et al: Impact of 2008 global economic crisis on suicide: time trend study in 54 countries. BMJ 347:f5239, 2013 24046155

Cohen MA, Tavares JL, Silberman S, et al: Economic insecurity for older adults in the presence of the COVID-19 pandemic: what can we learn from the most recent major economic downturn? (issue brief). Arlington, VA, National Council on Aging, April 2020. Available at: www.ncoa.org/article/economic-insecurity-for-older-adults-in-the-presence-of-the-covid-19-pandemic. Accessed July 7, 2021.

Congressional Research Service: Unemployment rates during the COVID-19 pandemic: in brief. Washington, DC, Congressional Research Service, December 7, 2020. Available at: https://crsreports.congress.gov/product/pdf/R/R46554/5. Accessed July 7, 2021.

Cutler DM, Summers LH: the COVID-19 pandemic and the $16 trillion virus. JAMA 324(15):1495–1496, 2020 33044484

Cutrona CE, Abraham WT, Russell DW, et al: Financial strain, inflammatory factors, and haemoglobin A1c levels in African American women. Br J Health Psychol 20(3):662–679, 2015 25327694

Davis K, Willink A: COVID-19 and affordability of coverage and care for Medicare beneficiaries. New York, Commonwealth Fund, Issue Briefs, September 3, 2020. Available at: www.commonwealthfund.org/publications/issue-briefs/2020/sep/covid-19-affordability-coverage-care-medicare-beneficiaries. Accessed July 7, 2021.

Encyclopedia.com: Elderly, impact of the Great Depression on the. Encyclopedia.com, 2019. Available at: www.encyclopedia.com/economics/encyclopedias-almanacs-transcripts-and-maps/elderly-impact-great-depression. Accessed July 7, 2021.

Farber HS: Employment, hours, and earning consequences of job loss: US evidence from the displaced workers survey. J Labor Econ 35(S1):S235–S272, 2017

Ferraro KF, Su Y: Financial strain, social relations, and psychological distress among older people: a cross-cultural analysis. J Gerontol B Psychol Sci Soc Sci 54(1):S3–S15, 1999 9934397

Garrett TA: Pandemic economics: the 1918 influenza and its modern-day implications. Federal Reserve Bank of St. Louis Review 90(2):75–93, 2008

Gémes K, Ahnve S, Janszky I: Inflammation a possible link between economical stress and coronary heart disease. Eur J Epidemiol 23(2):95–103, 2008 17985199

Johnson RW, Kawachi J: Job changes at older ages: effects on wages, benefits, and other job attributes. Washington, DC, Urban Institute, 2007. Available at: www.urban.org/sites/default/files/publication/46226/311435-Job-Changes-at-Older-Ages.PDF. Accessed July 7, 2021.

Kendzor DE, Businelle MS, Costello TJ, et al: Financial strain and smoking cessation among racially/ethnically diverse smokers. Am J Public Health 100(4):702–706, 2010 20167886

Kerr WC, Kaplan MS, Huguet N, et al: Economic recession, alcohol, and suicide rates: comparative effects of poverty, foreclosure, and job loss. Am J Prev Med 52(4):469–475, 2017 27856114

Kliff S, Silver-Greenberg J: A new item on your medical bill: the "Covid" fee. New York Times, November 8, 2020. Available at: nyti.ms/34WVJ9a. Accessed July 7, 2021.

Komazawa Y, Murayama H, Harata N, et al: Role of social support in the relationship between financial strain and frequency of exercise among older Japanese: a 19-year longitudinal study. J Epidemiol 31(4):265–271, 2021 32307351

LeadingAge: National survey of senior housing providers finds COVID-19 cases in majority of communities: financial strain and isolation identified as key concerns. Washington, DC, LeadingAge, October 1, 2020. Available at: https://leadingage.org/sites/default/files/Oct%202020%20affordable%20housing%20survey%20results%20summary%20Oct%2021%202020_0.pdf. Accessed July 7, 2021.

Li Y, Mutchler JE: Older adults and the economic impact of the COVID-19 pandemic. J Aging Soc Policy 32(4–5):477–487, 2020 32543304

Matthews RJ, Smith LK, Hancock RM, et al: Socioeconomic factors associated with the onset of disability in older age: a longitudinal study of people aged 75 years and over. Soc Sci Med 61(7):1567–1575, 2005 16005788

Nelson MC, Lust K, Story M, et al: Credit card debt, stress and key health risk behaviors among college students. Am J Health Promot 22(6):400–407, 2008 18677880

Osborn CY, Kripalani S, Goggins KM, et al: Financial strain is associated with medication nonadherence and worse self-rated health among cardiovascular patients. J Health Care Poor Underserved 28(1):499–513, 2017 28239015

Palta P, Szanton SL, Semba RD, et al: Financial strain is associated with increased oxidative stress levels: the Women's Health and Aging studies. Geriatr Nurs 36(2)(suppl):S33–S37, 2015 25784083

Pearlin LI, Lieberman MA, Menaghan EG, et al: The stress process. J Health Soc Behav 22(4):337–356, 1981 7320473

Prayogo E, Chater A, Chapman S, et al: Who uses foodbanks and why? Exploring the impact of financial strain and adverse life events on food insecurity. J Public Health (Oxf) 40(4):676–683, 2018 29145590

Roberts ET, Mehrotra A: Assessment of disparities in digital access among Medicare beneficiaries and implications for telemedicine. JAMA Intern Med 180(10):1386–1389, 2020 32744601

Samuel L, Szanton SL, Fedarko NS, et al: Leveraging naturally occurring variation in financial stress to examine associations with inflammatory burden among older adults. J Epidemiol Community Health 74(11):892–897, 2020 32665370

Scheidel W: The Great Leveler: Violence and the History of Inequality From the Stone Age to the 21st Century. Princeton, NJ, Princeton University Press, 2018

Shaw BA, Agahi N, Krause N: Are changes in financial strain associated with changes in alcohol use and smoking among older adults? J Stud Alcohol Drugs 72(6):917–925, 2011 22051205

Szanton SL, Allen JK, Thorpe RJ Jr, et al: Effect of financial strain on mortality in community-dwelling older women. J Gerontol B Psychol Sci Soc Sci 63(6):S369–S374, 2008 19092046

Tapia Granados JA, Diez Roux AV: Life and death during the Great Depression. Proc Natl Acad Sci U S A 106(41):17290–17295, 2009 19805076

Walker RJ, Garacci E, Campbell JA, et al: Relationship between multiple measures of financial hardship and glycemic control in older adults with diabetes. J Appl Gerontol 40(2):162–169, 2021 32167406

Whitehead BR, Torossian E: Older adults' experience of the COVID-19 pandemic: a mixed-methods analysis of stresses and joys. Gerontologist 61(1):36–47, 2021 32886764

Wilkinson LR: Financial strain and mental health among older adults during the Great Recession. J Gerontol B Psychol Sci Soc Sci 71(4):745–754, 2016 26843395

ETHICAL DILEMMAS AND RESOURCE SCARCITIES DURING PANDEMICS

Marilyn Price, M.D.
Donna M. Norris, M.D.
Samara E. Rainey, B.A.
Raya E. Kheirbek, M.D., M.P.H.

There are numerous ethical challenges for clinicians treating older adults during a pandemic. Early on in the coronavirus SARS-CoV-2 disease (COVID-19) pandemic, it became apparent that older adults were dying at vastly disproportionate rates, with 80% of COVID-19-related deaths occurring among adults ages 65 and older. The greatest risk for disability and death occurred within the population older than age 85, particularly those residing in skilled nursing facilities. Loneliness and isolation exacerbated by the pandemic increased risk factors for mental health concerns among persons in vulnerable populations, including older adults. From the onset, it has been apparent that Black and Hispanic groups have been similarly disproportionately affected. Treating patients under difficult circumstances gave rise to a significant burden of moral distress and moral injury among health care providers and others. In some parts of the world, health care professionals were forced to decide how to allocate scarce resources, such as ventilators and intensive care unit beds, as demand grew exponentially. In this chapter we provide an overview of likely ethical dilemmas and how to apply ethical principles to situations such as treatment priorities, isolation measures, and prioritizing experimental therapeutics and vaccine allocations to guide and facilitate sound ethical decision-making in the care of older adults.

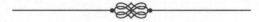

Vignette

Ms. P is an 88-year-old widow residing in a nursing home. She has moderate Alzheimer's disease but does not have an advance directive. Her family members struggle with surrogate decision-making because they never discussed her wishes with her before the onset of cognitive decline. Ms. P has contracted COVID-19, and her condition has deteriorated such that she needs to be placed on a respirator.

The discipline of health care ethics has developed over the years to protect the rights and ensure the safety of the most vulnerable. During the COVID-19 pandemic, numerous ethical issues came to the forefront as health care systems across the world struggled to meet an exponentially growing demand in the face of significant scarcity of health care resources. Within a short period of time, it became apparent that older adults were dying from the virus at vastly disproportionate rates (Farrell et al. 2020a, 2020b). The greatest risk for disability and death occurred in those older than age 80, with 41% of all COVID-19 deaths taking place in long-term care settings such as skilled nursing facilities (Girvan 2020; Panagiotou et al. 2021; Woolf et al. 2021).

Although, understandably, the focus has been on factors contributing to mortality, the growing concern is the impact of social isolation on seniors. Responding to the virus's rapid community spread and the lethal threat it posed to medically vulnerable individuals, public health officials implemented aggressive social distancing measures to lessen the risk of person-to-person spread. Family members were advised to maintain physical distance from their loved ones and, ideally, not to visit at all until the risk had been contained. The stay-at-home order may also have negatively affected health behaviors (Knell et al. 2020) of community-dwelling seniors who formerly enjoyed social activities and visits from family and friends. Scholars have speculated that pandemic-associated isolation may lead to increased rates of suicide among older adults (Wand et al. 2020). Hospitals and nursing homes implemented strict no-visitors policies, and many COVID-19 seniors died alone or with minimal social contact. The lack of family visits resulted in the most commonly reported fear among coronavirus patients: dying alone in an isolated environment, a process that not only is dehumanizing for the patient but also affects family members who are confronted with the realization that their loved one is suffering alone (Wakam et al. 2020).

Health care facilities, already struggling with understaffing and its attendant problems before the pandemic, found their resources further constrained. These circumstances have given rise to a plethora of ethical dilemmas on a scale not previously seen. Frontline health care workers experienced moral distress resulting from the perceived failure to fulfill their moral obligations and provide good patient care (Lai et al. 2020; Wu et al. 2009). Agonizing resource decisions had to be made as cases continued to surge, giving rise to significant moral distress and moral injury among health care providers (Borges et al. 2020; Silverman et al. 2021). The psychological consequences of this type of moral distress include negative feelings, decreased self-esteem, ambivalence, avoidance, frustration, anger, sadness, guilt, and shame (Austin et al. 2008; Hamric et al. 2006).

ETHICAL PRINCIPLES

Decision-making in geriatric psychiatry involves a careful balance of medical expertise and adherence to the ethical principles of medicine. Traditionally, these ethical principles include beneficence, nonmaleficence, autonomy and respect for persons, and justice and fairness. However, responding to the COVID-19 public health crisis demands a broader ethical perspective than the four-principle approach of traditional medical ethics. In pandemics, the collective interest of the society assumes the greatest relevance.

Beneficence

Beneficence refers to the principle of doing good or being helpful and can be applied to medical decision-making prior to care rationing (Ho and Neo 2021). Honoring the ethical principle of beneficence means that the provider is acting in order to be of benefit to the patient (McCormick 2018). A psychiatrist who recommends involuntary hospitalization is often acting on beneficence, believing that treatment—even over a patient's objection when that patient's judgment is impaired because of illness—may result in more benefit to the patient by preventing harm to the patient or others. Withholding care that is likely to be futile and to offer no clinical benefit to the patient also serves the principle of beneficence (Farrell et al. 2020a). During COVID-19, health care systems had to create capacity to accommodate a large number of COVID-19 patients in need. As a result, access to elective and routine services were curtailed. Protective gear had to be rationed and, in some cases, used for extended time periods because of shortages. Therefore, during the COVID-19 pandemic, beneficence to a single patient needed to be balanced by an urgent need to care for acutely ill patients.

Nonmaleficence

Nonmaleficence is the principle of avoiding harm and relates to the directive *primum non nocere*, that is, "first, do no harm" (Gillon 1985). The American Psychiatric Association (2020) notes that nonmaleficence may factor into discharge decisions. For example, an infectious patient may be quarantined rather than discharged to avoid inflicting harm on the patient's family or other caregivers. Nonmaleficence applies to both the individual and the community. It is what leads to public health measures of contact tracing, social distancing, and restrictive hospital visitation policies, such that the restriction is proportionate to the harm (Shearer 2020).

Nonmaleficence is also a duty to recognize the limitations of one's own clinical skills and to seek assistance when those limits are reached to augment or institute appropriate care. In pandemics, chaos ensues, and there is a rapid transition to a changed environment with an overwhelming number of patients. In this environment, health care professionals may be assigned to functions not normally within their responsibilities or may work in areas in which they are not trained or knowledgeable, and nonprofessionals may need to perform tasks that are normally the purview of professionals or assign professionals to work in areas for which they are not licensed or trained (World Health Organization 2007). Further, because of limited time for additional training (Silverman et al. 2021), harm may result, jeopardizing the principle of nonmaleficence. Failing to recognize and address the impact of health care disparities and inequity can result in a further violation of this principle; clinicians should maintain their knowledge of cultural disparities to ensure that their actions are consistent with nonmaleficence.

Autonomy and Respect for Persons

In geriatric psychiatry, one of the more challenging areas of ethics is the question of how best to honor principles of autonomy and respect for persons. The law protects an individual's right to refuse medical treatment, even during periods of incapacity. However, older people might internalize the idea that others (not themselves) know what is best for their well-being. Such paternalism can negatively affect their sense of autonomy and control. Ideally, competent adults would execute advance directives stating their wishes regarding the provision of medical care should they become incapacitated in the future. Do-not-resuscitate orders are among the most familiar of these directives, but advance care planning documents may also specify an individual's wishes regarding withdrawal of life support, provision of artificial nutrition and hydration, and decisions regarding life-sustaining treatment and the extent to which quality of life may be prioritized over longevity. Advance directives may also specify a desired substitute decision-maker who is authorized to make medical decisions on the patient's behalf should the patient be unable to do so.

Following a patient's advance directives honors the ethical principles of autonomy and respect for persons, even when the patient lacks the capacity to communicate such decisions (Curtis et al. 2020). The American Geriatrics Society (AGS) and others have stressed the critical importance of appropriate advance care planning to reduce potential ethical dilemmas in the treatment of older adults (Curtis et al. 2020; Farrell et al. 2020a). Unfortunately, only about half of adults older than age 60 have completed any advance directives regarding their health care preferences (Farrell et al. 2020a, 2020b). Clinicians can elicit the personal and moral values most important to the individual and encourage the completion of advance directives. In the vignette, if Ms. P had completed such an advance directive, her physicians could have honored her choices and preferences when her condition deteriorated.

The COVID-19 pandemic has raised multiple issues related to autonomy and competency. These issues include competence to refuse treatment, leave against medical advice, refuse testing, refuse vaccination, and even refuse wearing a mask. During a pandemic, the ethical issues involved in such decisions are complicated because it is not only the individual's well-being that may be at stake. The execution of advance care planning prior to serious acute illness is critical to avoid intensive life-sustaining treatments when unwanted by patients, avoid stressing the capacity of the health care system when intensive measures are not even desired, and, in the case of COVID-19, avoid unnecessary exposure of family members or health care workers (Curtis et al. 2020). It should be remembered that there is no ethically significant difference between decisions that withhold life-sustaining treatment and those that withdraw it. Physicians, however, may feel that there is a psychological difficulty in withdrawing treatment and may find it easier to suggest a time-limited trial of treatment.

Justice and Fairness

The ethical principle of justice relates to the equitable allocation of resources and fairness in the distribution of care:

> The foundational ethical principle of crisis standards of care is fairness: a transparent decision-making process must prioritize allocation stan-

> dards that are "recognized as fair" by all stakeholders. The resulting allocation scheme is based on medical need, not on extraneous demographic and social factors. The ethical framework for crisis standards of care requires that the ethical norms of a duty to care and a duty to steward resources be balanced against one another, with conflicts resolved through fair and transparent processes. (Garrett et al. 2020, p. 80)

Prioritizing wealthy or privileged individuals over those of limited economic means when allocating doses of a vaccine, for example, would violate the ethical principle of fairness (Spencer 2021; Wamsley 2020). Similarly, the AGS states that "[t]here is something particularly unjust about membership in a class, such as an age group, determining whether a person receives health care" (Farrell et al. 2020a). The American Psychiatric Association (2020) notes that considering the needs of caregivers and maintaining transparency regarding allocation of resources serve the principle of justice and equity. Strategies for equitable distribution need to ensure ease of access to resources for everyone in the population, including the most vulnerable. It is clear that Black people have been disproportionately affected by this pandemic, and they are also experiencing access barriers to registering for and obtaining COVID-19 vaccines (Morales 2021). These barriers include historic distrust in the medical community; the rapidity by which the vaccine was developed; and limited access to information, technology, and broadband internet access (Chatters et al. 2020; Morales 2021).

Older patients in disadvantaged neighborhoods or rural areas may not have the technological equipment or capability to negotiate a path to successful vaccination. A federal initiative plans to address this inequity by sending 1 million doses of the vaccines to retail pharmacies and community clinics (The White House 2021). However, many seniors live in "pharmacy deserts" (communities underserved by pharmacy services), so vaccine availability is still an issue for them, and lack of adequate transportation provides an additional challenge. Strategies to address these challenges include having teams go to the homes of vulnerable patients and establishing large public venues (e.g., stadiums, theaters, empty department stores) to offer greater opportunity to serve larger segments of the population. Nevertheless, these venues may be difficult to access and navigate for seniors who experience physical limitations.

The systems that should protect people have systematically discriminated against them (Gold et al. 2020; Millett et al. 2020; Price-Haywood et al. 2020). Confronting unequal treatment of the population we serve must be at the forefront of our work. Factors contributing to disparities need to be identified and addressed, including reduced access to care and lower health care utilization related to lower socioeconomics and lack of trust in the health care system, living in crowded places, inequalities in income, and lack of support for caregivers.

Other Ethical Principles and Theories

In the context of the COVID-19 pandemic, the ethical theory of consequentialism bears special importance, "with the ultimate aims of reducing suffering and maximizing the number of lives and life years saved" (Bruno and Rose 2020, pp. 20–21). The Advisory Committee on Immunization Practices (ACIP) recently highlighted the importance of five ethical principles to help guide decisions regarding allocation of the COVID-19 vaccines: maximizing benefits and minimizing harms, equity, justice, fairness, and transparency (Bell et al. 2020). Jeffrey (2020) also explored key challenges specific to COVID-19 in three domains, including ethics of isolation and social distancing, duty of care to patients, and access to treatment when in a resource-scarce environment.

SPECIFIC ETHICAL GUIDANCE

Pandemic and disaster planning guidance documents now routinely include sections that articulate the underlying ethical principles of the plan (Devereaux et al. 2008; Pape et al. 2010). The Institute of Medicine has supported numerous projects related to disaster planning that included both expert ethics consensus and community engagement efforts designed to elicit relevant values related to triage and allocation of scarce resources (Joint Centre for Bioethics 2005; World Health Organization 2007). Specific ethical guidance is available from several professional organizations, including the World Health Organization, American Medical Association (AMA), American College of Chest Physicians, and the American Psychiatric Association (APA).

Many resources have been developed by professional organizations to guide physicians in the ethical care of patients in the context of the COVID-19 pandemic (American Medical Association 2020a, 2020b), including the American Medical Association's (2021) COVID-19 resource center. The AMA Code of Medical Ethics, first drafted in the 1950s (Young 2020), forms the backbone of ethics in medicine in the United States. The code is built around nine core principles (Jeffrey 2020), which are listed in Table 14–1.

The American Psychiatric Association (2020) has also published timely recommendations on addressing risks to confidentiality when using new technology and exercising caution when working outside one's usual scope of practice. The document also stresses the impor-

Table 14–1.   Core principles of the American Medical Association's Code of Medical Ethics

A physician shall be dedicated to providing competent medical care, with compassion and respect for human dignity and rights.

A physician shall uphold the standards of professionalism, be honest in all professional interactions, and strive to report physicians deficient in character or competence, or engaging in fraud or deception, to appropriate entities.

A physician shall respect the law and also recognize a responsibility to seek changes in those requirements that are contrary to the best interests of the patient.

A physician shall respect the rights of patients, colleagues, and other health professionals and shall safeguard patient confidences and privacy within the constraints of the law.

A physician shall continue to study, apply, and advance scientific knowledge; maintain a commitment to medical education; make relevant information available to patients, colleagues, and the public; obtain consultation; and use the talents of other health professionals when indicated.

A physician shall, in the provision of appropriate patient care, except in emergencies, be free to choose whom to serve, with whom to associate, and the environment in which to provide medical care.

A physician shall recognize a responsibility to participate in activities contributing to the improvement of the community and the betterment of public health.

A physician shall, while caring for a patient, regard responsibility to the patient as paramount.

A physician shall support access to medical care for all people.

Source. Jeffrey 2020.

tance of self-care and emotional and spiritual support for psychiatrists, given the significant potential for moral injury when practicing in resource-constrained settings and highly stressful circumstances. An additional APA resource contains valuable principles to guide the geriatric psychiatrist to manage ethical dilemmas, including those that have arisen related to the COVID-19 pandemic (American Psychiatric Association 2013).

DEALING WITH RESOURCES THAT MAY BE LIMITED

The COVID-19 pandemic has revealed and highlighted several limitations in resources that have stressed and, in some cases, such as in Italy,

Brazil, and India, completely overwhelmed health care systems. We review these limitations in this section.

Medications and Vaccines

The pandemic has had an adverse impact on the availability of prescription medications (Unguru 2020). Supply chain problems began to emerge in 2020 when pharmacies experienced shortages of medications either due to higher-than-usual demand or due to the impact of the COVID-19 pandemic on staffing and operations in China, where many medications are produced.

COVID-19 vaccine distribution began in the United States on December 14, 2020. As of November 5, 2021, 78.1% of the U.S. population ages 12 and older had been vaccinated (https://covid.cdc.gov/covid-data-tracker/#datatracker-home). A larger proportion of those 65 years and older, 97.8%, had been vaccinated. Although pharmaceutical companies developed and released vaccines at an unprecedented pace, the initial distribution was slow, and early access was limited, such that determining how to allocate doses was an important ethical dilemma for public health officials. Persad et al. (2020) recommend that three ethical values be considered in vaccine prioritization. The first is that the vaccine must benefit people and prevent or limit harm. The second is prioritizing disadvantaged populations, including those who experience socioeconomic deprivation and oppression, higher risk of death, or medical vulnerability. Finally, "the third, equal concern precludes considering differences, such as gender, race, or religion, when doing so would not prevent harm or prioritize disadvantaged groups. Equal concern does not support treating differently situated individuals identically or ignoring relevant differences" (Persad et al. 2020, p. 1601). The Hastings Center also provided guidance for addressing ethical challenges in COVID-19 vaccine allocation (Berlinger et al. 2021).

Keeping these ethical principles in mind, the ACIP gave highest priority to the vaccination of frontline health care workers and residents of long-term care facilities (Berlinger et al. 2021). Prioritizing in-person health care professionals, also recommended by the National Academy of Medicine, lessens harm to workers, maintaining the workforce needed to care for the sick, and reduces the spread of the virus within health care facilities (Persad et al. 2020). Persad and colleagues (2020) noted the benefits of additionally prioritizing people engaged in essential high-risk jobs, such as food supply work, and those living in congregate housing situations (e.g., assisted living, nursing homes, prisons, detention facilities) or neighborhoods with high infection rates that are at increased risk of community spread. The World Health Organization and the National Academy of Medicine recommended that priority be given to persons who have health conditions that place them at increased risk of poor outcomes and death (Persad et al. 2020). The Hastings Center cautioned against expanding access to all persons older than age 65 before first providing access to those at highest risk, persons older than age 75, and those with multiple comorbidities (Berlinger et al. 2021).

Human Resources

Human resources are vital to the ethical provision of care, and the importance of protecting health care workers' physical and emotional welfare cannot be overstated. In a recent survey about resource limitations and patient care, a participant health care worker noted that human resources were among the resource limitations with the greatest impact: "The main limitation for a long time was really nursing, staffing.... Like everybody, we were worried about ventilator capacity, but that turned out to be sort of, at the end, not the main problem" (Butler et al. 2020, p. 7). Knowledge, skill, and expertise are among the human resources that may be limited; ethical dilemmas can arise easily when workers are reassigned because of need or are concerned that they may bring the infection home to family members.

The well-being of health care providers may be adversely affected by the working conditions experienced by many during the pandemic (American Psychiatric Association 2020). Treating patients in a time of human resources scarcity and extreme pressure carries special risks for older clinicians, many of whom are at higher risk themselves from COVID-19 (Buerhaus et al. 2020). Moral distress among clinicians has been reported as a significant concern (Dolgin et al. 2021). As human beings, health care personnel have limited stores of physical and emotional energy, and working under extreme pressure for prolonged periods of time carries a cost to the provider's well-being. Time caring for patients is time spent away from their own families.

Informal caregivers, such as a patient's family members, are also a limited human resource. Caregivers may be vulnerable to fatigue and depression, which can increase the risk for elder abuse and neglect (Storey 2020). Attending to the well-being of a patient's caregivers helps to uphold the ethical principles of beneficence and nonmaleficence. Family engagement improves health care outcomes (Crawford et al. 2002). Research demonstrates that family visits shorten length of stay, reduce delirium, and reduce medication errors (Kheirbek et al. 2021; Yoneyama et al. 2016). Further, family engagement improves acceptance and satisfaction with end-of-life care, palliative care, and care transitions. Innovative strategies to keep caregivers engaged through the use of technology have shown some promise (Calton et al. 2020).

Funding, Capital, and Socioeconomic Disparities

Financial resources may be limited not only by pandemic-related factors but also by preexisting socioeconomic disparities. For many individuals throughout the world, the option to practice social distancing is a luxury, and many American Indian reservations may not have running water or indoor plumbing. Many essential workers cannot work from home or take time off from work to isolate themselves, and many live in densely populated areas and share living quarters with others who also cannot stay home. Older adults living on a fixed income may not be able to afford broadband internet access, which may be needed for telehealth appointments (Nadkarni et al. 2020). Limited financial resources may also affect outcomes because of the need to access and purchase large quantities of personal protective equipment for face-to-face care.

Diagnostic Testing Capabilities

Routinely testing patients for COVID-19 may help to reduce risk, but diagnostic testing capabilities are finite. The American Psychiatric Association (2020) has not yet announced an official policy regarding the necessity (or lack thereof) of testing patients for COVID-19 prior to admission to psychiatric hospitalization. The organization also notes that COVID-19 tests are not infallible, as illustrated by high rates of false negatives, and that enhanced safety, hygiene, and physical distancing precautions are warranted even when treating patients who have tested negative for the virus (American Psychiatric Association 2020). The Substance Abuse and Mental Health Services Administration (2020) recommended that psychiatric hospitals conduct intake screening and testing when appropriate and, when possible, that "all new admissions be segregated until COVID-19 testing results are available." Self-testing and saliva-based testing options may offer added convenience and safety for older adults, and such tests usually are covered by Medicare or private insurance.

Treatment Technologies and Equipment

Initially, during the pandemic, there was significant concern about the scarcity of ventilators (Yahya and Khawaja 2020) and personal protective equipment (Woolley et al. 2020), both of which are critical to risk containment and patient care. In some areas, such as Italy during the initial spike in virus activity, ventilator shortages indeed led to serious ethical dilemmas for physicians (Le Couteur et al. 2020). However, limited resources in other forms of treatment equipment and technology have had a greater impact on access to care than was originally anticipated. For example, during spikes in the pandemic, when positive test rates were high in particular geographic areas, physicians' offices often closed temporarily, and elective surgeries were postponed to help contain risk. These measures, prudent from the perspective of virus risk containment, led to delays in care for many older adults, thereby raising the risk of morbidity and mortality from other causes. Additional ethical dilemmas may arise when health care professionals are faced with the prospect of providing care without ample personal protective equipment.

Time

Finally, time is a vital resource that may factor into ethical dilemmas in geriatric psychiatry. There is a need for research and education to help inform risk management, but staff who are busy providing clinical care to seriously ill patients have minimal time to devote to research and obtaining additional continuing medical education. Furthermore, in making care decisions for a patient who is critically ill, there may not be sufficient time for ethics consultations or detailed analysis of the pros and cons of various treatment options.

POTENTIAL ETHICAL DILEMMAS

One of the most challenging ethical dilemmas during the COVID-19 pandemic has been balancing risks to individuals against risks to the group or to the human population as a whole. In resource-limited settings, it is not uncommon for ethical principles to come into conflict. For example, the ethical principle of beneficence may prompt the psychiatrist to recommend life-sustaining treatment, whereas the ethical principle of autonomy and respect for persons may require the withdrawal of such treatment if the patient's advance directive requests it. As the American Psychiatric Association (2020, p. 2) explained, these ethical dilemmas relate to competing moral obligations:

> Ethical dilemmas arise when there are multiple ethical responsibilities that stand in tension with each other. During this pandemic, treating psychiatrists have competing obligations to their patients, to themselves and their families, and to the public good. Similarly, physicians have respon-

sibility for public health efforts, but at the same time must acknowledge that the health systems in which they are asked to serve are held accountable while making decisions under conditions of uncertainty.

Although it is not possible within the space of one chapter to analyze all potential ethical dilemmas that may arise for geriatric clinicians operating in resource-constrained settings, we present several examples of potential and common dilemmas.

Visitors and Isolation

In order to minimize the risk of community spread in congregate-care settings such as hospitals and nursing homes, many facilities adopted strict no-visitors policies during the COVID-19 pandemic. Such measures helped to decrease the risk of infection to staff and patients. However, these policies also further isolated vulnerable older adults whose families, friends, and spiritual care providers were now unable to visit them. Loneliness and social isolation pose significant risks not only to patients' mental health and emotional well-being but also to their physical health. Isolation can paradoxically increase the likelihood of frailty and associated problems that the containment measures were intended to prevent (Piccoli et al. 2020). Furthermore, strict enforcement of isolation-based containment strategies resulted in the heartbreaking reality that many older adults were left to die alone (Elsner 2021; Moore 2020). Infections and social isolation both have negative effects on neuropsychiatric functioning in older adults who have neurocognitive disorder (NCD) as well as those who do not (Manca et al. 2020). With respect to balancing the risks of isolation against the risks of greater infection spread, health care providers and facility administrators had no easy decisions during the pandemic.

Milieu and Treatment Setting

Closely related to the dilemma of risk containment and isolation is the difficulty of decisions regarding milieu and treatment setting, particularly for older adults with NCD. Because of frailty, nonpharmacological interventions are often preferred over medication to treat the behavioral and psychiatric symptoms of NCD; such interventions typically involve close contact with health care providers, other patients, and the patient's family and friends (Nkodo et al. 2020). However, the close physical proximity that functions as a therapeutic element in inpatient psychiatric treatment settings significantly increases the risk of person-to-person infection spread (Fahed et al. 2020). Similarly, allowing patients to ambulate and wander within the safety of a treatment environment can help to manage agitation (thereby lessening the need for nonpreferred psychopharmacological measures or physical restraints), but such freedom of movement increases the risk of infection spread (Nkodo et al. 2020). Special considerations may apply in correctional settings regarding the detention of nonviolent offenders whose medical conditions place them at higher risk for the adverse consequences of COVID-19 (Rubin 2020).

Capacity and Competency

Issues related to capacity and competency may pose ethical dilemmas. For example, some patients who retain the capacity for treatment decisions may decline COVID-19 testing, treatment (Fahed et al. 2020), or vaccines. Treatment providers and health care facility administrators may be placed in the difficult situation of having to decide whether to allow such patients into offices or hospitals for treatment, which may place staff and other patients at risk. Further complicating such decisions is the fact that patient hesitancy toward testing, vaccines, and treatment may be an entirely rational distrust of the health care system based on past injustices (Annesley 2020). The APA does not recommend forcible COVID-19 testing and advises instead that patients who decline such testing be maintained in quarantine for a period of time in order to protect others (American Psychiatric Association 2020). Other ethical dilemmas may arise in the care of patients with impaired capacity. For example, patients with major NCD may repeatedly remove masks because they are uncomfortable and may not understand or remember their purpose.

CULTURAL COMPETENCE

Ethical treatment during pandemics demands a blend of knowledge about culture, spiritual and religious beliefs, value systems, and human rights (Bennett and Carney 2010; Varghese 2010). Despite good intentions, health care providers may err because of a lack of awareness of religious or cultural backgrounds.

Disagreements

Disagreements are common sources of ethical dilemmas for clinicians. Disputes may arise between the patient and their loved ones regarding the appropriateness of hospitalization or placement in long-term residential care, for example. In the context of COVID-19, disagreements with patients or their families may arise regarding refusals to wear masks or practice social distancing. Disagreements may occur between supervisors or care setting administrators and clinicians when the administrator requires clinicians to provide face-to-face in-person care rather than services via telehealth (Borges et al. 2020). Another example is that of a psychiatric hospital that admits new COVID-19 patients without adequate physical distancing (American Psychiatric Association 2020). The psychiatrist may disagree with such a policy, but full recusal from service is unlikely to result in improved patient care; rather, one might approach such an ethical dilemma by continuing to advocate for institutional policy changes that help to improve infection control practices.

Case Triage, Resource Allocation, and Care Rationing

Case triaging, allocating scarce resources, and rationing care likely represent the most challenging ethical dilemmas for health care providers practicing under the constraints of the COVID-19 pandemic. Although these three concepts are similar and interrelated, they represent distinct practices:

> Firstly, the concept of allocation defines the distribution of all medical facilities, devices and resources disregarding the principle of scarcity. Secondly, the concept of rationing deals with the distribution of medical resources while considering the availability and sufficiency of resources to satisfy patients' needs. Thirdly, the concept of "triage" has a limited scope. It is used in healthcare field to focus on decision-making about distribution and utilization of scarce medical resources. (Jaziri and Alnahdi 2020, pp. 4–5)

Care rationing often results in policies and practices that prioritize patients most likely to survive following treatment (Elbaum 2020), meaning that elderly patients are less likely to receive scarce resources such as ventilators, a scenario that became reality during the case surge in Europe, where in Italy patients younger than age 65 were prioritized for ventilators (Le Couteur et al. 2020). Rockwood (2021) cautioned that approaches like care rationing should be applied judiciously and that, in some circumstances, these approaches have failed to take patients' preferences into account. Furthermore, in some settings, standardized tools for case triage and care rationing were recommended for widespread implementation without ensuring that clinicians using them had received adequate training in their use (Lewis et al. 2021). The AGS and others have recommended against the categorical use of age as a criterion for resource allocation because such policies may conflict with the ethical principle of justice (Farrell et al. 2020a; White and Lo 2020). Similarly, the American Society of Clinical Oncology recommends the use of multiprinciple frameworks to guide decision-making during times of severe shortages (Marron et al. 2020). The principles of beneficence and autonomy can be applied to treatment decisions before rationing care (Ho and Neo 2021).

Mandating Vaccination

The FDA initially approved three vaccines under emergency use authorizations (the Pfizer-BioNTech vaccine received full FDA approval in August 2021), and authorizing mandates can be ethically problematic because these authorizations do not require safety and efficacy data as stringent as what the FDA requires for biologics license application full approval (Gostin et al. 2021). Mello et al (2020) recommends that six trigger criteria should be present before considering a state mandate:

1. COVID-19 is not adequately contained in the state.
2. The ACIP has recommended vaccination for the groups to be covered by the mandate.
3. There is sufficient vaccine available to vaccinate all members of the mandated groups.
4. There has been transparent communication about the efficacy and side effects of the proposed vaccine.
5. The state has sufficient infrastructure to provide access without financial or logistic barriers, workers would receive compensation for side effects resulting from the vaccination, and the state would institute real-time surveillance of vaccine adverse events.
6. Voluntary vaccination among high-priority groups has not been at the levels required to prevent epidemic spread.

Quality and Preservation of Life

Clinicians must consider not only infection control practices but also the effect of policies and treatment recommendations on the emotional and spiritual well-being of the patients they care for as well as that of patients' loved ones. Potential conflicts may arise between COVID-19-targeted interventions (e.g., infection control, medical treatment of patients with the virus) and interventions aimed at treating a patient's psychiatric illness. For example, Bojdani (2021) reported a case in which an 86-year-old patient with bipolar disorder experienced a significant drop in valproic acid levels while being treated for COVID-19. Similarly, psychiatrists should be cognizant of the risk of drug-drug interactions, which is already heightened in older patients and may be especially pronounced in older patients with COVID-19 (Güngör et al. 2021).

Other Ethical Dilemmas

Additional ethical considerations include the need to balance patient confidentiality against the duty to protect other people. It may be appropriate for the provider to inform patients about the rationale for contact tracing and explain that they may be contacted by public health authorities for this reason (American Psychiatric Association 2020). In addition, patients or their families may request specific medications for which there is little or no evidence of efficacy for treating COVID-19 (El Rhazi and Adarmouch 2020).

RECOMMENDATIONS

Collaboration and Consultation

Collaborating and consulting with other professionals are important ethical practices in mental health in general (American Psychiatric Association 2020), regardless of whether one is practicing in the context of COVID-19 or other resource-limited settings. Palliative care specialists can inform treatment recommendations (Taylor-Clark et al. 2010), and ethics consultants may play a valuable role (Dolgin et al. 2021). Most patients and family members will feel distress when faced with treatment limitations or lack of effectiveness. Additional support resources should be made available to them. The AGS has stressed the value of interdisciplinary triage committees for ensuring sound ethical decision-making in the context of the COVID-19 pandemic and other periods of resource scarcities (Farrell et al. 2020a). The APA's Ethics Committee can respond to questions from APA members about the pandemic and relevant ethical dilemmas.

Using Existing Guidance and Education

Infection control practice guidelines and any ethical guidance published by relevant professional societies, such as the AMA, APA, and AGS, are valuable resources for frontline clinicians. Making time to stay current on emerging scientific knowledge regarding COVID-19 and its prevention and treatment is in keeping with the AMA Principles of Medical Ethics (Section 5) (American Medical Association 2016) and the APA's commentaries on their application to psychiatry: "A physician shall continue to study, apply, and advance scientific knowledge, maintain a commitment to medical education, make relevant information available to patients, colleagues, and the public, obtain consultation, and use the talents of other health professionals when indicated" (American Psychiatric Association 2013, p. 10).

Although ethicists find no difference between withholding and withdrawing life-sustaining treatments (Truog et al. 2008), health care providers feel differently, which presents an opportunity for education. Nevertheless, even with appropriate education, the emotional strain and moral distress associated with withdrawal of treatment should be addressed through counseling to prevent burnout.

Restructuring the Care Environment and Threat Containment

Restructuring the treatment milieu to minimize the risk of infection spread helps to serve the ethical principles of nonmaleficence and justice. To minimize infection risk, remote treatment options, such as telepsychiatry and remote patient monitoring, should be considered when feasible. Nkodo et al. (2020) recommend the use of dedicated cognitive-behavioral units specially designed to limit infection risks for treating patients with concurrent disruptive behavioral and psychiatric symptoms of major NCD and COVID-19.

Individualized Care Planning and Shared Decision-Making

Ho and Neo (2021) noted that many ethical dilemmas not associated with scarcity in the care of older patients during the COVID-19 pandemic can be resolved through informed and shared decision-making. Treatment recommendations should take a patient's values and quality of life into account and should be individualized and approached on a case-by-case basis (American Psychiatric Association 2020, p. 2). Individualized care planning performs a critical role—ideally, prior to the emergence of a crisis—in ensuring ethical care provision to older adults (Farrell et al. 2020a).

Standardized screening tools are being evaluated to inform decisions about care planning for vulnerable patients. For example, Huayanay and Luu (2020) reported a case in which the Clinical Frailty Scale was used for an 81-year-old Latina woman who had no advance directives. Other scholars have cautioned that there are significant drawbacks and ethical concerns related to the use of this scale and similar rating scales (Ho and Neo 2021; Lewis et al. 2021; Rockwood 2021). In general, triage systems based on even limited evidence are ethically preferable to those based on clinical judgment alone.

SUMMARY

Providing care to older adults in the context of a pandemic increases clinicians' uncertainty as well as patients' vulnerability and may, therefore, interfere with disciplined, ethical, and shared decision-making. Pandemics present numerous ethical challenges to clinicians caring for older adults. As we struggle to adapt to a rapidly changing world and the moral dilemmas that may arise, approaching issues with core ethical principles in mind may prove helpful. Unfortunately, however, ethics issues permeate virtually all aspects of pandemic and disaster response, and as the American Psychiatric Association (2020) noted, "there are no simple answers and psychiatrists are encouraged to seek consultation with colleagues and ethics resources to navigate these challenging times" (p. 2). In this chapter we aimed to address some of the most pressing issues. Our suggestions reflect the consensus of experts. We recognize, however, that our suggestions, including those related to end-of-life care, may benefit from continuing the dialogue on articulating values to guide health care decisions during disasters for sound ethical decision-making in the psychiatric care of older adults.

KEY POINTS

- In the United States, COVID-19 cases and deaths were disproportionately higher in older adults and in Black and Hispanic patients.

- Ethical and moral dilemmas occur when clinicians are placed in a position of allocating scarce health care resources during times of exponential demand.

- Clinicians should understand ethical principles when prioritizing treatment options, including vaccines and therapeutics.

QUESTIONS FOR REVIEW

1. The greatest risk of death from COVI-19 occurs in persons from which age group?

    A. 0–15 years old
    B. 15–25 years old
    C. 25–35 years old

    D. 35–45 years old

    E. Older than age 85

Answer: E.

2. Which of the following ethical principles has been described as *foundational* to crisis standards of care?

    A. Beneficence

    B. Nonmaleficence

    C. Autonomy and respect for persons

    D. Justice and fairness

    E. Consequentialism

Answer: D.

3. Roughly what percentage of adults over 60 have completed advance directives regarding their health care preferences?

    A. Less than 10%

    B. 25%

    C. 50%

    D. 75%

    E. 90%

Answer: C.

ADDITIONAL RESOURCES

American Geriatrics Society: COVID-19 information hub, www.american geriatrics.org/covid19

American Journal of Geriatric Psychiatry: Open-access articles on COVID-19, www.ajgponline.org/covid19

American Medical Association: AMA Journal of Ethics, COVID-19 ethics resource center (regularly updated), https://journalofethics.ama-assn.org/covid-19-ethics-resource-center

American Psychiatric Association Ethics Committee: apaethics@psych.org

Center for the Study of Traumatic Stress: COVID-19 pandemic response resources, www.cstsonline.org/resources/resource-master-list/coronavirus-and-emerging-infectious-disease-outbreaks-response

Hastings Center: Ethics guidance and resources on COVID-19, www.the-hastingscenter.org/news/ethics-guidance-and-resources-on-covid-19

Johns Hopkins University Coronavirus Resource Center: https://coronavirus.jhu.edu

White DB, Bernard L: A framework for rationing ventilators and critical care beds during the COVID-19 pandemic. JAMA 323(18):1773–1774, 2020 32219367

White DB, Halpern S: Allocation of scarce critical care resources during a public health emergency. Department of Critical Care Medicine, School of Medicine, University of Pittsburgh, April 15, 2020. Available at: https://ccm.pitt.edu/sites/default/files/UnivPittsburgh_ModelHospitalResourcePolicy_2020_04_15.pdf. Accessed July 13, 2021.

REFERENCES

American Medical Association: AMA Code of Medical Ethics: AMA principles of medical ethics. Chicago, IL, American Medical Association, 2016. Available at: www.ama-assn.org/sites/ama-assn.org/files/corp/media-browser/principles-of-medical-ethics.pdf. Accessed July 13, 2021.

American Medical Association: AMA Code of Medical Ethics: guidance in a pandemic. Chicago, IL, American Medical Association, April 14, 2020a. Available at: www.ama-assn.org/delivering-care/ethics/ama-code-medical-ethics-guidance-pandemic. Accessed July 13, 2021.

American Medical Association: Ethics guidance during a pandemic: an overview. Chicago, IL, American Medical Association, July 29, 2020b. Available at: www.ama-assn.org/delivering-care/ethics/ethics-guidance-during-pandemic-overview. Accessed July 13, 2021.

American Medical Association: COVID-19 ethics resource center. Chicago, IL, American Medical Association, 2021. Available at: https://journalofethics.ama-assn.org/covid-19-ethics-resource-center. Accessed July 13, 2021.

American Psychiatric Association: The Principles of Medical Ethics With Annotations Especially Applicable to Psychiatry, 2013 Edition. Arlington, VA, American Psychiatric Association, 2013. Available at: www.psychiatry.org/File%20Library/Practice/Ethics%20Documents/principles2013--final.pdf. Accessed July 13, 2021.

American Psychiatric Association: COVID-19 Related Opinions of the APA Ethics Committee. Washington, DC, American Psychiatric Association, May 29, 2020. Available at: www.psychiatry.org/File%20Library/Psychiatrists/Practice/Ethics/APA-COVID-19-Ethics-Opinions.pdf. Accessed July 13, 2021.

Annesley K: Connecting epistemic injustice and justified belief in health-related conspiracies. Ethics Med Public Health 15:100545, 2020

Austin W, Lemermeyer G, Goldberg L, et al: Moral distress in healthcare practice: the situation of nurses. Alta RN 64(4):4–5, 2008 18512614

Bell BP, Romero JR, Lee GM: Scientific and ethical principles underlying recommendations from the Advisory Committee on Immunization Practices for COVID-19 vaccination implementation. JAMA 324(20):2025–2026, 2020 33090194

Bennett B, Carney T: Law, ethics and pandemic preparedness: the importance of cross-jurisdictional and cross-cultural perspectives. Aust NZ J Public Health 34(2):106–112, 2010 23331351

Berlinger N, Wynia M, Powell T, et al: Ethical challenges in the middle tier of Covid-19 vaccine allocation: guidance for organizational decision-making. Garrison, NY, Hastings Center, January 15, 2021. Available at: www.the-hastingscenter.org/ethical-challenges-in-the-middle-tier-of-covid-19-vaccine-allocation/. Accessed July 13, 2021.

Bojdani E: Pharmacokinetic implications leading to marked valproic acid level-drop during COVID-19 treatment. Psychiatry Res 296:113701, 2021 33418460

Borges LM, Barnes SM, Farnsworth JK, et al: A contextual behavioral approach for responding to moral dilemmas in the age of COVID-19. J Contextual Behav Sci 17:95–101, 2020 32834968

Bruno B, Rose S: Patients left behind: ethical challenges in caring for indirect victims of the COVID-19 pandemic. Hastings Cent Rep 50(4):19–23, 2020 33448404

Buerhaus PI, Auerbach DI, Staiger DO: Older clinicians and the surge in novel coronavirus disease 2019 (COVID-19). JAMA 323(18):1777–1778, 2020 32227200

Butler CR, Wong SPY, Wightman AG, et al: US clinicians' experiences and perspectives on resource limitation and patient care during the COVID-19 pandemic. JAMA Netw Open 3(11):e2027315, 2020 33156349

Calton B, Shibley WP, Cohen E, et al: Patient and caregiver experience with outpatient palliative care telemedicine visits. Palliat Med Rep 1(1):339–346, 2020 34223495

Chatters LM, Taylor HO, Taylor RJ: Older Black Americans during COVID-19: race and age double jeopardy. Health Educ Behav 47(6):855–860, 2020 33090052

Crawford MJ, Rutter D, Manley C, et al: Systematic review of involving patients in the planning and development of health care. BMJ 325(7375):1263, 2002 12458240

Curtis JR, Kross EK, Stapleton RD: The importance of addressing advance care planning and decisions about do-not-resuscitate orders during novel coronavirus 2019 (COVID-19). JAMA 323(18):1771–1772, 2020 32219360

Devereaux AV, Dichter JR, Christian MD, et al: Definitive care for the critically ill during a disaster: a framework for allocation of scarce resources in mass critical care: from a Task Force for Mass Critical Care summit meeting, January 26–27, 2007, Chicago, IL. Chest 133(5)(suppl):51S–66S, 2008 18460506

Dolgin J, McLeod-Sordjan R, Markowitz W, et al: A novel ethical approach to moral distress during COVID 19 in New York. Clin Ethics 16(4):330–340, 2021

Elbaum A: Black lives in a pandemic: implications of systemic injustice for end-of-life care. Hastings Cent Rep 50(3):58–60, 2020 32596896

El Rhazi K, Adarmouch L: Ethical issues related to the hydroxychloroquine treatment prescription for Covid-19. Ethics Med Public Health 14:100547. Epub 17 June 2000 32835062

Elsner AM: After COVID-19: the way we die from now on. Camb Q Healthc Ethics 30(1):69–72, 2021 33371912

Fahed M, Barron GC, Steffens DC: Ethical and logistical considerations of caring for older adults on inpatient psychiatry during the COVID-19 pandemic. Am J Geriatr Psychiatry 28(8):829–834, 2020 32409192

Farrell TW, Ferrante LE, Brown T, et al: AGS position statement: resource allocation strategies and age-related considerations in the COVID-19 era and beyond. J Am Geriatr Soc 68(6):1136–1142, 2020a 32374440

Farrell TW, Francis L, Brown T, et al: Rationing limited healthcare resources in the COVID-19 era and beyond: ethical considerations regarding older adults. J Am Geriatr Soc 68(6):1143–1149, 2020b 32374466

Garrett JR, McNolty LA, Wolfe ID, et al: Our next pandemic ethics challenge? Allocating "normal" health care services. Hastings Cent Rep 50(3):79–80, 2020 32596905

Gillon R: "Primum non nocere" and the principle of non-maleficence. Br Med J (Clin Res Ed) 291(6488):130–131, 1985 3926081

Girvan G: Nursing homes and assisted living facilities account for 42% of COVID-19 deaths. Austin, TX, Foundation for Research on Equal Opportunity, May 7, 2020. Available at: http://freopp.org/the-covid-19-nursing-home-crisis-by-the-numbers-3a47433c3f70. Accessed July 13, 2021.

Gold JAW, Wong KK, Szablewski CM, et al: Characteristics and clinical outcomes of adult patients hospitalized with COVID-19—Georgia, March 2020. MMWR Morb Mortal Wkly Rep 69(18):545–550, 2020 32379729

Gostin LO, Salmon DA, Larson HJ: Mandating COVID-19 vaccines. JAMA 325(6):532–533, 2021 33372955

Güngör ES, Yalçın M, Tüzer MY, et al: Adverse drug reactions associated with concurrent acute psychiatric treatment and Covid-19 drug therapy. Int J Psychiatry Clin Pract 25(2):142–146, 2021 33143519

Hamric AB, Davis WS, Childress MD: Moral distress in health care professionals. Pharos Alpha Omega Alpha Honor Med Soc 69(1):16–23, 2006 16544460

Ho EP, Neo HY: COVID 19: prioritise autonomy, beneficence and conversations before score-based triage. Age Ageing 50(1):11–15, 2021 32975564

Huayanay I, Luu S: Tough decisions during the COVID 19 pandemic: a frail Latino patient. Gerontol Geriatr Med 6:2333721420970336, 2020 33225019

Jaziri R, Alnahdi S: Choosing which COVID-19 patient to save? The ethical triage and rationing dilemma. Ethics Med Public Health 15:100570, 2020 32837999

Jeffrey DI: Relational ethical approaches to the COVID-19 pandemic. J Med Ethics 46(8):495–498, 2020 32522813

Joint Centre for Bioethics: Stand on Guard for Thee: Ethical Considerations in Preparedness Planning for Pandemic Influenza: A Report. Toronto, ON, Canada, University of Toronto, Joint Centre for Bioethics, 2005

Kheirbek RE, Gruber-Baldini A, Shulman LM: Family engagement for hospitalized COVID-19 patients: policy with unintended consequences. Qual Manag Health Care 30(1):78–79, 2021 33230000

Knell G, Robertson MC, Dooley EE, et al: Health behavior changes during COVID-19 pandemic and subsequent "stay-at-home" orders. Int J Environ Res Public Health 17(17):E6268, 2020 32872179

Lai J, Ma S, Wang Y, et al: Factors associated with mental health outcomes among health care workers exposed to coronavirus disease 2019. JAMA Netw Open 3(3):e203976, 2020 32202646

Le Couteur D, Anderson R, Newman A: COVID-19 through the lens of gerontology. J Gerontol A Biol Sci Med Sci 75(9):e119–e120, 2020 32222763

Lewis EG, Breckons M, Lee RP, et al: Rationing care by frailty during the COVID-19 pandemic. Age Ageing 50(1):7–10, 2021 32725156

Manca R, De Marco M, Venneri A: The impact of COVID-19 infection and enforced prolonged social isolation on neuropsychiatric symptoms in older adults with and without dementia: a review. Front Psychiatry 11:585540, 2020 33192732

Marron JM, Joffe S, Jagsi R, et al: Ethics and resource scarcity: ASCO recommendations for the oncology community during the COVID-19 pandemic. J Clin Oncol 38(19):2201–2205, 2020 32343643

McCormick TR: Principles of bioethics. Seattle, Department of Bioethics and Humanities, University of Washington Medicine, 2018. Available at: https:// depts.washington.edu/bhdept/ethics-medicine/bioethics-topics/articles/ principles-bioethics. Accessed July 13, 2021.

Mello MM, Silverman RD, Omer SB: Ensuring uptake of vaccines against SARS-CoV-2. N Engl J Med 383(14):1296–1299, 2020 32589371

Millett GA, Jones AT, Benkeser D, et al: Assessing differential impacts of COVID-19 on Black communities. Ann Epidemiol 47:37–44, 2020 32419766

Moore B: Dying during Covid-19. Hastings Cent Rep 50(3):13–15, 2020 32596910

Morales C: Blacks and Latino Americans confront many challenges to vaccinations. New York Times, February 18, 2021. Available at: www.nytimes.com/2021/ 02/18/world/us-coronavirus-vaccine-minorities.html. Accessed July 13, 2021.

Nadkarni A, Hasler V, AhnAllen CG, et al: Telehealth during COVID-19—Does everyone have equal access? Am J Psychiatry 177(11):1093–1094, 2020 33135470

Nkodo JA, Camus V, Fougère B: Ethical issues in the management of patients with behavioral and psychological symptoms of dementia during COVID-19 containment: examples from institutions in France. Am J Geriatr Psychiatry 28(12):1332–1333, 2020 33077342

Panagiotou OA, Kosar CM, White EM, et al: Risk factors associated with all-cause 30-day mortality in nursing home residents with COVID-19. JAMA Intern Med 181(4):439–448, 2021 33394006

Pape JW, Rouzier V, Ford H, et al: The GHESKIO field hospital and clinics after the earthquake in Haiti—dispatch 3 from Port-au-Prince. N Engl J Med 362(10):e34, 2010 20164476

Persad G, Peek M, Emanuel EJ: Fairly prioritizing groups for access to COVID-19 vaccines. JAMA 324(16):1601–1602, 2020 32910182

Piccoli M, Tannou T, Hernandorena I, et al: Ethical approach to the issue of confinement of the elderly in the context of the COVID-19 pandemic: prevention of frailty versus risk of vulnerability [in French]. Ethics Med Public Health 14:100539, 2020 32835057

Price-Haywood EG, Burton J, Fort D, et al: Hospitalization and mortality among Black patients and white patients with Covid-19. N Engl J Med 382(26):2534–2543, 2020 32459916

Rockwood K: Rationing care in COVID-19: if we must do it, can we do better? Age Ageing 50(1):3–6, 2021 32939534

Rubin R: The challenge of preventing COVID-19 spread in correctional facilities. JAMA 323(18):1760–1761, 2020 32259189

Shearer J: Coronavirus and the ethics of quarantine-why information matters. BMJ Opinion, February 17, 2020. Available at: https://blogs.bmj.com/bmj/ 2020/02/17/coronavirus-and-the-ethics-of-quarantine-why-information-matters/. Accessed July 13, 2021.

Silverman HJ, Kheirbek RE, Moscou-Jackson G, et al: Moral distress in nurses caring for patients with Covid-19: a qualitative study. Nurs Ethics Apr 29, 2021 32939534 Epub ahead of print

Spencer T: Florida company accused of steering vaccines to rich donors. Huffington Post, January 6, 2021. Available at: www.huffpost.com/entry/morselife-florida-covid-19-vaccine_n_5ff639edc5b64e568bf3c574. Accessed July 13, 2021.

Storey JE: Risk factors for elder abuse and neglect: a review of the literature. Aggress Violent Behav 50:101339, 2020

Substance Abuse and Mental Health Services Administration: Covid19: interim considerations for state psychiatric hospitals. Rockville, MD, Substance Abuse and Mental Health Services Administration, May 8, 2020. Available at: www.samhsa.gov/sites/default/files/covid19-interim-considerations-for-state-psychiatric-hospitals.pdf. Accessed July 13, 2021.

Taylor-Clark KA, Viswanath K, Blendon RJ: Communication inequalities during public health disasters: Katrina's wake. Health Commun 25(3):221–229, 2010 20461607

Truog RD, Campbell ML, Curtis JR, et al: Recommendations for end-of-life care in the intensive care unit: a consensus statement by the American College of Critical Care Medicine. Crit Care Med 36(3):953–963, 2008 18431285

Unguru Y: Confronting medication scarcity in the era of COVID-19. Clin Ethics Published online 2020

Varghese SB: Cultural, ethical, and spiritual implications of natural disasters from the survivors' perspective. Crit Care Nurs Clin North Am 22(4):515–522, 2010 21095559

Wakam GK, Montgomery JR, Biesterveld BE, et al: Not dying alone—modern compassionate care in the Covid-19 pandemic. N Engl J Med 382(24):e88, 2020 32289215

Wamsley L: Stanford apologizes after vaccine allocation leaves out nearly all medical residents. NPR, December 18, 2020. Available at: www.npr.org/sections/coronavirus-live-updates/2020/12/18/948176807/stanford-apologizes-after-vaccine-allocation-leaves-out-nearly-all-medical-resid. Accessed July 13, 2021.

Wand APF, Zhong BL, Chiu HFK, et al: COVID-19: the implications for suicide in older adults. Int Psychogeriatr 32(10):1225–1230, 2020 32349837

White DB, Lo B: A framework for rationing ventilators and critical care beds during the COVID-19 pandemic. JAMA 323(18):1773–1774, 2020 32219367

The White House: Fact sheet: President Biden announces community health centers vaccination program to launch next week and another increase in states, tribes and territories' vaccine supply. Washington, DC, The White House, February 9, 2021. Available at: www.whitehouse.gov/briefing-room/statements-releases/2021/02/09/fact-sheet-president-biden-announces-community-health-centers-vaccination-program-to-launch-next-week-and-another-increase-in-states-tribes-territories-vaccine-supply. Accessed July 13, 2021.

Woolf SH, Chapman DA, Lee JH: COVID-19 as the leading cause of death in the United States. JAMA 325(2):123–124, 2021 33331845

Woolley K, Smith R, Arumugam S: Personal protective equipment (PPE) guidelines, adaptations and lessons during the COVID-19 pandemic. Ethics Med Public Health 14:100546, 2020 32835061

World Health Organization: Ethical considerations in developing a public health response to pandemic influenza. Geneva, World Health Organization, 2007. Available at: www.who.int/csr/resources/publications/WHO_CDS_EPR_GIP_2007_2c.pdf. Accessed July 13, 2021.

Wu P, Fang Y, Guan Z, et al: The psychological impact of the SARS epidemic on hospital employees in China: exposure, risk perception, and altruistic acceptance of risk. Can J Psychiatry 54(5):302–311, 2009 19497162

Yahya AS, Khawaja S: Medical ethics and ventilator allocation during the COVID-19 pandemic. Prim Care Companion CNS Disord 22(4):20com02687, 2020 32678525

Yoneyama S, Makita Y, Miyazu K, et al: The role of family variables in the length of stay of psychiatric in-patients. Clin Pract Epidemiol Ment Health 12:87–93, 2016 27867414

Young G: Toward a unified health work ethics code. Ethics Med Public Health 15:100590, 2020

Zhou Y, Stix G: COVID-19 is now the third leading cause of death in the U.S. Scientific American, October 8, 2020. Available at: www.scientificamerican.com/article/covid-19-is-now-the-third-leading-cause-of-death-in-the-u-s1. Accessed July 13, 2021.

CHAPTER 15

NEUROPSYCHIATRIC MANIFESTATIONS OF COVID-19

Rebecca Grossman-Kahn, M.D.
O. Joseph Bienvenu, M.D., Ph.D.

Older adults are the most likely to suffer serious illness as a result of coronavirus SARS-CoV-2 disease (COVID-19) infection. There is a growing body of literature documenting the neuropsychiatric manifestations of COVID-19. In the acute phase of illness, delirium, cerebrovascular disease, seizures, and other neurological disorders are common.

Vignette 1

A 71-year-old man with a history of coronary artery disease and hyperlipidemia is admitted to an internal medicine floor with shortness of breath and fatigue; he tests positive for COVID-19 on day 1 of admission. He is treated with oxygen and remdesivir, and his oxygen saturations improve. On hospital day 3, he is confused and agitated and tries to leave the hospital. On examination, he does not follow commands, his speech is soft and mumbling, and he is not oriented to place or date.

Vignette 2

A 67-year-old woman with a history of asthma presents to a primary care clinic for posthospital follow-up after an admission with symptomatic COVID-19. She did not require intensive care and was discharged after 5 days. She reports that her symptoms of headache, shortness of breath, and myalgias have resolved, but she is frequently tired and has difficulty completing small tasks around the house. She has not felt like herself since she was discharged and wonders if she could be depressed.

Vignette 3

A 69-year-old healthy business executive is transported via ambulance with severe COVID-19 and acute respiratory distress syndrome, requiring intubation in the emergency department, prone positioning, and a stay in the intensive care unit (ICU). In the ICU, he requires high doses of sedating medication and, eventually, neuromuscular blockade to preserve oxygen and prevent desynchronization from the mechanical ventilator. When he awakens, he appears frightened and recalls being imprisoned and tortured by "aliens." He believes his wife has left him and has difficulty resting when stepped down to an internal medicine ward.

COVID-19 AND OLDER ADULTS

COVID-19 is projected to affect a remarkably large proportion of the world's population. At the time of this writing, more than 242 million cases of COVID-19 infections have been reported globally (Johns Hopkins University and Medicine 2021). Although rates of infection are not higher for older adults, the geriatric population is at higher risk of being hospitalized with COVID-19, experiencing more severe disease, and experiencing chronic symptoms and functional impairment as a result of infection (Mueller et al. 2020). Since the beginning of the pandemic, patients in the United States ages 65 and older have accounted for 30%–52% of all COVID-19 hospitalizations (Centers for Disease Control and Prevention 2021a). Compared with that of young adults ages 18–29, the risk of hospitalization was 5 times higher for adults 65–74, 8 times higher for adults 75–84, and 13 times higher for adults 85 and older (Centers for Disease Control and Prevention 2021b). The lasting symptoms caused by severe COVID-19 disease requiring hospitalization disproportionately affect the geriatric population.

Much attention has been given to sequelae of COVID-19, including deconditioning, "long COVID" (Ladds et al. 2020) symptoms such as fatigue, and pulmonary complications, all of which will affect the geriatric population in the coming years. Additionally, a growing body of evidence supports the significant neuropsychiatric burden of COVID-19 infection. From delirium to strokes to anxiety, COVID-19 infection has been observed to affect the brain in varied and numerous ways. Older patients with underlying cognitive impairment or dementia may be particularly affected by the virus's neuropsychiatric manifestations. As a rising proportion of the geriatric patient population becomes exposed to the SARS-CoV-2 virus, it will be crucial for clinicians to have awareness of the neuropsychiatric burden of the infection.

In this chapter we summarize the extant literature as of January 2021 for the range of neuropsychiatric symptoms secondary to COVID-19 and how they may differentially manifest in older adults. We first address acute neurological manifestations, along with their hypothesized mechanisms, that may appear during hospitalization for coronavirus infection, even as the presenting symptom. The literature is skewed toward acute manifestations because January 2021 was still relatively early in the pandemic. We then summarize the existing data on subacute and chronic neuropsychiatric sequelae with proposed risk factors and mechanisms. In the final section we address the impact of the pandemic on the geriatric population as a whole, including the effects of policy measures such as social distancing on mental health and neurocognitive disorders.

ACUTE NEUROPSYCHIATRIC MANIFESTATIONS OF COVID-19

A wide range of neurological symptoms and conditions have been reported in patients in the acute phase of COVID-19 infection, and they are relatively common. Cohort studies of patients treated for COVID-19 identified a range of neuropsychiatric symptoms, affecting 22% (Nalleballe et al. 2020) to 84% (Helms et al. 2020) of patients; there may be an association of neuropsychiatric symptoms with more severe respiratory illness (Mao et al. 2020). Although most of the studies did not specifically study the geriatric population, geriatric patients are overrepresented in these studies given their proneness to symptomatic infections requiring hospitalization. The most frequent neurological manifestation was altered mental status, which comprises delirium and other forms of encephalopathy (e.g., coma).

In some cases, neurological symptoms (in particular, encephalopathy, stroke, and cognitive changes) were the presenting chief complaint. In other cases, neurological symptoms, including delirium and seizures, began only after hospitalization for COVID-19 symptoms (Pinna et al. 2020). When neurological complaints appear before respiratory or other COVID-19 symptoms, the illness tends to be less severe than in cases in which neuropsychiatric symptoms develop after respiratory symptoms (Pinna et al. 2020).

Proposed Mechanisms

Although the exact mechanisms by which COVID-19 causes neuropsychiatric symptoms have not yet been determined, evidence suggests several possible mechanisms. The virus may directly invade the central nervous system, possibly aided by inflammation-mediated breakdown of the blood-brain barrier. A target site of the virus, angiotensin converting enzyme 2, is expressed by neurons and glial cells, which may also explain neuroinvasion. A majority (up to 88%) of patients with COVID-19 report anosmia, supporting the idea that the virus directly invades the central nervous system via the olfactory nerves (Lechien et al. 2020). The virus and antibodies to it have been isolated from cerebrospinal fluid samples in some infected patients, although not from all that have been studied (Helms et al. 2020; Wu et al. 2020).

Another proposed mechanism through which the virus may cause neuropsychiatric symptoms is through secondary, systemic effects modulated by the immune response to the virus. Widespread inflammation and cytokine storm may lead to neuroinflammation. Markers of acute inflammation, including C-reactive protein, D-dimer, and ferritin, are often elevated in patients who experience neuropsychiatric symptoms (Beach et al. 2020; Ferrando et al. 2020; Radmard et al. 2020). In one study, a measure of increased immune system response was correlated with worse psychiatric outcomes (Mazza et al. 2020).

Other mechanisms by which the SARS-CoV-2 virus may affect the brain include the virus's tendency to cause coagulopathies, leading to disseminated intravascular coagulation and strokes. Because COVID-19 infection often causes breathing difficulties, lung injury, and even acute respiratory distress syndrome, prolonged hypoxia may cause brain damage as well as prime the brain for further neurological decline.

Altered Mental Status

Altered mental status is the most frequent neurological condition documented across several studies of patients with COVID-19 (Pinna et al. 2020; Varatharaj et al. 2020). In a recent meta-analysis using global data, altered mental status occurred in 8% of cases (Tsai et al. 2020), although other studies reported higher prevalences, from 20% to 69% of patients with COVID-19 requiring hospitalization (Beach et al. 2020; Helms et al. 2020; Kennedy et al. 2020; Liu et al. 2020; Varatharaj et al. 2020). Altered mental status is more common in older patients. Data from U.S. patients from March to November 2020 suggested prevalence of altered mental status was as high as 21% in hospitalized patients ages 65 and older, compared with just 3%–7% in younger adults (Centers for Disease Control and Prevention 2021a).

Clinicians caring for older adults must be particularly attuned to the potential for COVID-19 infection to manifest as altered mental status. In older adults, altered mental status may be the only presenting symptom of infection and may not be accompanied by shortness of breath or other typical COVID-19 symptoms (Kennedy et al. 2020). Patients with underlying dementia, in particular, can present with atypical symptoms of COVID-19 infection, including confusion, agitation, and refusal of food or care (Alonso-Lana et al. 2020). The risk factors for developing altered mental status from COVID-19 are similar to the risk factors for delirium from any infection: older age, use of psychotropic medication, residence in an assisted living or skilled nursing facility, vision or hearing loss, and history of stroke, Parkinson's disease, or dementia (Kennedy et al. 2020; Ticinesi et al. 2020).

Altered mental status may be due to a variety of underlying pathologies. In one study, of the patients who presented with altered mental status, 41% were eventually diagnosed with encephalitis or unspecified encephalopathy (Varatharaj et al. 2020). In one case of COVID-19-related encephalitis, the SARS-CoV-2 virus was isolated from cerebrospinal fluid (Moriguchi et al. 2020). Several studies have reported unspecified neurocognitive symptoms, including a dementia-like syndrome as well as short-term memory impairment (Pinna et al. 2020; Varatharaj et al. 2020) and a dysexecutive syndrome (Helms et al. 2020). However, some experts believe that these various descriptions of altered mental status likely represent delirium (Oldham et al. 2020).

Delirium

Delirium is the most common neuropsychiatric syndrome in hospitalized patients with COVID-19. Unsurprisingly, delirium is more common in patients older than age 65 and those with underlying cognitive impairment (Beach et al. 2020; Ticinesi et al. 2020). In adults older than age 65, the rate of delirium in patients hospitalized for COVID-19 is similar to or higher than that in other acute, severe illnesses: delirium is seen in at least 25% of all cases and two-thirds of severe cases (Oldham et al. 2020). In one case series of COVID-19-related delirium, in addition to the classic signs of delirium, several unusual clinical features were observed: multifocal myoclonus, rigidity, livedoid rash, anorexia, alogia, and akinetic mutism (Beach et al. 2020). The hyperactive variant of delirium, with prominent restlessness and agitation, has also been noted (Beach et al. 2020; Helms et al. 2020).

When managing delirium in older patients with COVID-19, a few points should be considered. Because family members and caretakers often cannot be present because of public health protocols, providers should consider technology to help delirious patients see and converse with their loved ones to help ameliorate confusion. Anecdotal evidence suggests that intubated patients with COVID-19 and delirium may require higher doses of sedation (Baller et al. 2020). Given the presence of rigidity in some cases, antipsychotics should be used even more cautiously than usual in older adults with COVID-19-related delirium because antipsychotics can worsen muscle rigidity. One approach involves initiating high-dose melatonin, followed by α_2 agonists, followed by cautious use of low-potency antipsychotics. Trazodone or valproic acid may be an effective option when antipsychotics cannot be used. Dopamine agonists such as amantadine and methylphenidate may be useful in cases of akinetic mutism (Baller et al. 2020).

Cerebrovascular Events

Cerebrovascular events are a relatively common complication of COVID-19. Coagulopathies and thrombotic events have been widely associated with COVID-19, leading to strokes and transient ischemic attacks. The rate of acute cerebrovascular events in hospitalized patients has been estimated at 1.0%–2.7% (Klok et al. 2020; Lodigiani et al. 2020; Nalleballe et al. 2020) but may be as high as 8% on the basis of a meta-analysis by Tsai et al. (2020). Patients older than age 60 are especially at risk of cerebrovascular events with COVID-19 infection (Varatharaj et al. 2020). Cases of intracerebral hemorrhage, subarachnoid hemorrhage, hypoxic ischemic brain injury, and subdural hematoma have all been reported in patients with COVID-19 (Pinna et al. 2020; Radmard et al. 2020).

Psychosis

New-onset psychosis has been observed in patients with COVID-19 across the world (Ferrando et al. 2020; Parra et al. 2020; Varatharaj et al. 2020). Psychosis may be a result of direct neurological involvement of the virus, immune system activation, and cross-reactive antibodies. Psychosis has been observed as the initial symptom (Ferrando et al. 2020), as well as developing up to 2 weeks after initial COVID-19 symptoms (Parra et al. 2020). In some cases, psychosis was the only presenting symptom, with COVID-19 tests coming back positive incidentally. In these cases, the acute phase reactants ferritin and C-reactive protein were elevated (Ferrando et al. 2020).

Fortunately, on the basis of existing studies, older adults do not appear to be at elevated risk of psychosis from infection. Some of the cases of new-onset psychosis may be due to the stress of the pandemic, triggering an initial episode of psychosis in patients with an underlying susceptibility. For older adults with a history of psychosis, the pandemic may prompt a recurrent episode.

The most common psychotic symptoms seen in patients with COVID-19 are delusions, particularly persecutory delusions and delusions of reference (Parra et al. 2020; Smith et al. 2020). Auditory hallucinations have also been reported, whereas visual hallucinations appear to be less common (Parra et al. 2020). Some patients with COVID-19-associated psychosis present with attention and orientation disturbances, so delirium must be ruled out carefully, particularly in older adults and those without prior psychiatric history. Importantly, drugs that were used to treat COVID-19, including hydroxychloroquine and corticosteroids, have known psychiatric side effects and may account for some of the instances of psychosis in patients with COVID-19 (García et al. 2020; Parra et al. 2020). Interestingly, geriatric patients do not seem to be at increased risk of psychiatric side effects from corticosteroids (Cerullo 2008).

Other Neurological Manifestations

Headaches and sleep disruption are common in both outpatients and inpatients with COVID-19 (Carfi et al. 2020; Nalleballe et al. 2020). Patients with COVID-19 are also at risk of new-onset seizures; status epilepticus has been the presenting symptom in some patients. Patients with underlying seizure disorders are at risk of seizures triggered by infection as well (Anand et al. 2020).

Case studies from around the world suggest the possibility of additional neurological presentations that may be related to COVID-19 infection. They include posterior reversible encephalopathy syndrome, gait ataxia, paresthesia, acute necrotizing hemorrhagic encephalopathy, Guillain-Barré syndrome, multifocal transverse myelitis, corticospinal tract signs, central nervous system vasculitis, dizziness, and polyneuropathy (Helms et al. 2020; Nalleballe et al. 2020; Pinna et al. 2020; Sedaghat and Karimi 2020; Sultana and Ananthapur 2020; Varatharaj et al. 2020).

COVID-19 infection may also exacerbate symptoms of other preexisting neurological diseases. In one study, patients with Parkinson's disease who contracted COVID-19 fared worse in the 3 months following infection compared with matched control subjects in both motor symptoms and nonmotor symptoms (Cilia et al. 2020).

SUBACUTE NEUROPSYCHIATRIC MANIFESTATIONS OF COVID-19

Psychiatric Sequelae

Although neurological syndromes are more common during the acute phase of COVID-19 infection, psychiatric syndromes dominate the subacute sequelae. Following COVID-19 infections, patients of all ages have developed psychiatric symptoms, including insomnia, mood lability, depression, anxiety, and PTSD. In one study of self-reported symptoms 1 month following hospitalization for COVID-19, 42% reported clinically significant symptoms of anxiety, 40% reported insomnia, 31% reported depression, 28% reported PTSD, and 20% reported obsessive-compulsive symptoms (Mazza et al. 2020). In a survey in the United Kingdom, in the period between 1 and 2.5 months after discharge from a COVID-19-related hospitalization, almost half of patients who received intensive care and nearly a quarter of those in the ward group reported symptoms of fatigue and psychological distress (Halpin et al. 2021).

In contrast to self-reports, receiving psychiatric diagnoses from health care providers was considerably less common: in the 2 weeks to 3 months following hospitalization for COVID-19, the rate of a new psychiatric diagnosis was 5.8% (compared with 2.5%–3.4% for control events such as hospitalization for influenza, skin infection, or kidney stones) (Taquet et al. 2021). Anxiety disorders were the most common diagnoses, followed by insomnia, depression, psychosis, and cognitive impairment. Patients with prior psychiatric diagnoses had higher rates of symptom flares following COVID-19 than after comparison health events (Taquet et al. 2021). However, when patients were diagnosed with COVID-19 but did not require hospital-level care, rates were lower. In a study of more than 40,000 patients, within 1 month of COVID-19 diagnosis, the prevalence of anxiety disorders was 4.6%, the prevalence of mood disorders was 3.8%, and 0.2% of patients reported suicidal ideation (Nalleballe et al. 2020). Because older adults are more likely to require hospitalization and intensive care, they are at higher risk of psychiatric sequelae in the weeks and months following infection.

Geriatric clinicians should also have a low threshold for cognitive screening after patients are infected with COVID-19. In one study, new cognitive impairments persisting 1 month after COVID-19 diagnosis occurred in 1.6% of patients older than age 65, in both outpatient and inpatient settings. The risk of developing cognitive impairment after COVID-19 was two to three times the risk after comparison illnesses (Taquet et al. 2021).

Post-ICU Psychiatric Distress: Learning From Other Critical Illnesses

Critical illnesses and intensive care are incredibly stressful (Bienvenu and Gerstenblith 2017). Patients in the ICU often face respiratory insufficiency, invasive procedures, systemic inflammation, hypothalamic-pituitary-adrenal axis activation with insufficient adrenal cortical response, high catecholamine levels (including exogenous administration), delirium with associated perceptual disturbances, communication difficulties, and very little autonomy. In this context, on the verge of death but unable to process what is happening, many patients develop memories of distorted facts (e.g., that they are being tortured) and have frightening nightmare-like experiences (e.g., seeing blood dripping down the walls) (Bienvenu and Gerstenblith 2017).

As with other intense stressors, psychiatric morbidity is quite common. Clinically significant symptoms of PTSD, depression, and nonspecific anxiety affect roughly 20% (Parker et al. 2015), 30% (Rabiee et al. 2016), and 35% (Nikayin et al. 2016) of survivors, respectively. Risk factors include prior psychiatric morbidity, higher sedative doses, and memories of frightening ICU experiences. Early post-ICU symptoms are potent predictors of persistent symptoms, and clinically significant symptoms from different domains tend to co-occur (Bienvenu et al. 2015, 2018).

Interventions to prevent long-term psychiatric morbidity are being developed, and many have shown promise, including in-ICU psychological interventions, ICU diaries (written to patients to help them process what occurred as they recover), mobile health interventions (which do not require that patients attend in-person appointments), physical exercise, and, most recently, virtual reality interventions (to help patients understand critical illnesses and intensive care interventions) (Cox et al. 2018; Jones et al. 2010; Peris et al. 2011; Vlake et al. 2021). This field is still young, with both negative and positive studies, but the future is promising (Bienvenu 2019).

LONG-TERM CONSIDERATIONS: CLUES FROM PAST PANDEMICS

At this time, the chronic impact of COVID-19 remains to be seen, and research is ongoing. However, there exists a body of literature on other severe coronavirus infections and psychiatric sequelae that may offer clues to what we might expect with COVID-19. In a meta-analysis that included studies of other coronaviruses such as severe acute respiratory syndrome (SARS) and Middle East respiratory syndrome (MERS), in the 6 weeks to 39 months following infection, patients reported depression, anxiety, fatigue, and PTSD. More than 15% of patients reported disrupted sleep, emotional lability, poor concentration, fatigue, and memory problems during this time period (Rogers et al. 2020). In SARS, psychiatric conditions persisted after physical symptoms resolved. Chronic fatigue and clinically significant psychiatric symptoms persisted up to 4 years after infection, even in patients with no psychiatric history prior to infection. The most common diagnoses were chronic fatigue syndrome, PTSD, somatoform pain disorder, and panic disorder (Lam et al. 2009).

For older adults, acquired neurocognitive deficits could have a lasting impact. Mild neurocognitive deficits have been shown to last 1–2 years following delirium caused by sepsis requiring an ICU stay (Chung et al. 2020). For patients with underlying neurodegenerative diseases, some researchers have predicted that COVID-19 will exacerbate these conditions, with worsening illness manifesting several months after initial COVID-19 infection (André et al. 2020; Cilia et al. 2020; Serrano-Castro et al. 2020).

POPULATION-LEVEL AND PUBLIC HEALTH CONSIDERATIONS

Although COVID-19 has a wide range of neuropsychiatric manifestations in infected persons, it must also be noted that the pandemic exacerbated psychiatric symptoms for many people in the general population who were never infected. Older adults who do not have symptomatic COVID-19 infection may still experience neuropsychiatric symptoms in the context of the pandemic.

The COVID-19 pandemic has led to social isolation, uncertainty about the future, cessation of usual activities, job losses, and financial stress, all of which can be risk factors for psychiatric conditions. For some people, the pandemic has exacerbated obsessive-compulsive symptoms, with the increased concern about infectious contamination (Fontenelle and Miguel 2020). Social isolation has also exacerbated existing mental health conditions and seems to have triggered new-onset depression and anxiety on the basis of recent survey data. For example, surveys of adults in the United States showed that participants were more than three times as likely to report symptoms of depressive or anxiety disorders than they were the year before. Between 30% and 40% of adults screened positive in spring 2020 for anxiety, depressive, or stressor- and trauma-related disorders related to the pandemic (Czeisler et al. 2020; Twenge and Joiner 2020). A little more than 13% reported increased substance use since the pandemic started, and more than 1 in 10 adults reported suicidal thoughts in the past month (Czeisler et al. 2020). In one study of adults with mild neurocognitive impairment, those living alone experienced higher rates of anxiety and sleep disturbances (Goodman-Casanova et al. 2020). These results suggest the need to screen all geriatric patients for mental health symptoms related to the pandemic.

For older adults with underlying dementia, changes in routines and separation from family and visitors may worsen dementia symptoms, including motor agitation, anxiety, apathy, insomnia, loss of appetite, and abnormal movements (Alonso-Lana et al. 2020; Simonetti et al. 2020). Even adjusting for expected declines in neuropsychiatric functioning due to progressive dementia, the pandemic appears to have accelerated or worsened memory and behavior impairments (Alonso-Lana et al. 2020). In one study of patients with Alzheimer's disease, the duration of confinement was positively correlated with worsening cognitive function and caregiver distress (Boutoleau-Bretonnière et al. 2020). Again, these studies suggest a need to consider worsening neuropsychiatric symptoms even in geriatric patients who avoid COVID-19 infection.

SUMMARY

The COVID-19 pandemic will disproportionately affect older adults. Although older adults do not account for a disproportionate number of cases, when they are infected, the consequences are often serious and long-lasting. Even those who are not infected are susceptible to psychiatric symptoms and worsening of underlying neurocognitive disorders. Although the chronic effects of the virus and pandemic remain to be seen, with this literature review we illustrated the neuropsychiatric impact of the SARS-CoV-2 virus. Ongoing data collection as the pandemic progresses will help elucidate the epidemiology of the syndromes described in this chapter, as well as any late-onset complications. Whether it is an acute stroke caused by hypercoagulation with COVID-19 or an acute episode of major depressive disorder brought on by social isolation, older adults are at risk of ongoing neuropsychiatric syndromes due to the pandemic. Clinicians who care for older adults must consider the neuropsychiatric burden of the pandemic in all patients.

KEY POINTS

- Neuropsychiatric manifestations are common in COVID-19 infections.
- Older adults are particularly susceptible to delirium as a result of COVID-19 infection.
- Psychiatric symptoms are common both in patients treated for infection and in the general population.

QUESTIONS FOR REVIEW

1. What is the most common acute neurological syndrome in COVID-19 infection?

   A. Stroke or transient ischemic attack
   B. Confusion and fluctuations in orientation and attention
   C. Headache
   D. Encephalitis

Answer: B.

2. The increased prevalence of psychiatric morbidity in the COVID-19 pandemic is due to which of the following?

   A. SARS-CoV-2 invasion of the brain
   B. Systemic inflammation in patients with COVID-19 infection
   C. Social isolation
   D. Financial distress
   E. All of the above

Answer: E.

3. Which of the following screening tools is least likely to identify neuropsychiatric sequelae in geriatric patients following a COVID-19 infection?

    A. Montreal Cognitive Assessment
    B. PHQ-9 for depressive symptoms
    C. GAD-7 for anxiety symptoms
    D. Geriatric 8 screening tool

Answer: A.

ADDITIONAL RESOURCE

Baller EB, Hogan CS, Fusunyan MA, et al: Neurocovid: pharmacological recommendations for delirium associated with COVID-19. Psychosomatics 61(6):585–596, 2020 32828569

REFERENCES

Alonso-Lana S, Marquié M, Ruiz A, et al: Cognitive and neuropsychiatric manifestations of COVID-19 and effects on elderly individuals with dementia. Front Aging Neurosci 12:588872, 2020 33192483

Anand P, Al-Faraj A, Sader E, et al: Seizure as the presenting symptom of COVID-19: a retrospective case series. Epilepsy Behav 112:107335, 2020 32739397

André A, Félix C, Corvacho M, et al: On the plausibility of late neuropsychiatric manifestations associated with the COVID-19 pandemic. J Neurol Sci 417:117060, 2020 32739501

Baller EB, Hogan CS, Fusunyan MA, et al: Neurocovid: pharmacological recommendations for delirium associated with COVID-19. Psychosomatics 61(6):585–596, 2020 32828569

Beach SR, Praschan NC, Hogan C, et al: Delirium in COVID-19: a case series and exploration of potential mechanisms for central nervous system involvement. Gen Hosp Psychiatry 65:47–53, 2020 32470824

Bienvenu OJ: What do we know about preventing or mitigating postintensive care syndrome? Crit Care Med 47(11):1671–1672, 2019 31609269

Bienvenu OJ, Gerstenblith TA: Posttraumatic stress disorder phenomena after critical illness. Crit Care Clin 33(3):649–658, 2017 28601139

Bienvenu OJ, Colantuoni E, Mendez-Tellez PA, et al: Cooccurrence of and remission from general anxiety, depression, and posttraumatic stress disorder symptoms after acute lung injury: a 2-year longitudinal study. Crit Care Med 43(3):642–653, 2015 25513784

Bienvenu OJ, Friedman LA, Colantuoni E, et al: Psychiatric symptoms after acute respiratory distress syndrome: a 5-year longitudinal study. Intensive Care Med 44(1):38–47, 2018 29279973

Boutoleau-Bretonnière C, Pouclet-Courtemanche H, Gillet A, et al: The effects of confinement on neuropsychiatric symptoms in Alzheimer's disease during the COVID-19 crisis. J Alzheimers Dis 76(1):41–47, 2020 32568211

Carfì A, Bernabei R, Landi F, et al: Persistent symptoms in patients after acute COVID-19. JAMA 324(6):603–605, 2020 32644129

Centers for Disease Control and Prevention: COVID-NET: laboratory-confirmed COVID-19-associated hospitalizations. Atlanta, GA, Centers for Disease Control and Prevention, 2021a. Available at: https://gis.cdc.gov/grasp/covidnet/COVID19_5.html. Accessed July 14, 2021.

Centers for Disease Control and Prevention: COVID-19: older adults: older unvaccinated adults are more likely to be hospitalized or die from COVID-19. Atlanta, GA, Centers for Disease Control and Prevention July 3, 2021b. Available at: www.cdc.gov/coronavirus/2019-ncov/need-extra-precautions/older-adults.html. Accessed July 14, 2021.

Cerullo MA: Expect psychiatric side effects from corticosteroid use in the elderly. Geriatrics 63(1):15–18, 2008 18257615

Chung HY, Wickel J, Brunkhorst FM, Geis C: Sepsis-associated encephalopathy: from delirium to dementia? J Clin Med 9(3):E703, 2020 32150970

Cilia R, Bonvegna S, Straccia G, et al: Effects of COVID-19 on Parkinson's disease clinical features: a community-based case-control study. Mov Disord 35(8):1287–1292, 2020 32449528

Cox CE, Hough CL, Carson SS, et al: Effects of a telephone- and web-based coping skills training program compared with an education program for survivors of critical illness and their family members. A randomized clinical trial. Am J Respir Crit Care Med 197(1):66–78, 2018 28872898

Czeisler MÉ, Lane RI, Petrosky E, et al: Mental health, substance use, and suicidal ideation during the COVID-19 pandemic—United States, June 24–30, 2020. MMWR Morb Mortal Wkly Rep 69(32):1049–1057, 2020 32790653

Ferrando SJ, Klepacz L, Lynch S, et al: COVID-19 psychosis: a potential new neuropsychiatric condition triggered by novel coronavirus infection and the inflammatory response? Psychosomatics 61(5):551–555, 2020 32593479

Fontenelle LF, Miguel EC: The impact of coronavirus (COVID-19) in the diagnosis and treatment of obsessive-compulsive disorder. Depress Anxiety 37(6):510–511, 2020 32383802

García CAC, Sánchez EBA, Huerta DH, et al: Covid-19 treatment-induced neuropsychiatric adverse effects. Gen Hosp Psychiatry 67:163–164, 2020 32636036

Goodman-Casanova JM, Dura-Perez E, Guzman-Parra J, et al: Telehealth home support during COVID-19 confinement for community-dwelling older adults with mild cognitive impairment or mild dementia: survey study. J Med Internet Res 22(5):e19434, 2020 32401215

Halpin SJ, McIvor C, Whyatt G, et al: Postdischarge symptoms and rehabilitation needs in survivors of COVID-19 infection: a cross-sectional evaluation. J Med Virol 93(2):1013–1022, 2021 32729939

Helms J, Kremer S, Merdji H, et al: Neurologic features in severe SARS-CoV-2 infection. N Engl J Med 382(23):2268–2270, 2020 32294339

Johns Hopkins University and Medicine: COVID-19 dashboard. Coronavirus Resource Center, 2021. Available at: https://coronavirus.jhu.edu/map.html. Accessed June 24, 2021.

Jones C, Bäckman C, Capuzzo M, et al: Intensive care diaries reduce new onset post traumatic stress disorder following critical illness: a randomised, controlled trial. Crit Care 14(5):R168, 2010 20843344

Kennedy M, Helfand BKI, Gou RY, et al: Delirium in older patients with COVID-19 presenting to the emergency department. JAMA Netw Open 3(11):e2029540, 2020 33211114

Klok FA, Kruip MJHA, van der Meer NJM, et al: Incidence of thrombotic complications in critically ill ICU patients with COVID-19. Thromb Res 191:145–147, 2020 32291094

Ladds E, Rushforth A, Wieringa S, et al: Persistent symptoms after Covid-19: qualitative study of 114 "long Covid" patients and draft quality principles for services. BMC Health Serv Res 20(1):1144, 2020 33342437

Lam MH, Wing YK, Yu MW, et al: Mental morbidities and chronic fatigue in severe acute respiratory syndrome survivors: long-term follow-up. Arch Intern Med 169(22):2142–2147, 2009 20008700

Lechien JR, Chiesa-Estomba CM, De Siati DR, et al: Olfactory and gustatory dysfunctions as a clinical presentation of mild-to-moderate forms of the coronavirus disease (COVID-19): a multicenter European study. Eur Arch Otorhinolaryngol 277(8):2251–2261, 2020 32253535

Liu K, Chen Y, Lin R, et al: Clinical features of COVID-19 in elderly patients: a comparison with young and middle-aged patients. J Infect 80(6):e14–e18, 2020 32171866

Lodigiani C, Iapichino G, Carenzo L, et al: Venous and arterial thromboembolic complications in COVID-19 patients admitted to an academic hospital in Milan, Italy. Thromb Res 191:9–14, 2020 32353746

Mao L, Jin H, Wang M, et al: Neurologic manifestations of hospitalized patients with coronavirus disease 2019 in Wuhan, China. JAMA Neurol 77(6):683–690, 2020 32275288

Mazza MG, De Lorenzo R, Conte C, et al: Anxiety and depression in COVID-19 survivors: role of inflammatory and clinical predictors. Brain Behav Immun 89:594–600, 2020 32738287

Moriguchi T, Harii N, Goto J, et al: A first case of meningitis/encephalitis associated with SARS-Coronavirus-2. Int J Infect Dis 94:55–58, 2020 32251791

Mueller AL, McNamara MS, Sinclair DA: Why does COVID-19 disproportionately affect older people? Aging (Albany NY) 12(10):9959–9981, 2020 32470948

Nalleballe K, Reddy Onteddu S, Sharma R, et al: Spectrum of neuropsychiatric manifestations in COVID-19. Brain Behav Immun 88:71–74, 2020 32561222

Nikayin S, Rabiee A, Hashem MD, et al: Anxiety symptoms in survivors of critical illness: a systematic review and meta-analysis. Gen Hosp Psychiatry 43:23–29, 2016 27796253

Oldham MA, Slooter AJC, Cunningham C, et al: Characterising neuropsychiatric disorders in patients with COVID-19. Lancet Psychiatry 7(11):932–933, 2020 33069307

Parker AM, Sricharoenchai T, Raparla S, et al: Posttraumatic stress disorder in critical illness survivors: a metaanalysis. Crit Care Med 43(5):1121–1129, 2015 25654178

Parra A, Juanes A, Losada CP, et al: Psychotic symptoms in COVID-19 patients: a retrospective descriptive study. Psychiatry Res 291:113254, 2020 32603930

Peris A, Bonizzoli M, Iozzelli D, et al: Early intra-intensive care unit psychological intervention promotes recovery from post traumatic stress disorders, anxiety and depression symptoms in critically ill patients. Crit Care 15(1):R41, 2011 21272307

Pinna P, Grewal P, Hall JP, et al: Neurological manifestations and COVID-19: experiences from a tertiary care center at the frontline. J Neurol Sci 415:116969, 2020 32570113

Rabiee A, Nikayin S, Hashem MD, et al: Depressive symptoms after critical illness: a systematic review and meta-analysis. Crit Care Med 44(9):1744–1753, 2016 27153046

Radmard S, Epstein SE, Roeder HJ, et al: Inpatient neurology consultations during the onset of the SARS-CoV-2 New York City pandemic: a single center case series. Front Neurol 11:805, 2020 32754113

Rogers JP, Chesney E, Oliver D, et al: Psychiatric and neuropsychiatric presentations associated with severe coronavirus infections: a systematic review and meta-analysis with comparison to the COVID-19 pandemic. Lancet Psychiatry 7(7):611–627, 2020 32437679

Sedaghat Z, Karimi N: Guillain Barre syndrome associated with COVID-19 infection: a case report. J Clin Neurosci 76:233–235, 2020 32312628

Serrano-Castro PJ, Estivill-Torrús G, Cabezudo-García P, et al: Impact of SARS-CoV-2 infection on neurodegenerative and neuropsychiatric diseases: a delayed pandemic? Neurologia (Engl Ed) 35(4):245–251, 2020 32364119

Simonetti A, Pais C, Jones M, et al: Neuropsychiatric symptoms in elderly with dementia during COVID-19 pandemic: definition, treatment, and future directions. Front Psychiatry 11:579842, 2020 33132939

Smith CM, Komisar JR, Mourad A, et al: COVID-19-associated brief psychotic disorder. BMJ Case Rep 13(8):e236940, 2020 32784244

Sultana S, Ananthapur V: COVID-19 and its impact on neurological manifestations and mental health: the present scenario. Neurol Sci 41(11):3015–3020, 2020 32865638

Taquet M, Luciano S, Geddes JR, et al: Bidirectional associations between COVID-19 and psychiatric disorder: retrospective cohort studies of 62 354 COVID-19 cases in the USA. Lancet Psychiatry 8(2):130–140, 2021 33181098

Ticinesi A, Cerundolo N, Parise A, et al: Delirium in COVID-19: epidemiology and clinical correlations in a large group of patients admitted to an academic hospital. Aging Clin Exp Res 32(10):2159–2166, 2020 32946031

Tsai ST, Lu MK, San S, et al: The neurologic manifestations of coronavirus disease 2019 pandemic: a systemic review. Front Neurol 11:498, 2020 32574246

Twenge JM, Joiner TE: U.S. Census Bureau-assessed prevalence of anxiety and depressive symptoms in 2019 and during the 2020 COVID-19 pandemic. Depress Anxiety 37(10):954–956, 2020 32667081

Varatharaj A, Thomas N, Ellul MA, et al: Neurological and neuropsychiatric complications of COVID-19 in 153 patients: a UK-wide surveillance study. Lancet Psychiatry 7(10):875–882, 2020 32593341

Vlake JH, van Bommel J, Hellemons ME, et al: Intensive care unit-specific virtual reality for psychological recovery after ICU treatment for COVID-19: a brief case report. Front Med (Lausanne) 7:629086, 2021 33614677

Wu Y, Xu X, Chen Z, et al: Nervous system involvement after infection with COVID-19 and other coronaviruses. Brain Behav Immun 87:18–22, 2020 32240762

CHAPTER 16

PSYCHOPHARMACO-LOGICAL CHALLENGES OF TREATING OLDER ADULTS WITH COVID-19

Badr Ratnakaran, M.B.B.S.
Daniel C. Dahl, M.D.

The coronavirus SARS-CoV-2 disease (COVID-19) pandemic has revealed unique challenges in prescribing psychotropic medications to older adults, who are vulnerable to severe illness from an infection by the COVID-19 virus. The steps taken to mitigate the spread of the virus also caused problems in caring for older adults. The multiorgan involvement in COVID-19 infection and the medications used to treat this illness need to be considered to prevent side effects from psychotropic medications. In this chapter we describe some of the challenges the pandemic posed to access to psychotropic medications during the COVID-19 pandemic and safely prescribing them in older adults experiencing a COVID-19 infection.

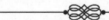

Vignette

In March 2020, Mr. B, a 70-year-old man with a history of schizophrenia, hypertension, and type 2 diabetes mellitus, was residing in a nursing home. He recently had a relapse of psychotic symptoms, and the dosage of previously prescribed oral clozapine was increased from 150 mg daily to 200 mg daily. However, following the increase in the dosage of clozapine, Mr. B became more sedated and confused at times, with new-onset tremors. As the COVID-19 pandemic had started to grip the nation, visitors, including physicians, were not allowed into the nursing home. The nursing home was not set up for care to be provided by telemedicine because of poor internet connections in the area. The nursing home staff were unsure whether Mr. B's symptoms were from side effects of clozapine or from a COVID-19 infection.

COVID-19 has multiple implications for geriatric psychopharmacology. In this chapter we briefly review some of the major considerations for geriatric psychopharmacology during the COVID-19 pandemic, including general psychopharmacology practice challenges, trouble initiating and continuing psychopharmacology during the pandemic, the impact of COVID-19 on psychotropic drug safety, and psychiatric considerations of COVID-19 treatments.

GENERAL PSYCHOPHARMACOLOGY PRACTICE CHALLENGES DURING COVID-19

During the COVID-19 pandemic, many of life's usual patterns were altered. Simple trips to any medical system were challenging. Fear of COVID-19 has been and still is real for patients, caregivers, and medical staff. COVID-19 news comes out daily, and it is impossible to avoid hearing that we are all at great risk of illness or dying. Older adults are now known to be at greater risk and should stay home, but the need to see loved ones can be overwhelming. In terms of medical care, staff have to face the realistic fear of going to work without adequate protection in places with increasing numbers of COVID-19 patients. Patients put off medical care, including trips to their mental health team, almost certainly worsening their mental health and well-being. Caregivers have become fearful not only for their own health but, even worse, of the possibility of transmitting the virus to others. The loss of an emotional support network may lead to depression or worsen already existing mental health issues. Many people's financial situation has deteriorated during the pandemic, and psychotropic medication may not make the list of affordable necessities or may be taken at lower doses or intermittently. The loss of psychotropics that softened agitation, insomnia, and aggression in patients may lead to intolerable behavior for caregivers, driving them away.

CHALLENGES IN INITIATING AND CONTINUING PSYCHOPHARMACOLOGY DURING COVID-19

Refusal by older adults to come in person for health care needs, including visits to health care providers and pharmacies; difficulties in arranging transportation; and restrictions of face-to-face encounters with patients by nursing homes, outpatient clinics, and pharmacies have created hardships for patients in obtaining the medications prescribed to them. The reduction of in-person encounters can also affect efforts at deprescribing in older adults (Elbeddini et al. 2021). Patients may self-adjust their medications without consulting their provider, leading to adverse drug-related events. Disruptions of the supply chain of drugs, workflow changes, shortages in staff (due to furloughs, working from home, or illness), and redeployment of health care personnel, including pharmacists and physicians, have caused delays in the availability of medications for patients. The number of long-acting antipsychotic injections administered during the pandemic was also found to be decreased (Ifteni et al. 2020). Further, therapeutic drug monitoring has been affected because laboratory testing needed for assessment for prescription of a drug can place patients and health care personnel at risk of COVID-19 infection.

To mitigate the exigencies caused by the pandemic, the answer proposed has been telehealth. In the United States, various steps were taken by federal and state governments at the beginning of the pandemic to help in the rapid implementation of telehealth. Medical licensure requirements were modified or waived by various state medical boards so that providers could see patients across state lines via telehealth (Brotman and Kotloff 2021). The Centers for Medicare and Medicaid Services helped with reimbursement for telehealth by making billing code adjustments for video and audio-only telehealth encounters (Hoffman 2020). Entities concerned with patient health information security and privacy, the Health Insurance Portability and Accountability Act (HIPAA), and Title 42 of the Code of Federal Regulations, part 2, reduced restrictions for various video platforms to provide care and communications via telehealth (Hoffman 2020). The Drug Enforcement Administration has been flexible regarding medication-assisted treatment with buprenorphine, including prescribing via telehealth and across state lines (Drug Enforcement Administration 2021). The U.S. Food and Drug Administration (2020c) provided updated guidance for medications covered by Risk Evaluation and Mitigation Strategy protections (including clozapine). The update recommended that health providers use their best clinical judgment in conducting the laboratory testing and imaging studies for continuing treatment during the pandemic.

Synchronous telehealth services through virtual clinic visits have helped health care providers directly engage with their patients. Patients could inform pharmacies and providers of their needs through secure messaging platforms provided by their health care facilities. In settings with limited internet access (rural and underserved urban areas) or when telehealth capabilities could not be integrated (e.g., because of lack of smartphone or computer or issues with video connectivity), audio-only telehealth (telephone) calls between providers and patients were used to ensure continuity of care. With telehealth, patients and providers need not adhere to universal masking during conversations, which reduces barriers in verbal communication and maintains nonverbal communication during video encounters. For older adults staying in community dwellings, retirement communities, independent living facilities, and nursing homes, home-based telehealth protects older adults against COVID-19 and infecting other high-risk individuals staying with them. Virtual geriatric clinics initiated during the pandemic in nursing homes and for community-dwelling older adults have been found to be beneficial in terms of patient satisfaction, cost-effectiveness, polypharmacy reviews, reducing waiting times, and reducing acute hospitalization rates (Murphy et al. 2020).

However, the use of telehealth with older adults has its unique challenges. Older adults may not have the equipment, bandwidth, or technical skills to make audiovisual sessions work. Decreased motivation or difficulties with the use of technology and cognitive and sensory impairments in older adults are important factors in accepting telehealth (Murphy et al. 2020). The ability to conduct a physical examination is limited via telehealth. Still, it can be supplemented by assistance from nursing home staff, readings of vital signs done by patients at home, and pictures and videos uploaded through secure messaging platforms provided for telehealth (Greenhalgh et al. 2020). Assessments by mental health providers in audio-only telehealth encounters are disadvantaged by the lack of observation of appearance and nonverbal cues (Lim et al.

2021). Ambient noise in the environment during telehealth encounters can create problems in communication in patients with hearing impairments. Obtaining collateral information to complement such assessments can also be problematic because many older adults live alone. Transfer of information between providers can be delayed if electronic medical records are different. For older adults who do not live alone, ensuring the privacy of the encounter can be an issue because of the risk of others overhearing conversations and situations of elder abuse (Sorinmade et al. 2020). For older adults who lack decision-making capacity to consent to treatment, care should be taken to ensure that legal guardians are present during telehealth encounters. These challenges can threaten the validity of telehealth assessments and decision-making when prescribing appropriate psychotropic medications in older adults.

IMPACT OF COVID-19 ON PSYCHOTROPIC DRUG SAFETY IN OLDER ADULTS

Age is considered an important risk factor for severe COVID-19 illness and has been associated with adverse health outcomes, including hospitalizations, intensive care unit stay, and mortality (Y. Chen et al. 2021). Older adults have increased likelihood of medical comorbidities such as hypertension, diabetes, obesity, cardiovascular disease, cerebrovascular disease, chronic kidney disease, and chronic pulmonary disease, which are also significant risk factors for severe illness, mortality, and morbidity from COVID-19 infection (Awortwe and Cascorbi 2020). The COVID-19 virus can affect multiple organs, and older adults are prone to organ damage from the virus, including acute respiratory distress syndrome, acute kidney injury, acute liver injury, and cardiac injury (Shahid et al. 2020).

The neuropsychiatric manifestations of the COVID-19 virus in the general population include depression, delirium, and psychosis (Brown et al. 2020). Symptoms of alcohol, sedative, and opioid withdrawal (nausea, diaphoresis, tremors, seizures, tachycardia, myalgias, and delirium) can mimic or worsen symptoms of COVID-19 illness. For these reasons, psychotropic medications are often prescribed to treat psychiatric symptoms in these patients. Because the virus can affect multiple organ systems, including the kidneys and liver, the metabolism and pharmacokinetic and pharmacodynamic factors of psychotropic medications are impaired. In older adults, age-related changes to perfusion of the kidneys and liver can decrease the renal and hepatic clearance of medications, resulting in increased accumulation and bioavailability of psychotropic medications (Reeve et al. 2017). Dose adjustment of psychotropic medications in older adults with COVID-19 becomes important because of the intrinsic safety concerns of psychotropic medications. Because of multiorgan involvement by the COVID-19 virus and the safety profile of psychotropic medications, multiple authors have recommended caution when prescribing psychotropic medications in patients with COVID-19 (Bilbul et al. 2020; Ostuzzi et al. 2020). We describe the major precautions to be taken and the reasons in Table 16–1.

Access to medications and laboratory testing for therapeutic drug monitoring (e.g., monitoring serum level of lithium and absolute neutrophil count [ANC] for clozapine) are cause for concern when prescribing medications. Experts have recommended continuing clozapine in patients with COVID-19-related leukopenia without neutropenia, reducing the frequency of monitoring ANC to every 3 months for patients who are hemodynamically stable and have been taking clozapine for more than a year with no problems (Gee et al. 2020; Siskind et al. 2020). Careful monitoring for adverse drug reactions and drug-drug interactions from psychotropic medications is required because they could lead to increased risk of hospitalization, prolonged length of stay, protracted recovery, and death. Initiation and continuation of psychotropic medication should be frequently assessed by regularly reviewing ongoing safety concerns and weighing the risks versus benefits of using the medication.

SAFETY AND PSYCHIATRIC CONSIDERATIONS OF COVID-19 TREATMENTS

Multiple treatments used for COVID-19 can lead to neuropsychiatric side effects and adverse interactions with common psychotropic medications. Some monoclonal antibody treatments have received emergency use authorization (EUA) from the FDA; these treatments are discussed later in this section. However, remdesivir is the only drug currently approved by the FDA for the treatment of COVID-19 (COVID-19 Treatment Guidelines Panel 2021). It inhibits RNA-dependent RNA polymerase, preventing viral replication. Remdesivir is a prodrug converted to an active metabolite. Serious adverse side effects include anaphylaxis, angioedema,

Table 16–1. Psychotropic safety concerns and recommendations related to organ systems involved in COVID-19

Organ system	Organ lesion and symptoms	Safety concerns of psychotropic medications	Precautions for prescribing psychotropic medications in patients with COVID-19
Hematological	Lymphopenia and leukopenia	Antipsychotics, TCAs, valproic acid, and carbamazepine are associated with neutropenia and risk of secondary infections.	Regular monitoring of CBC and coagulation factors for abnormalities (neutropenia, lymphopenia, thrombocytopenia, prolonged PT and aPTT) must be done. If abnormalities persist, weigh risk vs. benefit of continuing the psychotropic medication, decrease the dose, or switch to a safer psychotropic medication. Consider avoiding psychotropic medications that can suppress white blood cell production. If patient develops flu-like symptoms and fever, watch for signs of clozapine toxicity and consider decreasing the dose or stopping clozapine.
	Hypercoagulability	Antipsychotics are associated with increased risk of thromboembolism.	Caution is required in patients prescribed anticoagulants and immunosuppressants.
	Thrombocytopenia	Clozapine levels can increase in acute systemic infections, leading to clozapine toxicity.	Avoid psychotropic medications that can cause bleeding due to thrombocytopenia or impaired platelet aggregation.

Table 16-1. Psychotropic safety concerns and recommendations related to organ systems involved in COVID-19 (*continued*)

Organ system	Organ lesion and symptoms	Safety concerns of psychotropic medications	Precautions for prescribing psychotropic medications in patients with COVID-19
Hematological (*continued*)	Thrombocytopenia (*continued*)	SSRIs and SNRIs can cause impaired platelet aggregation. Valproic acid can cause thrombocytopenia.	
Cardiac	Arrhythmias, heart failure, acute cardiac injury, myocarditis, cardiomyopathy, and cardiac arrest	Antipsychotics, TCAs, stimulants, SSRIs (e.g., citalopram), and SNRIs (e.g., venlafaxine) have intrinsic QTc-prolonging properties. They can interact with medications used to treat COVID-19 (antivirals, chloroquine, hydroxychloroquine, azithromycin) and cause QTc prolongation.	Obtain baseline ECG for QTc and monitor for risk factors for prolongation of QTc (drug interactions, electrolyte abnormalities, cardiovascular comorbidities). Avoid psychotropic medications that are at high risk of prolonging QTc intervals. If QTc is prolonged, monitor daily ECG and reduce risk factors. Weigh risk vs. benefit of continuing the psychotropic medication, decrease the dose, or switch to a safer psychotropic medication.
Hepatic	Acute liver injury	Chlorpromazine, duloxetine, valproic acid, and carbamazepine are considered high risk for causing drug-induced liver injury.	Avoid drugs that are high risk for causing drug-induced liver injury.

Table 16–1. Psychotropic safety concerns and recommendations related to organ systems involved in COVID-19 *(continued)*

Organ system	Organ lesion and symptoms	Safety concerns of psychotropic medications	Precautions for prescribing psychotropic medications in patients with COVID-19
	Hepatic dysfunction (elevated liver enzymes and bilirubin)	Second-generation antipsychotics, TCAs, and SNRIs can cause elevated liver enzymes.	Obtain hepatic function tests. In hepatic dysfunction, make dose adjustment of psychotropic medication if necessary.
Renal	Acute kidney injury	Lithium can be nephrotoxic, and dehydration can increase lithium levels.	Hold lithium or switch to a safer psychotropic medication in acute kidney injury.
	Renal dysfunction	Psychotropic medications such as lithium, venlafaxine, bupropion, pregabalin, gabapentin, topiramate, and paliperidone are excreted by the kidneys.	Obtain renal function tests. In renal dysfunction, consider dose adjustment of psychotropic medications excreted by the kidneys. Monitor lithium levels and renal function with increased frequency until patient recovers.
Neurological	Delirium, impaired consciousness, vertigo, headache, anosmia, ageusia, ataxia, vision abnormalities, myelitis, ADEM, muscle injury	Benzodiazepines, lithium, and psychotropic medications with anticholinergic properties (TCAs, paroxetine, low-potency antipsychotics, benztropine, and diphenhydramine) can cause or exacerbate delirium.	Deliriogenic psychotropic medications should be avoided or used with caution. Avoid or taper dose of benzodiazepines in patients with delirium.

Table 16–1. Psychotropic safety concerns and recommendations related to organ systems involved in COVID-19 (*continued*)

Organ system	Organ lesion and symptoms	Safety concerns of psychotropic medications	Precautions for prescribing psychotropic medications in patients with COVID-19
Neurological (*continued*)	Seizures	Lithium, clozapine, quetiapine, olanzapine, first-generation antipsychotics, bupropion, and TCAs can lower seizure threshold.	Avoid psychotropic medications that can lower seizure threshold.
	Stroke	Antipsychotics are associated with increased cerebrovascular events in older adults.	Weigh risk vs. benefit of using antipsychotic medications in patients at high risk for cerebrovascular disease or presenting with stroke.
Pulmonary	Cough, dyspnea, pneumonia, acute respiratory distress syndrome	Respiratory drive can be decreased by benzodiazepines.	Weigh risk vs. benefit of using benzodiazepines for anxiety in patients with respiratory symptoms.

Note. ADEM=acute disseminated encephalomyelitis; aPTT=activated partial thromboplastin time; CBC=complete blood count; COVID-19=coronavirus SARS-CoV-2 disease; ECG=electrocardiogram; PT=prothrombin time; SNRI=serotonin-norepinephrine reuptake inhibitors; SSRI=selective serotonin reuptake inhibitor; TCA=tricyclic antidepressant.

infusion reactions, elevated alanine transaminase or aspartate transaminase, seizures, and acute kidney injury (U.S. Food and Drug Administration 2021f). Because of the possibility of elevated liver function tests, care should be taken with psychotropics known to increase them such as valproic acid (Bilbul et al. 2020).

Hydroxychloroquine is used for malaria, systemic lupus erythematosus, and rheumatoid arthritis. It was initially used to treat COVID-19, but its EUA was revoked on June 15, 2020 (U.S. Food and Drug Administration 2020a), because of its lack of efficacy for this illness and the risk of serious side effects. The exact mechanism of action for the drug is unknown. There are multiple potential serious reactions, including, but not limited to, seizures, bronchospasm, Stevens-Johnson syndrome, toxic epidermal necrolysis, fulminant hepatic failure, cardiomyopathy, ventricular arrhythmias, QT prolongation, torsades de pointes, and increased risk of suicide (U.S. Food and Drug Administration 2021d). Neuropsychiatric side effects include psychosis, delirium, depression, anxiety, personality changes, aggression, and compulsive impulses. Hydroxychloroquine is metabolized by cytochrome P450 3A4 (CYP3A4), leading to interactions with CYP3A4 inhibitors such as fluvoxamine and CYP3A4 inducers such as carbamazepine, oxcarbazepine, and modafinil (Bilbul et al. 2020).

Tocilizumab binds to and inhibits interleukin-6 receptors. It is a humanized recombinant monoclonal antibody that may help with cytokine storms seen in seriously ill COVID-19 patients. The National Institutes of Health (NIH) recommend tocilizumab in combination with dexamethasone for hospitalized patients with COVID-19 exhibiting rapid respiratory decompensation (COVID-19 Treatment Guidelines Panel 2021). Tocilizumab has a black box warning for chronic or recurrent infections such as tuberculosis (TB), invasive fungal infections, and other opportunistic infections, which were higher for patients ages 65 and older (U.S. Food and Drug Administration 2019d). Before initiation of tocilizumab, clinicians should screen for risk factors for TB such as being in close contact with persons with active or suspected TB, being born in countries with high TB risk, frequent or recent travel to high-risk countries, or working with high-risk populations, including homeless populations and drug and alcohol abusers (Cantini et al. 2015). Latent as well as active TB should be screened and patients should be monitored for infections during and after treatment with tocilizumab. Serious neuropsychiatric adverse reactions include demyelinating CNS disease such as multiple sclerosis and chronic demyelinating polyneuropathy. No major psychotropic drug interactions have been reported (Bilbul et al. 2020).

Favipiravir is an antiviral drug used for influenza in Japan and inhibits RNA-dependent RNA polymerase, preventing viral replication (Joshi et al. 2021). It is under study and has been approved for use in mild to moderate COVID-19 in Japan, Russia, Saudi Arabia, Thailand, Kenya, and parts of India (Joshi et al. 2021). There is little information available regarding neuropsychiatric side effects. It may cause QTc prolongation, so it should be used with caution with psychotropic drugs known to prolong the QTc interval (Bilbul et al. 2020).

Lopinavir/ritonavir is a combination product that binds to the active site of HIV protease, preventing mature virus particle formation. It was repurposed to treat COVID-19 infection because it had been found useful in treating severe acute respiratory syndrome (caused by SARS-CoV-1) and Middle East Respiratory Syndrome–related coronavirus infection (Cao et al. 2020). However, current studies do not show efficacy for hospitalized patients with COVID-19 (COVID-19 Treatment Guidelines Panel 2021). Side effects include Stevens-Johnson syndrome, diabetes mellitus, QTc prolongation, pancreatitis, neutropenia, hepatotoxicity, and chronic kidney disease (U.S. Food and Drug Administration 2019c). Neuropsychiatric side effects include agitation, anxiety, confusion, and emotional lability. Lopinavir/ritonavir is extensively metabolized by the CYP450 system, with increased concentrations of CYP3A4 and CYP2D6 substrates and decreased concentrations of CYP1A2 and CYP2B6 substrates (U.S. Food and Drug Administration 2019c). It is contraindicated in use with pimozide, lurasidone, midazolam, and triazolam because of potentiation of side effects. If benzodiazepines are needed, consider lorazepam, oxazepam, or temazepam because they are not dependent on the CYP system for metabolism. Lopinavir/ritonavir will lower the concentration of bupropion, methadone, lamotrigine, and valproate and increase concentrations of quetiapine, trazodone, and fentanyl by CYP system metabolism. Caution is indicated with potentially hepatotoxic psychotropics because there is increased risk for elevated aminotransferase levels (alanine transaminase) and psychotropic drugs that prolong the QTc interval.

Convalescent plasma therapy contains antibodies to COVID-19 and may help suppress SARS-CoV-2 and modify the inflammatory response (Wang et al. 2020). The FDA issued an EUA on August 23, 2020, granting convalescent plasma emergency use (U.S. Food and Drug Administration 2020b). There are infrequent serious adverse reactions, but risks include transfusion-transmitted infections, anaphylaxis, acute lung injury, and hemolytic reactions (U.S. Food and Drug Administration 2020b). No specific neuropsychiatric effects or interactions with psychotropics have been reported (Bilbul et al. 2020).

Bamlanivimab, etesevimab, casirivimab, and imdevimab are neutralizing monoclonal antibodies that bind to SARS-CoV-2, blocking entry into host cells. The FDA issued an EUA on February 9, 2021, for bamlanivimab plus etesevimab for mild to moderate COVID-19 outpatients at high risk for progression to severe disease (U.S. Food and Drug Administration 2021a). Casirivimab plus imdevimab also received an FDA EUA on November 21, 2020, for similar indications (U.S. Food and Drug Administration 2021b). Reactions include anaphylaxis and infusion-related reactions. No neuropsychiatric side effects have been reported. Currently, there are no known psychotropic drug interactions (Bilbul et al. 2020).

Azithromycin binds to the 50S ribosomal subunit inhibiting protein synthesis and has some immunomodulatory action. There was initial interest in its use as a treatment for COVID-19, but it is currently not included in NIH treatment guidelines for COVID-19 infections (COVID-19 Treatment Guidelines Panel 2021). Neuropsychiatric side effects include aggression, anxiety, headaches, dizziness, somnolence, and vertigo (U.S. Food and Drug Administration 2019a). Azithromycin can also cause QTc prolongation, torsades de pointes, hepatotoxicity, pancreatitis, and Stevens-Johnson syndrome, among other serious reactions. Elderly patients may be more likely to develop torsades de pointes. No specific psychotropic interactions have been reported (Bilbul et al. 2020).

Corticosteroids, including dexamethasone, inhibit multiple inflammatory cytokines and produce multiple glucocorticoid and mineralocorticoid effects. The NIH recommends dexamethasone use for patients hospitalized with COVID-19 who require supplemental oxygen alone or through a high-flow device, ventilation, or extracorporeal membrane oxygenation (COVID-19 Treatment Guidelines Panel 2021). The half-life of dexamethasone is 36–72 hours. Serious reactions include adrenal insufficiency, psychosis, mania, diabetes mellitus, seizures, emotional lability, insomnia, anxiety, agitation, catatonia, depersonalization, delirium, dementia, depression, and thromboembolism (U.S. Food and Drug Administration 2019b). Neuropsychiatric side effects tend to occur early and tend to be dose related, with the greatest risk at more than 40 mg/day prednisone equivalents (Dubovsky et al. 2012). Corticosteroids are inconsistently reported to be weak CYP3A4 and CYP2C19 inducers, and caution should be exercised with psychotropics known to lower seizure thresholds, such as bupropion (Bilbul et al. 2020).

Interferons bind to interferon receptors and activate tyrosine kinase, producing antiviral, antiproliferative, and immunomodulatory effects. The NIH does not recommend the use of interferons for the treatment of patients with COVID-19 (COVID-19 Treatment Guidelines Panel

2021). Interferon alfa-2b has a black box warning for causing or aggravating fatal or life-threatening neuropsychiatric, autoimmune, ischemic, and infectious disorders (U.S. Food and Drug Administration 2021e). Serious neuropsychiatric reactions include suicidal ideation, homicidal ideation, depression, suicidality, and seizures (U.S. Food and Drug Administration 2021e). Other serious reactions include lymphopenia, neutropenia, leukopenia, hepatotoxicity, hypothyroidism, hyperthyroidism, and congestive heart failure. There is a potential for bone marrow suppression, so caution must be exercised with psychotropics such as carbamazepine, valproate, and clozapine (Bilbul et al. 2020; U.S. Food and Drug Administration 2021e). Interferon may also lower the seizure threshold, so caution is indicated with psychotropics that lower the seizure threshold.

Fluvoxamine, an antidepressant of the selective serotonin reuptake inhibitor class with high σ_1 receptor agonism, has been found in a clinical trial to prevent clinical deterioration when given during mild COVID-19 illness (Lenze et al. 2020). Fluvoxamine is considered to decrease the inflammatory damage from the COVID-19 virus by regulating the cytokine production via its interaction with the endoplasmic reticulum stress sensor inositol-requiring enzyme 1α. The clinical trial was limited by its small sample size ($N=152$) and short follow-up period of study.

Three highly effective COVID-19 vaccines are now FDA approved or available for emergency use in the United States: Pfizer-BioNTech, Moderna, and Janssen (U.S. Food and Drug Administration 2021c). Vaccination has been recommended for all people ages 5 years and older in the United States. Seniors with multiple health problems, including mental illnesses, and health care workers are prioritized to receive the vaccine. The vaccines have been considered to be effective and safe in trials (Pormohammad et al. 2021). The common side effects of the vaccines include mild local reactions of pain, swelling, and/or redness at the injection site and mild systemic reactions of headache and fatigue (M. Chen et al. 2021). Severe adverse events from the vaccines are rare and include reports of anaphylactic shock, faciplegia, myocarditis, cerebral venous thrombosis, and vaccine-induced immune thrombotic thrombocytopenia. (Bozkurt et al. 2021; Castells and Phillips 2021; Sharifian-Dorche et al. 2021). There is a concern that medications metabolized by the liver (e.g., antiepileptics) can be affected by the vaccines because of the reduced expression of CYP450 enzymes by the increased production of cytokines such as interferon gamma elicited by the vaccines (Kow and Hasan 2021). Vaccine safety surveillance over time will be needed to monitor long-term vaccine-related adverse events.

SUMMARY

The COVID-19 pandemic caused disruption of the supply chain of medications, reduced access to health care for older adults, and caused barriers to therapeutic drug monitoring of psychotropic medications. Widespread adoption of telehealth and relaxation of related federal and state regulations in an expedited manner did help to overcome barriers in providing care to older adults with mental illness. However, older adults might not be ready to use telemedicine because of a lack of experience with technology and/or disability caused by cognitive and sensory impairments. Physical assessment of older adults via telehealth is limited, which can be a further impediment to assessment for safely prescribing psychotropic medications. Vigilance to emerging side effects is needed when prescribing psychotropic medications in older adults with COVID-19 infection because of the multiple organ systems affected by the virus and drug interactions with medications used to treat COVID-19 infection.

KEY POINTS

- Measures taken to contain the spread of COVID-19 infection have caused disruptions in access to care and medications for older adults.

- Unreadiness of older adults to use telehealth and limitations of physical examination via telehealth can be barriers to proper assessment for prescribing medications.

- Caution is needed to safely prescribe psychotropic medications to older adults with COVID-19 infection because of multiorgan involvement by the virus and potential drug-drug interactions with medications used for treatment of COVID-19 infection.

QUESTIONS FOR REVIEW

1. Systemic infections, including COVID-19 infection, can increase the drug levels of which of the following psychotropic medications?

    A. Carbamazepine
    B. Nortriptyline
    C. Clozapine
    D. Valproic acid

Answer: C.

2. Because of acute kidney injury and dehydration occurring in patients with COVID-19 infection, which of the following psychotropic drug levels should be closely monitored?

    A. Lithium
    B. Valproic acid
    C. Carbamazepine
    D. Clozapine

Answer: A.

3. Which of the following benzodiazepines can be used safely in patients being prescribed ritonavir for COVID-19 infection?

    A. Midazolam
    B. Diazepam
    C. Chlordiazepoxide
    D. Lorazepam

Answer: D.

REFERENCES

Awortwe C, Cascorbi I: Meta-analysis on outcome-worsening comorbidities of COVID-19 and related potential drug-drug interactions. Pharmacol Res 161:105250, 2020 33059010

Bilbul M, Paparone P, Kim AM, et al: Psychopharmacology of COVID-19. Psychosomatics 61(5):411–427, 2020 32425246

Bozkurt B, Kamat I, Hotez PJ: Myocarditis with COVID-19 mRNA vaccines. Circulation 144(6):471–484, 2021 34281357

Brotman JJ, Kotloff RM: Providing outpatient telehealth in the United States: before and during coronavirus disease 2019. Chest 159(4):1548–1558, 2021 33245875

Brown E, Gray R, Lo Monaco S, et al: The potential impact of COVID-19 on psychosis: a rapid review of contemporary epidemic and pandemic research. Schizophr Res 222:79–87, 2020 32389615

Cao B, Wang Y, Wen D, et al: A trial of lopinavir-ritonavir in adults hospitalized with severe Covid-19. N Engl J Med 382(19):1787–1799, 2020 32187464

Castells MC, Phillips EJ: Maintaining safety with SARS-CoV-2 vaccines. N Engl J Med 384(7):643–649, 2021 33378605

Chen M, Yuan Y, Zhou Y, et al: Safety of SARS-CoV-2 vaccines: a systematic review and meta-analysis of randomized controlled trials. Infect Dis Poverty 10(1):94, 2021 34225791

Chen Y, Klein SL, Garibaldi BT, et al: Aging in COVID-19: vulnerability, immunity and intervention. Ageing Res Rev 65:101205, 2021 33137510

COVID-19 Treatment Guidelines Panel: Coronavirus disease 2019 (COVID-19) treatment guidelines. Bethesda, MD, National Institutes of Health, July 8, 2021. Available at: www.covid19treatmentguidelines.nih.gov/about-the-guidelines/whats-new/. Accessed July 15, 2021.

Drug Enforcement Administration: COVID-19 information page. Springfield, VA, Drug Enforcement Administration, 2021. Available at: www.deadiversion. usdoj.gov/coronavirus.html. Accessed January 31, 2021.

Dubovsky AN, Arvikar S, Stern TA, et al: The neuropsychiatric complications of glucocorticoid use: steroid psychosis revisited. Psychosomatics 53(2):103–115, 2012 22424158

Elbeddini A, Prabaharan T, Almasalkhi S, et al: Barriers to conducting deprescribing in the elderly population amid the COVID-19 pandemic. Res Social Adm Pharm 17(1):1942–1945, 2021 32499161

Gee S, Gaughran F, MacCabe J, et al: Management of clozapine treatment during the COVID-19 pandemic. Ther Adv Psychopharmacol 10:2045125320928167, 2020 32542111

Greenhalgh T, Koh GCH, Car J: Covid-19: a remote assessment in primary care. BMJ 368:m1182, 2020 32213507

Hoffman DA: Increasing access to care: telehealth during COVID-19. J Law Biosci 7(2):lsaa043, 2020 32843985

Ifteni P, Dima L, Teodorescu A: Long-acting injectable antipsychotics treatment during COVID-19 pandemic—a new challenge. Schizophr Res 220:265–266, 2020 32349886

Joshi S, Parkar J, Ansari A, et al: Role of favipiravir in the treatment of COVID-19. Int J Infect Dis 102:501–508, 2021 33130203

Kow CS, Hasan SS: Potential interactions between COVID-19 vaccines and antiepileptic drugs. Seizure 86:80–81, 2021 33578259

Lenze EJ, Mattar C, Zorumski CF, et al: Fluvoxamine vs placebo and clinical deterioration in outpatients with symptomatic COVID-19: a randomized clinical trial. JAMA 324(22):2292–2300, 2020 33180097

Lim EC, Chen CY, Tan EK: Remote prescription during pandemic: challenges and solutions. Arch Med Res 52(4):450–452, 2021 33500154

Murphy RP, Dennehy KA, Costello MM, et al: Virtual geriatric clinics and the COVID-19 catalyst: a rapid review. Age Ageing 49(6):907–914, 2020 32821909

Ostuzzi G, Papola D, Gastaldon C, et al: Safety of psychotropic medications in people with COVID-19: evidence review and practical recommendations. BMC Med 18(1):215, 2020 32664944

Pormohammad A, Zarei M, Ghorbani S, et al: Efficacy and safety of COVID-19 vaccines: a systematic review and meta-analysis of randomized clinical trials. Vaccines (Basel) 9(5):467, 2021 34066475

Reeve E, Trenaman SC, Rockwood K, et al: Pharmacokinetic and pharmacodynamic alterations in older people with dementia. Expert Opin Drug Metab Toxicol 13(6):651–668, 2017 28460576

Shahid Z, Kalayanamitra R, McClafferty B, et al: COVID-19 and older adults: what we know. J Am Geriatr Soc 68(5):926–929, 2020 32255507

Sharifian-Dorche M, Bahmanyar M, Sharifian-Dorche A, et al: Vaccine-induced immune thrombotic thrombocytopenia and cerebral venous sinus thrombosis post COVID-19 vaccination; a systematic review. J Neurol Sci 428:117607, 2021 34365148

Siskind D, Honer WG, Clark S, et al: Consensus statement on the use of clozapine during the COVID-19 pandemic. J Psychiatry Neurosci 45(4):200061, 2020 32242646

Sorinmade OA, Kossoff L, Peisah C: COVID-19 and telehealth in older adult psychiatry-opportunities for now and the future. Int J Geriatr Psychiatry 35(12):1427–1430, 2020 32729632

U.S. Food and Drug Administration: Azithromycin prescribing information. Silver Spring, MD, U.S. Food and Drug Administration, 2019a. Available at: www.accessdata.fda.gov/drugsatfda_docs/label/2019/050693s031,05 0730s041lbl.pdf. Accessed March 13, 2021.

U.S. Food and Drug Administration: Dexamethasone tablets prescribing information. Silver Spring, MD, U.S. Food and Drug Administration, 2019b. Available at: www.accessdata.fda.gov/drugsatfda_docs/label/2004/ 11664slr062_decadron_lbl.pdf. Accessed March 13, 2021.

U.S. Food and Drug Administration: Lopinavir/ritonavir prescribing information. Silver Spring, MD, U.S. Food and Drug Administration, 2019c. Available at: https://www.accessdata.fda.gov/drugsatfda_docs/label/2013/ 021251s046_021906s039lbl.pdf Accessed March 13, 2021.

U.S. Food and Drug Administration: Tocilizumab prescribing information. Silver Spring, MD, U.S. Food and Drug Administration, 2019d. Available at: www.accessdata.fda.gov/drugsatfda_docs/label/2010/125276lbl.pdf. Accessed March 4, 2021.

U.S. Food and Drug Administration: Coronavirus (COVID-19) update: FDA revokes emergency use authorization for chloroquine and hydroxychloroquine (FDA News Release). Silver Spring, MD, June 15, 2020a. Available at: www.fda.gov/news-events/press-announcements/coronavirus-covid-19-update-fda-revokes-emergency-use-authorization-chloroquine-and. Accessed March 4, 2021.

U.S. Food and Drug Administration: COVID-19 plasma therapy emergency use authorization. Silver Spring, MD, U.S. Food and Drug Administration, 2020b. Available at: https://www.fda.gov/media/141480/download. Accessed March 13, 2021.

U.S. Food and Drug Administration: FDA provides update on patient access to certain REMS drugs during COVID-19 public health emergency. Silver Spring, MD, U.S. Food and Drug Administration, March 22, 2020c. Available at: www.fda.gov/news-events/press-announcements/coronavirus-covid-19-update-fda-provides-update-patient-access-certain-rems-drugs-during-covid-19. Accessed January 31, 2021.

U.S. Food and Drug Administration: Bamlanivimab and etesevimab emergency use authorization (EUA). Silver Spring, MD, U.S. Food and Drug Administration, 2021a. Available at: www.fda.gov/media/145802/download. Accessed March 13, 2021.

U.S. Food and Drug Administration: Casirivimab and imdevimab emergency use authorization (EUA). Silver Spring, MD, U.S. Food and Drug Administration, 2021b. Available at: www.fda.gov/media/143891/download. Accessed October 26, 2021.

U.S. Food and Drug Administration: COVID-19 vaccines. Silver Spring, MD, U.S. Food and Drug Administration, 2021c. Available at: www.fda.gov/ emergency-preparedness-and-response/coronavirus-disease-2019-covid-19/covid-19-vaccines. Accessed October 27, 2021.

U.S. Food and Drug Administration: Hydroxychloroquine prescribing information. Silver Spring, MD, U.S. Food and Drug Administration, 2021d. Available at: www.accessdata.fda.gov/drugsatfda_docs/label/2019/009768Orig1s051lbl.pdf. Accessed October 27, 2021.

U.S. Food and Drug Administration: Interferon alfa-2b prescribing information. Silver Spring, MD, U.S. Food and Drug Administration, 2021e. Available at: https://www.accessdata.fda.gov/drugsatfda_docs/label/2014/103132s5190lbl.pdf. Accessed March 13, 2021.

U.S. Food and Drug Administration: Remdesivir prescribing information. Silver Spring, MD, U.S. Food and Drug Administration, 2021f. Available at: www.accessdata.fda.gov/drugsatfda_docs/label/2021/214787s005lbl.pdf. Accessed March 4, 2021.

Wang X, Guo X, Xin Q, et al: Neutralizing antibodies responses to SARS-CoV-2 in COVID-19 inpatients and convalescent patients. Clin Infect Dis 71(10):2688–2694, 2020 32497196

CHAPTER 17

CHALLENGING TIMES

Consultation-Liaison Psychiatry in the Era of COVID-19

Farah Tabaja, M.D.

Paul B. Hill, M.D.

Maintaining adequate mental health services in the general hospital setting was crucial during the coronavirus SARS-CoV-2 disease (COVID-19) pandemic and posed unique challenges to the practice of consultation-liaison psychiatry (CLP). Challenges included personnel constraints, concerns about exposing staff and patients to the virus, and scarcity of resources. These challenges necessitated adaptations to the usual practice of hospital psychiatry, such as workflow changes, remote consultations, and rapid implementation of telemedicine technologies. Patients in the general hospital setting had more acute psychiatric needs because of the impact of the pandemic on the mental health system at large and the added stress of a novel, potentially life-threatening disease. Emerging neuropsychiatric findings in infected patients required special attention, and managing psychiatric sequelae of COVID-19 was critical to improving health outcomes in these patients. The lack of availability of usual services and resources complicated the management approach, placed an additional burden on staff, and often posed ethical dilemmas.

Vignette

Mr. E, a 65-year-old Jamaican-born man, presented for medical clearance prior to commitment to a state psychiatric hospital. He had engaged in homicidal speech and self-injurious behavior on the day leading to his evaluation. The police were called to the Mississippi River port where Mr. E was wading into the river speaking of cleansing himself and wanting to harm his wife and adult children with a baseball bat. He was screaming "Blood of Jesus!" and "I feel like I am dying inside!" The police were able to take Mr. E to an emergency department, where he eloped and required force to take him to the county crisis assessment center. Mr. E was found to be COVID-19 positive. No psychiatric facility would accept him for further evaluation and treatment at that time, so he was admitted to the COVID-19 unit in the general hospital, where he received a medical evaluation and a psychiatric consultation.

On evaluation, Mr. E was found to have poor grooming, a flat affect, auditory hallucinations, religious delusions of both grandiosity and persecution, and thought disorder. He was fully oriented and able to provide demographic information. Collateral information was collected from Mr. E's wife, who reported that he had a family history of a brother and paternal grandmother with a similar mental illness. He achieved typical developmental milestones and had never been medically or neurologically ill or injured. He was raised in a lower-middle-class, Christian home and had not experienced childhood trauma. He had begun to have delusions of reference in his 30s, with preoccupations with the Bible and with purity. He dropped out of junior college, worked in a local warehouse, and spent much of his time reading the Bible in isolation. Mr. E had no history of prior psychiatric evaluation or treatment. He had never used alcohol or drugs.

Mr. E was diagnosed with schizophrenia, and medical and psychiatric management was initiated with the consent of his wife because he was deemed not to have capacity to make medical decisions. He was started on haloperidol 5 mg twice a day and benztropine 1 mg at bedtime. He did receive several doses of ziprasidone 10 mg IM and lorazepam 2 mg when he was agitated, disinhibited, and threatening and refused to take haloperidol orally. He needed to be restrained for safety on several occasions. He was supported by a sitter and unit security. His family communicated with him by telephone.

Mr. E was treated for minor medical complications of COVID-19, pneumonitis, and dehydration. His basic laboratory results and imaging were unremarkable, with negative computed tomography of the head, urine drug screen, and serological testing for infection with syphilis and HIV. Thyroid-stimulating hormone, C-reactive protein, and erythrocyte sedimentation rate were normal. Mr. E had a mild increase in creatine phosphokinase, possibly from his restraint and taser shock. He was given zinc, antibiotics (piperacillin, ciprofloxacin), intravenous fluids, and oxygen by nasal cannula. After medical stabilization, he completed his quarantine period with continued psychiatric management, and he was transferred to a state psychiatric hospital after testing COVID-19 negative.

The role of the CLP team is to evaluate psychiatric symptoms, clarify the diagnosis, and provide treatment in a general hospital setting while communicating with and supporting primary hospital providers. This is essential to the stabilization of patients and disposition planning. Early in the course of the COVID-19 pandemic, the importance of maintaining adequate mental health services for medically admitted patients became apparent because physical isolation of patients, lack of family availability in the hospital, and anxiety about this unknown illness took their toll. In addition, neuropsychiatric manifestations of COVID-19 required special attention and the expertise of CLP providers for management.

EXPLORING THE PROBLEM: SYSTEM CAPACITY, STAFF TRAINING, AND SAFETY ISSUES

The COVID-19 pandemic created unprecedented challenges for CLP teams. The need to decrease exposure of health care workers and trainees led to staffing constraints, with some members of CLP teams working remotely and others (such as medical students) unable to participate in clinical care. In some settings, psychiatrists or psychiatric residents were redeployed to other medical settings with dire need for physicians. Ancillary staff members such as social workers and case managers frequently worked remotely or were redeployed. CLP providers occasionally found themselves having to care for patients who required psychiatric admission but had to be maintained on medical floors because of their COVID-19-positive status. This further increased patient case load and presented safety concerns for patients and staff. All these challenges necessitated fundamental changes to the practice of hospital psychiatry, and CLP teams across the country had to adapt in innovative ways to continue providing care to patients.

PATIENT EVALUATION IN THE ERA OF COVID-19: USE OF NOVEL APPROACHES, INCLUDING TELEMEDICINE

Given the increase in patient numbers, the increasing severity of COVID-19 symptoms, and the decrease in staffing during the pandemic, it was vital to be prepared to quickly evaluate COVID-19-positive patients with comorbid psychiatric symptoms or substance use disorders and to initiate safety and treatment plans. Safety of the patient, staff, and public was of paramount importance in evaluating COVID-19-positive patients. Collaboration between providers across teams and disciplines was invaluable to ensure proper evaluation and management of patients. This necessitated employing creative modifications to the ways psychiatric consultations were performed to address staffing, safety, and patient care concerns (Morris and Hirschtritt 2020).

In order to ensure the safety of health care providers and patients, to slow the spread of the virus, and to conserve personal protective equipment (PPE), there was a push to limit the number of staff members interacting with COVID-positive patients (Centers for Disease Control and Prevention 2020). One strategy in hospital psychiatry was to create different teams within the same consultation-liaison (CL) service, with certain providers being on-site and others working virtually (Shalev and Shapiro 2020).

The patient interview is one of the cornerstones of the consultation psychiatry evaluation. In the era of COVID-19, the classic bedside psychiatric interview was not always possible, and there were often barriers to effective communication with the patient. Telemedicine technology emerged as a popular alternative form of interacting with patients, and many hospitals saw a quick transition to adoption of telemedicine for the CL service.

In the hospital setting, CLP teams often resorted to hybrid consultation models. Decisions regarding whether to evaluate the patient in person or by telemedicine were made on a case-by-case basis after a risk-benefit analysis (Funk et al. 2020). In such hybrid models, consultations were divided into three types: e-consultations, telemedicine consultations, and traditional in-person consultations. Proper triage was essential, with emphasis placed on safety. The guiding principle was to minimize risk of exposure to the virus by performing virtual evaluations whenever possible while keeping in mind that in-person evaluations were sometimes necessary (Bojdani et al. 2020).

The first type of evaluation, e-consultations (sometimes called curbside or chart consultations), were performed when the patient interview and examination were deemed unlikely to yield additional information, such as in cases of intubated or delirious patients. Here, the CL psychiatrist gathered history by speaking with the consulting provider and by reviewing the medical record and collecting collateral information if needed. Recommendations were then provided without the psychiatrist having interacted with the patient.

When a patient interview was crucial for diagnosis but an in-person interview was deemed unnecessary, the CL provider often resorted to a telemedicine interview. This interview was done via telephonic or video technology depending on the availability in a particular setting. This method provided the psychiatrist with the ability to actually gather firsthand history from the patient and assess the components of the mental status examination available to the examiner, all while avoiding exposure to provider and patient. The presence of electronic medical records with built-in telemedicine platforms facilitated rapid transition to virtual evaluations, and there were reports of some institutions transitioning to a primarily virtual consultation workflow (Kalin et al. 2020).

Challenges to this form of consultation included limited availability of the needed technologies, such as phones, computers, tablets, and reliable internet connection. Hospital rooms often lacked these essential telemedicine resources. When they were not available in the patient's room, it was necessary to identify someone to bring them to the patient. This required coordination with a staff member who would don PPE, bring the needed items to the patient, and disinfect them after use. Often, frontline nursing staff had to bear this additional responsibility of facilitating telehealth visits, which required close interdisciplinary collaboration (Kalin et al. 2020).

Another challenge with virtual interviews was the proper evaluation of patients who had particular difficulty cooperating with telemedicine technology, such as patients with cognitive impairments or agitation. Also challenging were paranoid patients, who were sometimes suspicious of technology and at risk of becoming agitated when interviewed remotely.

The third approach, in-person psychiatric evaluation, was necessary when an adequate history could not be obtained via telemedicine technology or provider collaboration. It was especially needed for patients with complex histories and presentations, catatonic patients who required a physical exam, and patients for whom decisions of informed consent or involuntary commitment necessitated an in-person interview. Although this method was theoretically the closest to a classic CL interview, the restrictions imposed by the pandemic significantly hindered interaction with the patient. The connection with the patient was affected by the face mask and face shield, which distorted voice tone and facial expressions (Goldenberg et al. 2020). One strategy to overcome these difficulties was relying on summarization and reflection to ensure mutual understanding of the content of the conversation by patient and interviewer (Kaplan et al. 2021). It was also common to see providers taping pictures of themselves to their gowns in order to improve the patient connection and build rapport. The need for physical distancing was often challenging in a hospital room where space was limited, and sometimes clear plastic barriers were installed in patient rooms for the protection of staff, creating an additional barrier between provider and patient. Furthermore, physical distancing often necessitated louder speech, which raised concerns about privacy and ran the risk of deterring patients from disclosing personal or delicate information. Of the three methods of patient evaluation discussed, telepsychiatry interviews were often the preferred method, minimizing safety concerns for the CLP team and the patient while allowing for more comfortable and natural patient-clinician interactions, unhindered by PPE.

MAKING THE DIAGNOSIS: COMMON PSYCHIATRIC PRESENTATIONS DURING THE PANDEMIC

As always, making a diagnosis during the pandemic required collecting a personal and psychiatric history, and collateral information was often the key to completing this process. It was especially important when patients had delirium, psychosis, or other presentations that prevented them from providing an accurate history.

During the pandemic, communication with outpatient doctors' offices and mental health providers was compromised by offices being closed and staff being unavailable, which interfered with the ability to collect useful collaborative history. Furthermore, with visitor restrictions in place at most hospitals, family members or caretakers who would otherwise be at a patient's bedside were forced to stay home and were thus less accessible for CLP providers for history gathering.

Diagnoses commonly seen in the hospital during the pandemic included mood disorders, schizophrenia spectrum disorder, personality disorders, substance use disorders, and delirium associated with manifestations of medical or neurological disorders. The disruption in outpatient mental health resources, along with the additional social stressors of the pandemic, meant that patients were at higher risk of psychiatric decompensation. This was particularly true for patients with severe mental illnesses and substance use disorders. A survey of U.S. adults in June 2020 showed a considerable increase in reported symptoms of anxiety and depression, substance use, and suicidal ideation compared with the same time period 1 year earlier (Czeisler et al. 2020). This increase resulted in CLP teams being asked to evaluate a greater number of acutely ill medical patients, including suicidal and agitated patients in both the COVID-19 and non-COVID-19 groups.

This notable increase in anxiety and stress symptoms in admitted patients (Horn et al. 2020; Parker et al. 2021) was attributed to the psychological impact of isolation and the fear of this new life-threatening illness in an already medically vulnerable patient population (Shalev and Shapiro 2020). The absence of visitors in the hospital likely exacerbated the situation because patients were forced to face the entirety of their hospitalization alone. Facilitation of communication between patients and their family members and social supports by medical staff were helpful in mitigating this stress. This was especially important for elderly patients who were at an increased risk of delirium and required frequent reorientation and reassurance, a task facilitated by the presence of family members at the bedside in the prepandemic setting.

A host of neuropsychiatric manifestations resulting from COVID-19 infection were identified, and they required special attention. Delirium, often associated with severe agitation, was particularly common (Rogers et al. 2020), potentially interfering with medical care and leading to adverse outcomes. This topic is discussed in more detail in Chapter 15, "Neuropsychiatric Manifestations of COVID-19."

Patients with substance use disorders presented an additional challenge because they were at a heightened risk of infection with COVID-19 and its sequelae. Furthermore, societal disruptions related to the lockdown limited their access to substances, thus increasing their risk of going into withdrawal (Spagnolo et al. 2020). The paucity of in-person outpatient resources during the pandemic also worsened outcomes for these patients, increasing the likelihood of medical complications and hospitalization.

MANAGEMENT OF PSYCHIATRIC PATIENTS IN THE GENERAL HOSPITAL SETTING IN THE ERA OF COVID-19

After a diagnosis of a psychiatric disorder was established, early and aggressive management was imperative to achieve good control of symptoms and arrive at a disposition. Patients with substance use disorders required early intervention and detoxification to prevent potentially life-threatening withdrawal syndromes. Use of longer-acting scheduled medications was preferred over *as-needed* symptom-triggered protocols because the former strategy decreased the need for frequent reassessments and thus decreased provider exposure, conserving PPE (Shenouda and Desan 2020).

Delirium associated with COVID-19 infection was often difficult to treat and made care more complicated, especially when agitation was present. For patients in intensive care units with multiple lines and tubes, hyperactive delirium interfered with care and presented a challenge to nursing staff who were already stretched thin because of high patient volumes (Shalev and Shapiro 2020). Moreover, delirium sometimes precluded the weaning of patients off ventilators, which were a precious commodity during the pandemic. Thus, early identification and management of delirium were imperative, and it was important to rule out other causes of altered mental status, such as adverse medication effects, withdrawal from substances, untreated pain, untreated underlying psychosis (Altman et al. 2020), and neurological complications such as strokes or seizures (Baller et al. 2020).

Pharmacological interventions were key for treatment of delirium in acute and intensive care settings. Although there were no clear guidelines for pharmacological treatment of COVID-19 delirium, anecdotal evidence and expert recommendations suggested preferentially using α_2 agonists and antipsychotic agents (Baller et al. 2020). These medications could be titrated to an effective dosage, with special attention to QTc interval monitoring and drug-drug interactions, which was especially important given the polypharmacy used in such acutely ill patients. Physical restraint was sometimes unavoidable when agitation interfered with critical medical care or posed a danger to the patient or staff. In such circumstances it was necessary to don PPE prior to intervening. Frequent reassessment was necessary to ensure that restraint was discontinued at the earliest opportunity.

Given the complexity of managing delirium in the setting of COVID-19 infection, prevention was particularly important. This was especially relevant because usual delirium-preventing measures such as frequent patient reorientation by staff and having family members available at the bedside were not possible because of pandemic restrictions. Whenever feasible, arranging for telephone or video visits between patients and families could be helpful, especially in the setting of decreased frequency of patient-provider interaction and the barrier of extensive PPE. Sleep promotion and optimization of the patient environment could still be used for delirium prevention for all patients.

Another challenging class of patients was those with significant psychiatric symptoms and co-occurring COVID-19 infection precluding their transfer to psychiatric facilities. This group included patients with decompensated severe mental illness, patients at risk of harming themselves or others, patients who had attempted suicide, and acutely psychotic patients. In some settings, admission of COVID-19-positive patients to psychiatric wards was not possible until they were medically cleared and no longer deemed contagious, and the CLP teams had to manage these patients for extended periods of time in the general hospital. This sometimes meant holding patients in the hospital involuntarily because of the lack of psychiatric beds, resulting in an increased need for mechanical or chemical restraints and close safety monitoring and supervision. As a result, some changes in protocol were needed because the general hospital is not equipped with the same staffing and safety features as a psychiatric facility.

For patients at risk of self-harm, a detailed risk assessment was required to determine the imminence of the risk. The usual practice of placing a staff member in the patient room to continuously observe the patient (sometimes called a sitter) was not necessarily the default recommendation with COVID-19-positive patients. There was a higher threshold to initiating a 1:1 observer because of concerns about staff and patient exposure to infection. Some adaptations implemented when 1:1 supervision was deemed necessary included having the staff member sit outside the room and observe the patient through a glass panel, a window, or the open door, whichever was available. Another approach was using video monitoring, with the staff member available to respond immediately if any risky behaviors were noted. This latter approach required rooms equipped with video-monitoring capability as well as clear protocols about where the observing staff member should be located while monitoring the video (e.g., right outside the room, on the same unit) and who would be responsible to respond if needed. One prior study looking at virtual monitoring in the general hospital and emergency department reported no adverse events and concluded that it is a feasible option for select patients with low risk of impulsive behaviors (Kroll et al. 2020).

Another consideration with suicidal or psychotic patients in the CL setting was the safety of the hospital room environment. Safety was especially crucial for patients with an extended length of stay in the general hospital because of the unavailability of psychiatric beds for COVID-19-positive patients. It was important to remove sharp objects, including medical equipment, as well as unnecessary cords and tubes and even utensils. Nursing staff often had to be trained how to manage these patients, including when and how to use restraints and as-needed psychotropic medications. Initiating psychopharmacological treatments and optimizing dosing fell to the CL providers because they were no longer merely in charge of stabilization and transfer but were actively managing the patients as though they were admitted to the psychiatry unit.

CAPACITY EVALUATIONS AND ETHICAL AND LEGAL CONSIDERATIONS

Capacity evaluations are common consultation requests on most CLP services, and they are usually related to determining a patient's capacity to make medical decisions. During the COVID-19 pandemic there was a notable increase in capacity consultations, especially for COVID-19-positive patients, who were not able to have family at the bedside to help foster communication and ease the decision-making process (Rasimas 2020).

The public health concerns related to the pandemic and the duty of health care providers to promote not only a patient's individual health but also community health sometimes resulted in ethical dilemmas requiring the balancing of different ethical principles. Autotomy, beneficence, nonmaleficence, and justice might be at odds when resources are limited. This was especially important when COVID-19-positive patients requested to leave the hospital against medical advice and there was concern about their judgment and potential to infect others. CL psychiatrists were often involved in this analysis and in determining the contribution of mental illness to the patient's impaired judgment (Shalev and Shapiro 2020). The threshold of capacity increases with the gravity of the decision, and in the case of COVID-19-positive patients, impact on health care resources, public health, and staff safety were all important considerations. Consultation with the hospital ethics committee or medical-legal team was sometimes helpful in such situations.

STAFF SUPPORT

In addition to evaluating and managing patients, the CL psychiatric provider has an integral role in the support of fellow staff members in times of collective stress such as during a pandemic. Several surveys of health care workers during the COVID-19 pandemic indicated a high prevalence of symptoms of psychological distress, including acute stress, depression, and anxiety (Lai et al. 2020; Shechter et al. 2020).

Frontline health care workers faced the uncertainty of managing this new disease, longer work hours, shortage of PPE and medical supplies, and the looming risk of being infected with the virus themselves or bringing it home to their loved ones (Horn et al. 2020). CL providers were in the unique position of being able to relate to the struggles of their colleagues and also to provide psychological support, psychoeducation, and referral to wellness and mental health resources when needed. This was achieved by impromptu rounds on nursing and medical staff, creation of more formal forums and spaces targeting emotional support, and initiatives promoting wellness and self-care. Health care teams across the country witnessed exceptional teamwork, communication, and kindness directed toward patients during this difficult time. Case managers, nurses, social workers, chaplains, therapists, administrators, and other physicians were able to discuss and collaborate with a clear understanding of the complex mission to protect and serve the patients and the community.

SUMMARY

The COVID-19 pandemic created a parallel mental health crisis, and psychiatrists were at the forefront of managing this crisis, especially in the general hospital setting. The limitations to the usual practice of CL psychiatry imposed by the pandemic necessitated innovation in practice, including implementation of novel evaluation models, and treatment planning was adapted to meet available resources. During this time of exceptional uncertainty, interdisciplinary collaboration and support of staff at all levels of practice ensured the continued ability to deliver the best care to patients while ensuring staff and public health safety. As our research base on the manifestations and sequelae of the novel coronavirus expands, the practice of CL psychiatry will undoubtedly continue to grow and evolve, incorporating evidence-based practices to further enhance patient care.

KEY POINTS

- Application of fundamental CL practice during a novel pandemic necessitates innovation in assessment and management of patients.
- COVID-19-infected patients presented with various psychiatric symptoms, including neuropsychiatric manifestations, and disposition planning was complicated by the public health emergency.

- Treatment plans should be designed to prioritize the safety of patients and staff members, minimize exposure risk, and balance ethical and legal considerations.

QUESTIONS FOR REVIEW

1. What are the principles of medical ethics involved in the practice of CLP?

    A. Autonomy and justice
    B. Beneficence and nonmaleficence
    C. Resource management and rationing
    D. A and B
    E. B and C

Answer: D.

2. What is the most effective alternative to being present with the psychiatric patient in a medical setting?

    A. Telepsychiatry
    B. Telephone
    C. Collaborative care
    D. Chart review and suggestions

Answer: A.

3. Safety is vital to the care of psychiatric patients in a medical setting. Which of the following is correct?

    A. Mechanical restrains can be used in a medical setting to prevent self-injury prevent elopement, and protect the delivery of care.
    B. Chemical restraint is sometimes necessary for the safety of patients and staff.
    C. Having a sitter is a safe way to monitor a patient for safety.
    D. All of the above

Answer: D.

ADDITIONAL RESOURCES

American Psychiatric Association: Diagnostic and Statistical Manual of Mental Disorders, 5th Edition. Arlington, VA, American Psychiatric Association, 2013

Levenson JL: The American Psychiatric Association Publishing Textbook of Psychosomatic Medicine and Consultation-Liaison Psychiatry, 3rd Edition. Washington, DC, American Psychiatric Association Publishing, 2019

Lyketsos CG, Chisolm MS: Systematic Psychiatric Evaluation: A Step-by-Step Guide to Applying the Perspectives of Psychiatry. Baltimore, MD, Johns Hopkins University Press, 2012

McHugh PR, Slavney PR: The Perspectives of Psychiatry, 2nd Edition. Baltimore, MD, Johns Hopkins University Press, 1998

Stern TA, Freudenreich O, Smith FA, et al: Massachusetts General Hospital Handbook of General Hospital Psychiatry, 7th Edition. New York, Elsevier, 2018

REFERENCES

Altman S, Faeder M, Fishman D, et al: Consultation liaison psychiatry Covid-19 service manual. Bethesda, MD, Academy of Consultation-Liaison Psychiatry, 2020. Available at: www.clpsychiatry.org/wp-content/uploads/University-of-Pittsburgh-Medical-Center-COVID19-CL-COVID-MANUAL-032620.pdf. Accessed July 16, 2021.

Baller EB, Hogan CS, Fusunyan MA, et al: Neurocovid: pharmacological recommendations for delirium associated with COVID-19. Psychosomatics 61(6):585–596, 2020 32828569

Bojdani E, Rajagopalan A, Chen A, et al: COVID-19 pandemic: impact on psychiatric care in the United States. Psychiatry Res 289:113069, 2020 32413707

Centers for Disease Control and Prevention: Interim infection prevention and control recommendations for healthcare personnel during the coronavirus disease 2019 (COVID-19) pandemic. Atlanta, GA, Centers for Disease Control and Prevention, February 23, 2020. Available at: www.cdc.gov/coronavirus/2019-ncov/hcp/infection-control-recommendations.html#minimize. Accessed July 16, 2021.

Czeisler MÉ, Lane RI, Petrosky E, et al: Mental health, substance use, and suicidal ideation during the COVID-19 pandemic—United States, June 24–30, 2020. MMWR Morb Mortal Wkly Rep 69(32):1049–1057, 2020 32790653

Funk MC, Beach SR, Shah SB, et al: Consultation-liaison psychiatry in the age of COVID-19: reaffirming ourselves and our worth. Psychosomatics 61(5):571–572, 2020 32439183

Goldenberg MN, Gerkin JS, Penaskovic KM, et al: Being reactive: assessing affect in the COVID-19 era. Acad Psychiatry 44(6):682, 2020 32761314

Horn M, Granon B, Vaiva G, et al: Role and importance of consultation-liaison psychiatry during the Covid-19 epidemic. J Psychosom Res 137:110214, 2020 32798833

Kalin ML, Garlow SJ, Thertus K, et al: Rapid implementation of telehealth in hospital psychiatry in response to COVID-19. Am J Psychiatry 177(7):636–637, 2020 32605442

Kaplan A, Smith CM, Toukolehto O, et al: Psychiatric care in a novel federal COVID-19 treatment center: development of a consultation-liaison psychiatry service at the Javits New York Medical Station. Mil Med 186(5–6):129–131, 2021 33386851

Kroll DS, Stanghellini E, DesRoches SL, et al: Virtual monitoring of suicide risk in the general hospital and emergency department. Gen Hosp Psychiatry 63:33–38, 2020 30665667

Lai J, Ma S, Wang Y, et al: Factors associated with mental health outcomes among health care workers exposed to coronavirus disease 2019. JAMA Netw Open 3(3):e203976, 2020 32202646

Morris NP, Hirschtritt ME: Telepsychiatry, hospitals, and the COVID-19 pandemic. Psychiatr Serv 71(12):1309–1312, 2020 32933415

Parker C, Shalev D, Hsu I, et al: Depression, anxiety, and acute stress disorder among patients hospitalized with coronavirus disease 2019: a prospective cohort study. J Acad Consult Liaison Psychiatry 62(2):211–219, 2021 33198962

Rasimas JJ: Capacity and the COVID-19 surge. Psychosomatics 61(6):852–853, 2020 32798054

Rogers JP, Chesney E, Oliver D, et al: Psychiatric and neuropsychiatric presentations associated with severe coronavirus infections: a systematic review and meta-analysis with comparison to the COVID-19 pandemic. Lancet Psychiatry 7(7):611–627, 2020 32437679

Shalev D, Shapiro PA: Epidemic psychiatry: the opportunities and challenges of COVID-19. Gen Hosp Psychiatry 64:68–71, 2020 32279023

Shechter A, Diaz F, Moise N, et al: Psychological distress, coping behaviors, and preferences for support among New York healthcare workers during the COVID-19 pandemic. Gen Hosp Psychiatry 66:1–8, 2020 32590254

Shenouda R, Desan P: Psychiatric consultation service: special guidelines for patients with definite or possible highly contagious infectious disease. Bethesda, MD, Academy of Consultation-Liaison Psychiatry, 2020. Available at: www.clpsychiatry.org/wp-content/uploads/YNHH-Psychiatric-Consultation-Service-Guidelines-112520.pdf. Accessed July 16, 2021.

Spagnolo PA, Montemitro C, Leggio L: New challenges in addiction medicine: COVID-19 infection in patients with alcohol and substance use disorders—the perfect storm. Am J Psychiatry 177(9):805–807, 2020 32660296

INDEX

Page numbers printed in **boldface** type refer to tables and figures.